Women's Health Updates

Edited by Julio Elito Júnior
and Edward Araujo Júnior

Published in London, United Kingdom

Women's Health Updates
http://dx.doi.org/10.5772/intechopen.1003568
Edited by Julio Elito Júnior and Edward Araujo Júnior

Contributors
Alfredo Guillermo Chong Viteri, Amanda Rumondang, Angélica María Apolo Montero, Anshula Deshpande, Arminda Eugenio, Ayşe Figen Türkçapar, Ayşe Topcu Akduman, Dalenda Chelli, Edward Araujo Júnior, Enrique Valdés Rubio, Eya Kristou, Fathi Mraihi, Germania Elizabeth Yugcha Andino, Germán Arturo Vélez Sáenz, Igor Solev, Iva Duval, Jessica Paken, Jiaxin Li, Jimmy Emmanuel Ramos Valencia, Jingyi Wu, Joel Paul Vargas Caicedo, Jose Chidassicua, Julio Elito Júnior, Junna Ye, Kyoo Kim, Lucas Almeida das Chagas, Magnolia Ngcobo-Sithole, Marcelo Graziano Custodio, Martha Cecilia Jaramillo Cardona, Martin Downes, María Eugenia Ugarte Vega, María Fernanda Calderón León, Mathieu Leboeuf, Medha Wadhwa, Mehrad Rafiei, Montacer Hafsi, Moraima Elizabeth Pazmiño Iñiga, Nataly del Carmen Quisiguiña Jarrín, Nathalia Isabella Muskitta, Neeraj Deshpande, Nomawonga Msutwana, Paula Andrea Vásquez Jaramillo, Pulkit Kalyan, Qi Yu, Rabeea F. Omar, Rosiane Mattar, Rosângela Maria Lopes de Sousa, Salma Chidassicua, Sylvie Trottier, Thabisa Mabusela, Tommaso Simoncini, Yizhu Lin, Yuditiya Purwosunu, Yujuan Wang, Zhuochao Zhou

First published in London, United Kingdom, 2025 by IntechOpen
IntechOpen is the global imprint of INTECHOPEN LIMITED, registered in England and Wales, registration number: 11086078, 167-169 Great Portland Street, London, W1W 5PF, United Kingdom

For EU product safety concerns: IN TECH d.o.o., Prolaz Marije Krucifikse Kozulić 3, 51000 Rijeka, Croatia, info@intechopen.com or visit our website at intechopen.com.

British Library Cataloguing-in-Publication Data
A catalogue record for this book is available from the British Library

Women's Health Updates
Edited by Julio Elito Júnior and Edward Araujo Júnior
p. cm.

This title is part of the Public Health Book Series, Volume 5
Series Editor: José Antonio Mirón Canelo

Print ISBN 978-1-83634-344-8
Online ISBN 978-1-83634-343-1
eBook (PDF) ISBN 978-1-83634-345-5
ISSN 3049-8872

IntechOpen Book Series

Public Health

Volume 5

Aims and Scope of the Series

Public health is what we as a society do collectively to contribute to and ensure the health and social conditions for the enjoyment of health as a resource for life. It can also be defined as science and research that promotes health, prevents disease, and improves populations' well-being and quality of life. Its objective is to know the risk factors that determine and condition the populations' health levels at present. At the end of the 20th century and the beginning of the 21st century, it is unjustifiable and regrettable that morbimortality according to age plays a leading role when the causes are mostly well known and therefore preventable, such as obesity, AIDS, cirrhosis, diabetes mellitus, addictions and cancer associated with the consumption of tobacco and alcohol, etc. In short, public health is science based on epidemiology and biostatistics, and currently, new technologies and artificial intelligence must be incorporated to identify patterns and trends in what we do collectively as a society to ensure living conditions and prevent risk factors that affect individual and population health. For all these reasons, it is essential to scientifically investigate and act on the determinants that impede the well-being and quality of life related to the health of people, patients, and populations in general, given that to control the determinants of diseases, it is important to control the environment and genetics. Consequently, the current fight for public health must prioritize the control of the environment, such as atmospheric and biological pollution and environmental and social biodiversity, promoting the sensitivity and training of society and its individuals by empowering them to make free and appropriate decisions about these aspects to lead healthy lifestyles based on motivation and responsibility in the face of the challenges they cope with from an individual point of view, such as dealing with the addictions that exist in today's complex world. Public health also requires an ethical vision and incorporates strategies to reduce social inequality.

Meet the Series Editor

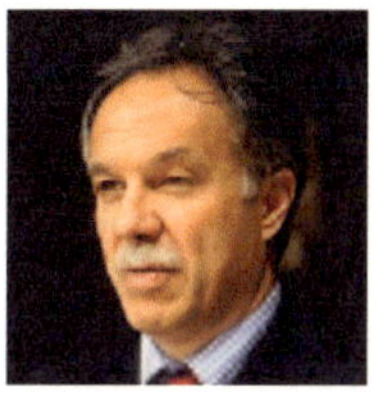

José Antonio Mirón Canelo is a physician, doctor, and professor of Preventive Medicine and Public Health at the Faculty of Medicine and Dentistry of the University of Salamanca with over 30 years of experience. He is the director of the USAL's Expert Degree in Health Management, currently in its 13th edition. Prof. Mirón Canelo directs a research group at the Research Institute of Biomedical Sciences (IBSAL) of the University of Salamanca focused on addressing the challenges and care needs of vulnerable people and patients such as the elderly with multiple pathologies and people with disabilities and dependence. As a teacher, he has been recognized for excellence in teaching three times in a period of five years.

Meet the Volume Editors

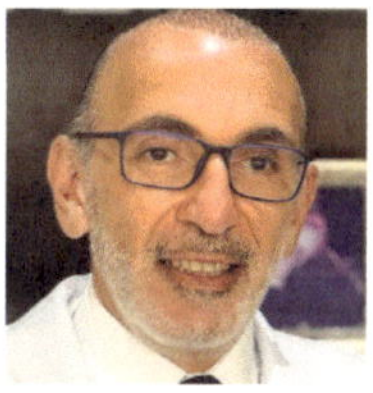

Julio Elito Júnior received his M. D. and Ph. D. degrees from the Paulista School of Medicine at the Federal University of São Paulo (EPM-UNIFESP) in 1995 and 1997, respectively. He is a specialist in Laparoscopy and Reproductive Medicine. In 2006, he was appointed Associate Professor in the Department of Obstetrics at EPM-UNIFESP. He is currently head of the Obstetric Pathology Department at the same university. Dr. Elito has published several journal articles and book chapters and has edited several books. He is a reviewer for several international journals and has presented at national and international congresses. He has been nominated several times as an "Honored Professor" by his students at the EPM-UNIFESP.

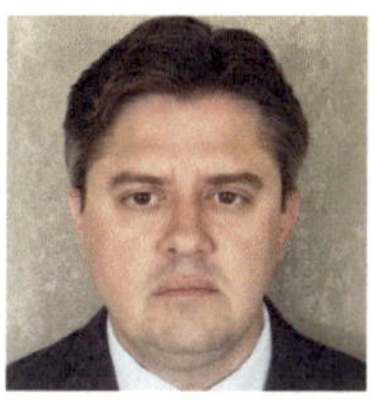

Edward Araujo Júnior holds a degree in Medicine from the Federal University of Triângulo Mineiro (UFTM) (2000). He completed his residency in Obstetrics and Gynecology at the Hospital of Clinics, Faculty of Medicine of Ribeirão Preto – University of São Paulo (FMRP-USP) (2003). He earned his Master's degree (2006), Doctorate (2007), and Specialization in Maternal-Fetal Medicine (2008), followed by a Postdoctoral Fellowship (2008) at the Department of Obstetrics, Paulista School of Medicine – Federal University of São Paulo (EPM-UNIFESP). Dr. Araujo Júnior further pursued postdoctoral fellowships in Fetal Therapy at the Department of Obstetrics and Gynecology, Katholieke Universiteit Leuven (Belgium) (2011), in Fetal Cardiology at the Department of Obstetrics and Gynecology, Baylor College of Medicine (USA) (2012), and in Fetal Therapy at the Department of Obstetrics, Leiden University (The Netherlands) (2015). He is currently an Associate Professor in the Discipline of Fetal Medicine at the Department of Obstetrics, Paulista School of Medicine – Federal University of São Paulo (EPM-UNIFESP).

Contents

Preface **XV**

Section 1
Contraceptive Methods **1**

Chapter 1 **3**
Contraception during Disaster and Pandemic Periods: Challenges and Strategies
by Ayşe Topcu Akduman and Ayşe Figen Türkçapar

Chapter 2 **19**
Interprofessional Collaboration to Enhance Contraceptive Uptake among School-Going Adolescents in South Africa
by Thabisa Mabusela, Nomawonga Msutwana and Magnolia Ngcobo-Sithole

Section 2
Maternal-Fetal Medicine **37**

Chapter 3 **39**
Diet as a Risk Factor for the Development of Gestational Diabetes Mellitus: A Narrative Review
by Lucas Almeida das Chagas, Rosângela Maria Lopes de Sousa, Rosiane Mattar, Julio Elito Júnior and Edward Araujo Júnior

Chapter 4 **49**
Normal Prolonged Labor: Do Calcium and Thyroid Have a Role?
by Yuditiya Purwosunu, Amanda Rumondang and Nathalia Isabella Muskitta

Chapter 5 **65**
Oral Health Status among Pregnant and Breastfeeding Women
by Medha Wadhwa, Pulkit Kalyan, Anshula Deshpande and Neeraj Deshpande

Chapter 6 **77**
Pregnancy: A Comprehensive Review
by Junna Ye, Jiaxin Li, Yizhu Lin, Yujuan Wang, Jingyi Wu and Zhuochao Zhou

Chapter 7 99
Tunisian Pregnant Women Benefiting from Cervical Ripening in the Third Trimester
by Montacer Hafsi, Eya Kristou, Fathi Mraihi and Dalenda Chelli

Chapter 8 119
Efficacy and Safety of Metformin Use in Pregestational Insulin Resistance Pregnant Women and in Gestational Diabetes Mellitus in Perinatal Outcome: An Update
by Enrique Valdés Rubio

Section 3
Gynecological Cancer 131

Chapter 9 133
Management of Cervical Cancer and Human Papillomavirus in Pregnancy
by María Fernanda Calderón León, María Eugenia Ugarte Vega, Germania Elizabeth Yugcha Andino, Paula Andrea Vásquez Jaramillo, Germán Arturo Vélez Sáenz, Joel Paul Vargas Caicedo, Moraima Elizabeth Pazmiño Iñiga, Alfredo Guillermo Chong Viteri, Angélica María Apolo Montero and Nataly del Carmen Quisiguiña Jarrín

Chapter 10 145
The Need for Audiological Care for Cervical Cancer Patients in South Africa
by Jessica Paken

Chapter 11 165
Understanding Cervical Cancer in Mozambique: Insights from Patients, Partners, and Families
by Iva Duval, Salma Chidassicua, Arminda Eugenio and Jose Chidassicua

Section 4
Gynecology Endocrinology 185

Chapter 12 187
Empowering Women in Priority Attention Zones of Tijuana: A Transdisciplinary Participatory Intervention to Address Socioeconomic and Cultural Vulnerabilities and Promote Gender Equity
by Jimmy Emmanuel Ramos Valencia and Martha Cecilia Jaramillo Cardona

Chapter 13 207
Perspective Chapter: Oral Condition and Lifetime Hormonal Fluctuations
by Mehrad Rafiei

Chapter 14 227
The Impact of Estrogen Deficiency Symptoms on Health-Related Quality of Life in Menopausal-Aged Women in China
by Martin Downes, Kyoo Kim, Marcelo Graziano Custodio, Igor Solev, Tommaso Simoncini and Qi Yu

Chapter 15 **243**
Women-Controlled Universal Vaginal Protection against STIs and Unintended Pregnancy
by Rabeea F. Omar, Sylvie Trottier and Mathieu Leboeuf

Preface

Women's health care has come a long way in the past 50 years. The introduction of the birth control pill, the use of estrogen to treat menopausal symptoms, and improved prenatal care for the maternal-fetal binomial are just a few of the breakthroughs. During this time, women have made significant progress in society, overcoming prejudice, entering the workforce, and improving their quality of life. This book also covers current topics in women's health care, such as the treatment of obstetric pathologies, induction of labor, new contraceptive methods, and the treatment of menopausal symptoms. This textbook is of great importance to both undergraduate students and professionals in various healthcare fields who wish to improve their knowledge of women's healthcare at all ages. Finally, I would like to thank the publisher, IntechOpen, for the opportunity to edit this book, which I believe will be of great importance to those who wish to work in global women's health care.

Julio Elito Júnior and Edward Araujo Júnior
Department of Obstetrics,
Paulista School of Medicine,
Federal University of São Paulo,
São Paulo, Brazil

Section 1

Contraceptive Methods

Chapter 1

Contraception during Disaster and Pandemic Periods: Challenges and Strategies

Ayşe Topcu Akduman and Ayşe Figen Türkçapar

Abstract

Disasters and pandemics have profound impacts on healthcare systems, significantly affecting the efficiency and accessibility of Sexual and Reproductive Health (SRH) services, thereby increasing the risks to women's reproductive health. Contraceptive methods and tools are among the most crucial factors that help individuals manage their reproductive health. Although there is growing recognition that SRH care is an integral component of disaster response, this issue often fails to receive the necessary attention during crises. This chapter aims to address gaps in knowledge regarding the improvement of contraceptive services during disaster and pandemic periods, review current practices, and fill knowledge gaps in this field.

Keywords: contraception, sexual and reproductive health, disaster, pandemic, epidemic

1. Introduction

Family planning is a process designed to enable individuals to have the desired number of children at their preferred time [1]. Contraception, on the other hand, encompasses various methods used to reduce or entirely eliminate the risk of pregnancy. These methods can be classified as hormonal methods (birth control pills, injections), barrier methods (condoms), natural methods (calendar-based methods), and surgical methods (tubal ligation) [2]. Contraception plays a key role in helping individuals effectively manage their sexual and reproductive health, with the primary goal of preventing unintended pregnancies. Access to contraceptive services becomes especially critical during disasters and pandemics, as it helps safeguard health and prevent unwanted pregnancies. In such situations, the sustainability of family planning practices is essential for community rebuilding and improving individuals' quality of life.

The desire to have children represents a complex and multidimensional facet of human existence. Throughout history, childbirth has been viewed as one of the most crucial events in life, and despite the associated risks, fertility has continued unabated under various circumstances [3]. In ancient civilizations, including those of the Egyptians, Romans, and Greeks, numerous methods—such as herbal mixtures, vaginal sponges, and other techniques—were utilized to manage fertility and prevent pregnancies [4]. The increased understanding of human anatomy and the reproductive system during the Renaissance period laid the foundation for the advancement of contraceptive practices. The groundbreaking approval of the first oral contraceptive by the Food and Drug Administration (FDA) in 1960 represented a significant transformation in the field of family planning [5]. In the last 60 years, progress in this area has been remarkably swift and effective, resulting in the creation of safer and more diverse hormonal contraceptives (HCs) [2]. Nevertheless, with nearly half of all pregnancies globally still being unintended, there is a clear necessity for further innovations and improvements in family planning services.

The accessibility and sustainability of family planning services are of paramount importance for safeguarding individuals' reproductive rights and enhancing overall societal well-being [6]. In many countries, these services are shaped by legal frameworks that align with societal needs and national policies. However, during times of crisis, such as pandemics and natural disasters, family planning services often experience significant disruptions, which can have serious adverse effects on public health. The COVID-19 pandemic, which began in 2019, along with the global response to it, has clearly illustrated the worldwide disruptions faced by various cultural, ethnic, and socioeconomic groups in accessing reproductive health services and how these services have been affected [7].

The World Health Organization defines disasters as events that exceed local capacity and significantly disrupt the functioning of a community, necessitating national or international assistance [8]. Disasters can be categorized into two main types: natural (such as earthquakes, floods, hurricanes, droughts, and pandemics) and human-made (including chemical spills and wars). In recent years, events like the 2020 Australian bushfires, the floods in Turkey and Europe in 2021, and the major earthquakes in Turkey and Morocco in 2023 have left profound impacts on humanity. Notably, the earthquake centered in Kahramanmaraş, Turkey, in 2023 resulted in substantial loss of life and severely affected healthcare services and infrastructure in the region [9]. Similarly, pandemics can trigger global health crises. Over the past decade, pandemics such as COVID-19 (2019-present), Ebola (2014–2016, 2018-present), Zika virus (2015–2016), and HIV have had significant global repercussions. Moreover, studies indicate that it typically takes around 23 months to fully reveal the impacts of pandemics on perinatal health, underscoring the seriousness of these situations [10]. Large-scale disasters lead to interruptions in the overall structure of healthcare services, resulting in critical challenges that severely affect sexual and reproductive health (SRH) services. The repercussions are particularly profound and extensive for vulnerable groups, such as women and children [11]. It is essential for individuals, healthcare teams, hospitals, and health systems to be adequately prepared to effectively manage such crises and to develop robust strategies in this regard.

This section will address the fundamental issues that may arise in reproductive health services, particularly in contraception, during times of disaster and pandemic. The challenges faced during significant recent disasters and pandemics will be examined through examples from the literature. Additionally, the section will evaluate approaches that could be integrated into strategic plans to prevent similar adverse outcomes in the future. It will also focus on the necessary measures, policy recommendations, and ways to optimize healthcare services to ensure the effective provision of contraceptive services during crisis periods.

2. The importance of contraceptive services during epidemics and disasters

During crisis periods such as pandemics and disasters, safeguarding sexual and reproductive health is crucial for both individual and public health. Sexual and reproductive health services should encompass not only prenatal care, skilled delivery, and postpartum care but also comprehensive abortion services and family planning (FP) services. It is essential that these services continue uninterrupted throughout all phases, including emergencies [12]. Disruptions in family planning services can lead to an increase in unintended pregnancies, subsequently raising maternal and neonatal morbidity and mortality rates.

The uncertainty, mental health issues, and adverse living conditions brought about by crisis periods can increase women's tendencies to avoid pregnancy. However, the heightened burden on health systems often leads to the limitation of contraceptive resources and makes access to services more challenging, resulting in a further rise in unintended pregnancies [13]. For instance, an assessment of the impact of the Ebola outbreak on health systems and community health in Sierra Leone revealed an increase in adolescent pregnancies following the epidemic [14]. Unintended pregnancies are associated with negative outcomes such as unsafe abortions, miscarriages, pregnancy complications, HIV and other sexually transmitted infections, post-traumatic stress disorder, depression, suicide, and partner violence.

Evidence indicates that disasters can have both short- and long-term effects on pregnancy outcomes. For instance, a study conducted in Sumatra revealed that improvements in maternal and infant mortality rates stagnated following a major earthquake, during which there was an increase in child mortality and stillbirth rates [15]. Additionally, following the gas leak incident in Bhopal, India, a high incidence of spontaneous abortions was reported, aside from congenital anomalies [16]. It was noted that the destruction of crops after Hurricane Gilbert led to a decrease in folic acid intake, which was associated with an increase in neural tube defects [17]. These findings demonstrate that disasters can adversely affect pregnancy outcomes in various ways. Women may unintentionally become pregnant, or a planned pregnancy can turn into an unwanted situation. It is well-established that desired and planned pregnancies result in more favorable outcomes for both maternal and child health.

In addition to the negative impacts on services provided during epidemic periods, uncertainties regarding transmission routes of the virus, its fetal and maternal effects during pregnancy, and the efficacy and safety of treatments and vaccines significantly influenced the behaviors of women planning pregnancies or who are already pregnant. Similarly, the Zika virus (ZIKV) outbreak clearly illustrates the effects of disasters on pregnancy [18]. The Zika virus epidemic, which began in 2015, created a major public health crisis in Brazil, exposing women of reproductive age to a range of potentially serious risks concerning their pregnancies and their children's health. During this period, uncertainties surrounding the virus's transmission, its fetal and maternal impacts, and the lack of available vaccines and treatments significantly affected the behaviors of women considering pregnancy or those already expecting. Research indicates that while women may wish to delay their pregnancy plans, there exists a notable disconnect between their fertility desires and their behaviors. One of the most prominent reasons for this disconnect is the challenges women face in accessing sexual and reproductive health services [19, 20].

Disasters often have a disproportionately greater impact on women compared to men. The tsunami disaster that occurred in December 2004 exemplifies this situation dramatically, as it revealed that the highest mortality rates were among women and girls. This finding underscores the exacerbation of gender inequality during crisis periods, placing women at greater risk. The obstacles women face in accessing healthcare highlight the critical importance of protecting sexual and reproductive health. The 2004 tsunami serves as a stark reminder of the gender-based violence and increasing incidents of sexual harassment experienced by displaced women in affected countries [21]. During this process, deficiencies in women's sanitation needs, secure living spaces, and access to contraception became evident, leading to an increase in unintended pregnancies and a heightened need for protection.

The importance of safeguarding sexual and reproductive health becomes particularly evident during crises, especially concerning the additional risks faced by pregnant individuals. During infectious disease outbreaks, pregnant populations are often more susceptible to infections compared to other demographic groups. The physiological changes associated with pregnancy can render these individuals more vulnerable to infections, potentially increasing the risk of severe illness [22]. Furthermore, there are risks related to vertical transmission and adverse pregnancy outcomes. Pathological processes, particularly placental abnormalities, can lead to intrauterine growth restrictions, stillbirths, preterm births, and congenital anomalies, significantly adversely affecting both maternal and fetal health.

For instance, infants born to women infected with the H1N1 virus are more likely to experience preterm birth, low birth weight (LBW), and lower Apgar scores [23]. The Ebola virus disease (EVD) outbreak in 2014 was associated with maternal mortality rates ranging from 39 to 42%. Additionally, nearly 80% of EVD cases resulted in spontaneous miscarriages and stillbirths [24]. During the Zika virus outbreak from 2015 to 2016, which affected over 50 countries, the prevalence of congenital microcephaly was reported to be approximately 3% [25]. There has been limited research on the perinatal health impacts of MERS-CoV, first identified in 2012 and primarily affecting Middle Eastern countries, which later spread to Asia, Africa, Europe, and other regions of the United States. The main observed perinatal outcomes include stillbirth, preterm birth, and maternal mortality [26]. Systematic reviews of neonatal outcomes for infants born to mothers with COVID-19 during pregnancy indicate an increase in rates of preterm birth, low birth weight (LBW), and small for gestational age (SGA) outcomes [27].

Pandemics and disasters place significant pressure on health systems, directly affecting access to essential family planning services. During such crises, women face various barriers related to healthcare worker shortages, supply chain disruptions, and access to health services. The experiences during the COVID-19 pandemic demonstrate that these challenges are likely to recur in future pandemic or disaster situations. According to UNFPA's report on *The Impact of COVID-19 on Family Planning and Ending Gender-based Violence*, disruptions of this nature are anticipated. This underscores the need for proactive strategies to ensure the continuity of family planning services during crisis periods [28].

Table 1 summarizes the primary effects of the COVID-19 pandemic on family planning and suggests that similar effects can be expected in other epidemic or disaster scenarios:

Furthermore, instances of gender-based violence have increased during the pandemic, with UNFPA estimating that if service interruptions persist for six months, there could be an additional 31 million cases. Similarly, programs combating female

Key effects of COVID-19 on family planning	Challenges
Healthcare worker shortages	The focus of clinical staff on the pandemic prevents them from allocating time to family planning services.
Closure of health facilities	Many facilities are closing or restricting family planning services.
Access restrictions	Women avoid visiting health facilities due to fear of exposure to COVID-19 or movement restrictions.
Supply chain disruptions	Supply chain interruptions limit contraceptive availability in many places, leading to stock depletion.
Inability to use preferred methods	Product shortages and lack of access to trained healthcare providers may lead women to use less effective methods or abandon contraceptive use entirely.
Increase in unintended pregnancies	If disruptions continue for six months, an additional 7 million unintended pregnancies are expected.

Table 1.
The impact of COVID-19 on family planning: Key effects and associated challenges.

genital mutilation and child marriage have been severely disrupted, with millions of new cases anticipated by 2030 [28].

These effects are not limited to the COVID-19 pandemic; similar disruptions and challenges are expected in future pandemics or disasters. It is crucial for health systems to plan necessary strategies in advance to sustain family planning services during such crises.

3. Challenges in providing contraceptive services during crises

This section will address the fundamental challenges faced in providing contraceptive services under crisis conditions and discuss the negative impacts of these challenges on women's and community health.

3.1 Logistical barriers: Supply chain disruptions, medication and material shortages

Disaster and epidemic situations significantly restrict access to healthcare services. Supply chain disruptions, along with shortages of materials and personnel, pose logistical challenges that hinder the provision of sexual and reproductive health services. Interruptions in access to essential healthcare, particularly concerning contraceptive and pregnancy-related emergency services, increase the risk of unwanted pregnancies and health complications.

The COVID-19 pandemic impacted access to healthcare services, including contraceptive services. A study conducted in South Africa and Zambia involved a survey of 537 women and in-depth interviews with 39 participants. The findings indicated that while there was no significant change in contraceptive use among the participants, barriers to access were reported, including long wait times, shortages of supplies, and fears related to COVID-19 [29].

The World Health Organization defines inequities in access to reproductive health services as unjust differences both within and between groups [30]. Access to contraceptive services is particularly crucial for disadvantaged groups, such as migrants.

Research in Europe has shown that immigrant and refugee women experience higher rates of unwanted pregnancies and abortions compared to their non-immigrant counterparts [31, 32].

Displacements following disasters and epidemics are fraught with various logistical barriers that significantly affect immigrants' access to sexual and reproductive health services. Disruptions in the supply chain, along with shortages of medications and materials, complicate the delivery of these essential services. In migrant camps, healthcare is often constrained by inadequate infrastructure and limited resources. Delays in procuring necessary contraceptive supplies during emergencies increase the risk of unwanted pregnancies and associated health complications. A study conducted in Oslo, Norway, revealed that the contraceptive needs of Somali immigrant women are not adequately met, with knowledge gaps regarding the safety and accessibility of modern contraceptive methods identified as significant barriers [33]. This situation is considered one of the contributing factors to the high rates of unwanted pregnancies and abortions among immigrant women in Europe.

Zika virus infection is associated with adverse pregnancy outcomes, including miscarriage, intrauterine growth restriction, and congenital brain abnormalities. As of 2016, Puerto Rico reported the highest number of Zika virus cases among the United States and its territories, highlighting the need for effective and accessible contraceptive methods for women living in these areas who do not wish to become pregnant. Reports indicate that approximately two-thirds of women of reproductive age in Puerto Rico experience unintended pregnancies, with significant restrictions in access to contraceptive methods [34].

In environments with limited financial resources, providing healthcare services during disaster periods becomes significantly more challenging. The inherent burden that disasters place on healthcare systems is compounded by financial pressures, adversely affecting the capacity to deliver essential services. Among the groups most impacted by these challenges are women and children [14]. For instance, a study examining the effects of the 2010 Haiti earthquake on women's reproductive health found that increased earthquake intensity led to a decrease in the use of injections, the most common modern contraceptive method in Haiti, resulting in a rise in unwanted pregnancies. Furthermore, the study noted that the severity of the earthquake intensified the unmet need for family planning among women and reduced their access to condoms [35].

3.2 Shortage of healthcare workers and services: Interruptions in healthcare personnel and clinical services

During disasters and pandemics, there is often a widespread lack of information and education regarding sexual health and contraceptive methods. Disruptions in educational and informational activities can hinder individuals from acquiring sufficient knowledge about contraceptive options. This limitation can subsequently restrict both the demand for contraceptive services and their effective utilization.

For instance, during the Ebola outbreak, nurses and midwives in Sierra Leone continued to provide care driven by various motivations, including their professional responsibilities, community obligations, and religious beliefs. This situation serves as a significant example of the continuity of healthcare services [36]. Similarly, a study examining access to contraceptives and changes in contraceptive methods before and after the 2006 earthquake in Indonesia found a decrease in the use of injections and implants within a year following the disaster, alongside an increase in the use of oral contraceptives. Additionally, the prevalence of coitus interruptus as a contraceptive method significantly rose post-disaster, and participants facing difficulties accessing contraceptive methods exhibited higher rates of unintended pregnancies. The extensive damage to healthcare facilities in Yogyakarta is believed to have restricted the abilities of nurses and midwives to perform intrauterine device insertions, implant placements, or administer injections, contributing to the observed outcomes [11].

These examples illustrate how the challenges faced by healthcare workers during disasters and pandemics affect access to sexual health and contraceptive services. A notable critical factor that emerges is the lack of education, which poses a significant threat to the continuity of these services.

3.3 Cultural and social barriers: Increased societal pressures, security concerns, and misinformation during crises

Socio-cultural barriers encompass various factors that hinder women's use of modern contraceptive methods, including religious beliefs, societal norms, social pressures, and opposition from partners to the use of such methods [33].

Studies conducted in Europe indicate that unwanted pregnancy and abortion rates are notably higher among immigrant and refugee women, many of whom do not utilize modern contraceptive methods. For instance, a study involving Somali immigrant women in Oslo identified systemic and socio-cultural barriers, such as language difficulties, inadequate information, religious beliefs, gender roles, and social pressures, that complicate access to contraceptive methods for these women. The research highlighted that although a significant portion of Somali women expressed a willingness to maintain their desired birth spacing, these barriers impede their ability to use modern contraceptive methods [33].

Religion is a significant component of the socio-cultural fabric in many societies, with religious leaders playing a crucial role in either facilitating or hindering the adoption of contraceptive methods. For instance, in Nigeria, the prevalence of modern contraceptive use remains alarmingly low at 9.8%. A study assessing the impact of exposure to family planning messages from religious leaders found that women exposed to these messages were 70% more likely to utilize modern contraceptive methods (odds ratio = 1.70; 95% confidence interval, 1.54–1.87; $P < 0.001$) [37].

The widespread sexual violence directed at women and girls displaced due to disasters, coupled with inadequate gender-sensitive health services and unsafe living conditions, has been documented as creating camp environments that expose women to an increased risk of harassment by undermining cultural norms [21].

3.4 Psychological and social factors

Disasters and pandemics can profoundly impact individuals' psychosocial wellbeing. Psychological factors such as stress, trauma, and anxiety can indirectly lead to adverse outcomes in sexual and reproductive health. In particular, Post-Traumatic Stress Disorder (PTSD) and other psychiatric conditions can significantly influence sexual health behaviors and the use of contraceptives during these periods. The pressures created by psychosocial issues negatively shape attitudes toward and access to contraceptive services.

During periods of disaster and pandemics, women's fertility preferences are influenced by psychosocial factors such as heightened anxiety and uncertainty. A study conducted in Turkey examined how COVID-19 affected women's pregnancy plans;

it found that some women postponed their plans due to the anxiety generated by the pandemic, while others decided to pursue pregnancy due to increased free time and a desire for closeness with their partners. This indicates that pandemics can influence not only fertility preferences but also decisions regarding contraception [18].

During disaster periods, although there is a general decline in quality of life, cultural norms supporting extended family structures persist. This situation emerges as a deterrent factor in the use of contraception. Women, in particular, experience peer pressure from other women and mothers, leading to encouragement for those with fewer children to have more. These social norms and peer pressure are significant contributors to the low utilization of contraceptive methods [33].

Male partners' resistance to family planning also presents a significant barrier to contraceptive use. For instance, studies conducted with refugees have revealed that women often fear their husbands may seek another partner if they do not bear a sufficient number of children [33]. Similarly, a study conducted in Tanzania found that women who used contraception without their husbands' consent faced the risk of violence or divorce [38].

During the COVID-19 pandemic, migrant women faced structural barriers to accessing healthcare, compounded by fears of discrimination. Concerns about health and safety became significant factors influencing their contraception and pregnancy choices. A study conducted in New York revealed how economic hardships and health anxieties during the pandemic shaped migrant women's reproductive health decisions [39].

3.5 Political and economic factors: Changes in government policies and lack of funding

Disasters and pandemics can significantly exacerbate economic challenges, which in turn restrict individuals' access to contraceptive products. Loss of income and economic crises can limit personal health expenditures, reducing the allocation of resources to essential healthcare services such as contraception. Low-income individuals and communities are particularly vulnerable to these adverse effects.

The high cost of modern contraceptive methods has been reported as a major barrier to their use. For instance, a study by Gele et al. on Somali immigrant women in Oslo identified the high cost of modern contraception as a key obstacle to contraceptive use [33].

4. Strategies for ensuring continuity of contraceptive services during crises

4.1 Telemedicine: The use of remote health services

Pandemics and disasters often lead to interruptions in access to healthcare services. In this context, telemedicine has emerged as an effective strategy to ensure the continuity of contraceptive services. The COVID-19 pandemic, in particular, posed significant challenges to young people's timely access to sexual and reproductive health (SRH) services, highlighting the need for telemedicine solutions. A study by Sturgiss et al. (2022) found that international innovations aimed at improving SRH access for young people, and services provided through telemedicine, have been instrumental in raising awareness about gender-based violence [40].

During the COVID-19 pandemic, the use of telemedicine for contraceptive services rapidly increased. In a study conducted with open-ended responses from 546 contraceptive providers in the United States, it was noted that telemedicine facilitated continuous access and overcame challenges posed by in-person visits. Providers emphasized the importance of telemedicine in reaching young people, especially when schools were closed. However, challenges such as lack of awareness about available services and limited access to technology were also reported. Additionally, concerns were raised about reduced personal connection and privacy issues during virtual consultations [41].

In conclusion, while telemedicine is a vital tool, it is essential to address the challenges encountered during crises and develop hybrid care models to ensure effective service delivery.

4.2 International collaboration and support: The role of international organizations and non-governmental organizations

Access to SRH services becomes crucial for saving women's lives during periods of crisis and disaster. In this context, international and non-governmental organizations play a vital role in ensuring the continuity of SRH services, particularly in the face of emergencies such as pandemics and natural disasters. These entities provide essential guidelines and standards for maintaining SRH services in times of crisis, supporting women's access to critical healthcare, including safe childbirth and family planning services, and facilitating the uninterrupted delivery of these essential services.

The 1978, Alma-Ata Declaration emphasized that access to healthcare is a fundamental human right, which can be achieved through primary healthcare (PHC) systems [42]. Sexual and reproductive health (SRH) services represent a core component of both primary and secondary healthcare, and their continuity in disaster-affected regions is of paramount importance, especially through international collaboration and support. The World Health Organization (WHO) and other global actors actively promote the preservation of these critical services and develop policies and programs to ensure sustained access at the PHC level.

To underscore the significance of these efforts, it is important to note that the United Nations Population Fund (UNFPA) projected in 2015 that two-thirds of maternal deaths worldwide occur in countries affected by humanitarian crises or vulnerable conditions [43]. The Global Strategy for Women's and Children's Health, implemented by the United Nations between 2010 and 2015, has saved millions of lives and made progress toward achieving the Millennium Development Goals (MDGs). However, by the end of this period, women, children, and adolescents in disaster and crisis-affected areas continued to face significant challenges in accessing essential healthcare services. To address this issue, the Global Strategy for Women's, Children's, and Adolescents' Health for the period 2016–2030 was developed, aiming to ensure access to health services for women and children, even in the context of humanitarian crises and challenging environments [44].

In this regard, it is crucial for national governments to strengthen the resilience of their health systems to reduce maternal mortality and ensure access to universal health services. The European Sexual and Reproductive Health Action Plan emphasizes the importance of improving access to contraception services for disadvantaged groups, such as migrants [45].

In addition to efforts conducted by international organizations, numerous local initiatives are also ongoing. For instance, a research project supported by the Government of Bangladesh's National Institute of Population Research and Training (NIPORT) includes operational research aimed at improving sexual and reproductive health services in remote and disaster-prone areas. This project seeks to identify feasible interventions for Menstrual Regulation (MR) and Post-Abortion Care (PAC) that can be implemented in hard-to-reach healthcare facilities in the Barisal and Sylhet regions [46].

5. Case studies of best practices

5.1 Successful strategies

Strategies that have been effectively implemented during pandemics and disaster periods play a critical role in ensuring the continuity of sexual and reproductive health services. One notable example is the Z-CAN (Zika Contraception Access Network) program, which was launched in Puerto Rico during the Zika virus outbreak. This initiative provided a comprehensive approach to preventing unintended pregnancies by offering a variety of contraceptive methods, including long-acting reversible contraceptives (LARC), at no cost. The program was a collaborative effort involving federal and local health agencies, the private sector, and non-governmental organizations. Between 2016 and 2017, Z-CAN served over 21,000 women, enabling them to access their chosen contraceptive methods on the same day. This resulted in a significant increase in the utilization of LARC methods. The Z-CAN model is regarded as an effective solution for enhancing access to contraceptive services in future outbreaks and disasters [47].

5.2 Regional and global experiences

Another successful initiative involves postpartum family planning (FP) strategies. Emergency postpartum family planning (EPPFP) interventions can contribute to the prevention of over 30% of maternal deaths and hold significant importance during humanitarian crises. In 2014, Save the Children incorporated postpartum intrauterine devices (IUDs) into their emergency family planning package, followed by the inclusion of implants in 2017. Countries with high-intensity EPPFP implementations have reported a notable increase in the adoption of IUDs or implants among women within the first 48 hours post-delivery. These findings indicate a strong demand for long-acting reversible contraceptives (LARC) in humanitarian settings [48].

During epidemics and disaster periods, the significance of self-administered contraceptive methods for women increases. The World Health Organization's (WHO) "Family Planning: A Global Handbook for Providers," specifically in the "Providing Family Planning Services During an Epidemic" section, highlights that various contraceptive methods can be safely and effectively used without direct support from healthcare providers. **Table 2** provides essential information regarding these self-administered methods [49].

Enhancing the accessibility of these methods will help protect women's health and facilitate their access to necessary services. It is crucial to remember that the self-administration of contraceptives is a vital strategy for ensuring women's access to health services.

Contraceptive methods	Usage method	Notes
Combined oral contraceptives (COCs)	Taken orally on a daily basis	Safe and effective; suitable for self-administration.
Progestin-only pills (POPs)	Taken orally on a daily basis	Safe and effective; suitable for self-administration.
Emergency contraceptive pills (ECPs)	Taken orally as soon as possible after unprotected intercourse	Provides rapid solutions in emergency situations.
Spermicides	Inserted into the vagina prior to intercourse	Easily applied by users; provides a barrier to sperm.
Diaphragms	Inserted into the vagina prior to intercourse	Must be used with spermicide; effective barrier method.
Condoms (male and female)	Worn during intercourse	Safe and effective; widely used; provides dual protection against STIs.

Table 2.
Self-care for contraception: Primary contraceptive methods used by women during epidemics.

6. Conclusion and recommendations

Ensuring the continuity of contraceptive services during disasters and pandemics necessitates significant advance planning and preparedness. This process involves identifying material and personnel requirements and developing strategic preparations for emergency scenarios. Additionally, training programs aimed at increasing the knowledge and awareness of healthcare workers and communities regarding contraception can promote the effective and appropriate use of services.

Collaboration between international and local health organizations can enhance the accessibility of contraceptive services by optimizing resource management. Community-supported approaches can also contribute to the dissemination of these services. Emergency contraception is a critical component in safeguarding sexual and reproductive health, and the strategies and solutions developed during this process can improve access to and effectiveness of health services, thereby mitigating the adverse health impacts of emergencies.

Author details

Ayşe Topcu Akduman* and Ayşe Figen Türkçapar
Department of Obstetrics and Gynaecology, Gulhane Training and Research Hospital, Gulhane Faculty of Medicine, Health Science University, Ankara, Turkey

*Address all correspondence to: drayse58@gmail.com

References

[1] World Health Organization. Family Planning. 2022. Available from: https://www.who.int/news-room/fact-sheets/detail/family-planning

[2] Genazzani AR, Fidecicchi T, Arduini D, Giannini A, Simoncini T. Hormonal and natural contraceptives: A review on efficacy and risks of different methods for an informed choice. Gynecological Endocrinology. 2023;**39**(1):2247093. DOI: 10.1080/09513590.2023.2247093

[3] Price NL, Hawkins K. A conceptual framework for the social analysis of reproductive health. Journal of Health, Population, and Nutrition. 2007;**25**(1):24-36

[4] Christin-Maitre S. History of oral contraceptive drugs and their use worldwide. Best Practice & Research. Clinical Endocrinology & Metabolism. 2013;**27**(1):3-12. DOI: 10.1016/j.beem.2012.11.004

[5] Tyrer L. Introduction of the pill and its impact. Contraception. 1999;**59**(1 Suppl):11S-16S. DOI: 10.1016/s0010-7824(98)00131-0

[6] World Health Organization. Family planning/Contraception. 2018. Available from: http://www.who.int/mediacentre/factsheets/fs351/en/

[7] Riley T, Sully E, Ahmed Z, Biddlecom A. Estimates of the potential impact of the COVID-19 pandemic on sexual and reproductive health In low- and middle-income countries. International Perspectives on Sexual and Reproductive Health. 2020;**16**(46):73-76. DOI: 10.1363/46e9020

[8] World Health Organization. Emergency and Essential Surgical Care: Disasters and Emergencies. Available from: http://www.who.int/surgery/challenges/esc_disasters_emergencies/en/ [Accessed: October 30, 2017]

[9] Balikuddembe JK, Reinhardt JD, Vahid G, Di B. A scoping review of post-earthquake healthcare for vulnerable groups of the 2023 Turkey-Syria earthquakes. BMC Public Health. 2024;**24**(1):945. DOI: 10.1186/s12889-024-18395-z

[10] Malange VNE, Hedermann G, Lausten-Thomsen U, Hoffmann S, Voldstedlund M, Aabakke AJM, et al. The perinatal health challenges of emerging and re-emerging infectious diseases: A narrative review. Frontiers in Public Health. 2023;**5**(10):1039779. DOI: 10.3389/fpubh.2022.1039779

[11] Hapsari ED, Widyawati, Nisman WA, Lusmilasari L, Siswishanto R, Matsuo H. Change in contraceptive methods following the Yogyakarta earthquake and its association with the prevalence of unplanned pregnancy. Contraception. 2009;**79**(4):316-322. DOI: 10.1016/j.contraception.2008.10.015

[12] United Nations Population Fund (UNFPA). Sexual and Reproductive Health and Rights: An Essential Element of Universal Health Coverage. New York: UNFPA; 2020

[13] Aly J, Choi L, Christy AY. The impact of coronavirus on reproduction: Contraceptive access, pregnancy rates, pregnancy delay, and the role of vaccination. F&S Reviews. 2022;**3**(3):190-200. DOI: 10.1016/j.xfnr.2022.05.002

[14] Azmat SK, Ali M, Siddiqui FJ, Tirmizi SFA, Kiarie J. Scoping

review on the impact of outbreaks on sexual and reproductive health services: Proposed frameworks for pre-, intra-, and Postoutbreak situations. BioMed Research International. 2021;**8**(2021):9989478. DOI: 10.1155/2021/9989478

[15] Djafri D, Chongsuvivatwong V, Geater A. Effect of the September 2009 Sumatra earthquake on reproductive health services and MDG 5 in the city of Padang, Indonesia. Asia-Pacific Journal of Public Health. 2015;**27**(2):NP1444-NP1456

[16] Kapoor R. Fetal loss and contraceptive acceptance among the Bhopal gas victims. Social Biology. 1991;**38**:242-248

[17] Duff EM, Cooper ES. Neural tube defects in Jamaica following hurricane Gilbert. American Journal of Public Health. 1994;**84**:473-476

[18] Akduman AT, Türkçapar AF, İçöz T, Özdemir Ö, Karaşahin KE. Fertility preferences of Turkish married women during the COVID-19 pandemic. Eastern Mediterranean Health Journal. 2023;**26**(11):885-893. DOI: 10.26719/emhj.23.110

[19] Chen HL, Tang RB. Why Zika virus infection has become a public health concern? Journal of the Chinese Medical Association. 2016;**79**(4):174-178. DOI: 10.1016/j.jcma.2016.03.001

[20] Marteleto LJ, Weitzman A, Coutinho RZ, Alves SV. Women's reproductive intentions and Behaviors during the Zika epidemic in Brazil. Population and Development Review. 2017;**43**(2):199-227. DOI: 10.1111/padr.12074

[21] Pittaway E, Bartolomei L, Rees S. Neglected issues and voices. Asia-Pacific Journal of Public Health. 2007;**19**(69):69. DOI: 10.1177/101053950701901S11

[22] Sappenfield E, Jamieson DJ, Kourtis AP. Pregnancy and susceptibility to infectious diseases. Infectious Diseases in Obstetrics and Gynecology. 2013;**2013**:752852. DOI: 10.1155/2013/752852

[23] Newsome K, Alverson CJ, Williams J, McIntyre AF, Fine AD, Wasserman C, et al. Outcomes of infants born to women with influenza a(H1N1)pdm09. Birth Defects Research. 2019;**111**(2):88-95. DOI: 10.1002/bdr2.1445

[24] Bebell LM, Oduyebo T, Riley LE. Ebola virus disease and pregnancy: A review of the current knowledge of Ebola virus pathogenesis, maternal, and neonatal outcomes. Birth Defects Research. 2017;**109**(5):353-362. DOI: 10.1002/bdra.23558

[25] Martins MM, Alves da Cunha AJL, Robaina JR, Raymundo CE, Barbosa AP, Medronho RA. Fetal, neonatal, and infant outcomes associated with maternal Zika virus infection during pregnancy: A systematic review and meta-analysis. PLoS One. 2021;**16**(2):1-26. DOI: 10.1371/journal.pone.0246643

[26] Alserehi H, Wali G, Alshukairi A, Alraddadi B. Impact of Middle East respiratory syndrome coronavirus (MERS-CoV) on pregnancy and perinatal outcome. BMC Infectious Diseases. 2016;**2**(16):105. DOI: 10.1186/s12879-016-1437-y

[27] Chi H, Chiu NC, Tai YL, Chang HY, Lin CH, Sung YH, et al. Clinical features of neonates born to mothers with coronavirus disease-2019: A systematic review of 105 neonates. Journal of Microbiology, Immunology, and Infection. 2021;**54**(1):69-76. DOI: 10.1016/j.jmii.2020.07.024

[28] UNFPA. The Impact of COVID-19 on Family Planning, Gender-Based Violence, Female Genital Mutilation, and Child Marriage. Glastonbury, CT: Avenir Health; Baltimore, MD: Johns Hopkins University; Melbourne, Australia: Victoria University; 2020

[29] Callahan RL, Cartwright AF, Beksinska M, Kasaro M, Tang JH, Milford C, et al. Contraceptive access and use before and during the COVID-19 pandemic: A mixed-methods study in South Africa and Zambia. Gates Open Research. 2024;**18**(7):61. DOI: 10.12688/gatesopenres. 14590.1

[30] Leeners B, Bieli S, Huang D, Tschudin S. Why prevention of repeat abortion is so challenging: Psychosocial characteristics of women at risk. The European Journal of Contraception & Reproductive Health Care. 2017;**22**(1):38-44. DOI: 10.1080/13625187.2016.1258053

[31] Raben LAD, van den Muijsenbergh METC. Inequity in contraceptive care between refugees and other migrant women?: A retrospective study in Dutch general practice. Family Practice. 2018;**35**(4):468-474. DOI: 10.1093/fampra/cmx133

[32] Bruckner TA, Mortensen LH, Catalano RA. Social and demographic drivers of trend and seasonality in elective abortions in Denmark. BMC Pregnancy and Childbirth. 2017;**17**(1):214. DOI: 10.1186/s12884-017-1397-2

[33] Gele AA, Musse FK, Shrestha M, Qureshi S. Barriers and facilitators to contraceptive use among Somali immigrant women in Oslo: A qualitative study. PLoS One. 2020;**15**(3):e0229916. DOI: 10.1371/journal.pone.0229916

[34] Tepper NK, Goldberg HI, Bernal MI, Rivera B, Frey MT, Malave C, et al. Estimating contraceptive needs and increasing access to contraception in response to the Zika virus disease outbreak--Puerto Rico. MMWR. Morbidity and Mortality Weekly Report. 2016;**65**(12):311-314. DOI: 10.15585/mmwr.mm6512e1

[35] Behrman JA, Weitzman A. Effects of the 2010 Haiti earthquake on Women's reproductive health. Studies in Family Planning. 2016;**47**(1):3-17. DOI: 10.1111/j.1728-4465.2016.00045.x

[36] Jones S, Sam B, Bull F, Pieh SB, Lambert J, Mgawadere F, et al. 'Even when you are afraid, you stay': Provision of maternity care during the Ebola virus epidemic: A qualitative study. Midwifery. 2017;**52**:19-26. DOI: 10.1016/j.midw.2017.05.009

[37] Adedini SA, Babalola S, Ibeawuchi C, Omotoso O, Akiode A, Odeku M. Role of religious leaders in promoting contraceptive use in Nigeria: Evidence from the Nigerian urban reproductive health initiative. Global Health: Science and Practice. 2018;**6**(3):500-514. DOI: 10.9745/GHSP-D-18-00135

[38] Schuler SR, Rottach E, Mukiri P. Gender norms and family planning decision-making in Tanzania: A qualitative study. The Journal of Public Health in Africa. 2011;**2**(2):e25. DOI: 10.4081/jphia.2011.e25

[39] Samari G, Wurtz HM, Desai S, Coleman-Minahan K. Perspectives from the pandemic epicenter: Sexual and reproductive health of immigrant women in New York City. Perspectives on Sexual and Reproductive Health. 2024;**56**(2):136-146. DOI: 10.1111/psrh.12260

[40] Sturgiss E, Dut GM, Matenge S, Desborough J, Hall Dykgraaf S, Mazza D,

et al. COVID-19 and access to sexual and reproductive healthcare for young people: An overview of the international literature and policy. Australian Journal of General Practice. 2022;**51**(4):271-277. DOI: 10.31128/AJGP-10-21-6206

[41] Rao L, Comfort AB, Dojiri SS, Goodman S, Yarger J, Shah N, et al. Telehealth for contraceptive services during the COVID-19 pandemic: Provider perspectives. Womens Health Issues. 2022;**32**(5):477-483. DOI: 10.1016/j.whi.2022.05.001

[42] ICPHC. (International Conference on Primary Health Care). Declaration of Alma-Ata. Geneva: World Health Organization; 1978. Available from: https://www.who.int/docs/default-source/documents/almaata-declaration-en.pdf [Accessed: February 15, 2023]

[43] UNFPA (United Nations Population Fund). Maternal Mortality in Humanitarian Crises and in Fragile Settings. New York: United Nations Population Fund; 2015. Available from: https://www.unfpa.org/resources/maternal-mortality-humanitarian-crises-and-fragile-settings [Accessed: November 12, 2015]

[44] Every Woman Every Child. The Global Strategy for Women's, Children's and Adolescents' Health (2016-2030): Survive, Thrive, Transform. 2015. Available from: https://www.gavi.org/global-health-development/unsg-global-strategy [Accessed: May 25, 2024]

[45] World Health Organization. Action Plan for Sexual and Reproductive Health: Towards Achieving the 2030 Agenda for Sustainable Development in Europe–Leaving No One behind. Geneva: WHO; 2016

[46] Ray-Bennett NS, Ekezie W, Biswas I, Choudhary NI, Cowie D, Dissanayake L, et al. Sexual and reproductive service interventions for menstrual regulation, safe abortion, and post-abortion care and their effectiveness during disaster response: A global systematic review. International Journal of Disaster Risk Science. 2024;**15**:359-373. DOI: 10.1007/s13753-024-00565-7

[47] Lathrop E, Romero L, Hurst S, Bracero N, Zapata LB, Frey MT, et al. The Zika contraception access network: A feasibility programme to increase access to contraception in Puerto Rico during the 2016-17 Zika virus outbreak. The Lancet Public Health. 2018;**3**(2):e91-e99. DOI: 10.1016/S2468-2667(18)30001-X

[48] Gallagher MC, Morris CN, Fatima A, Daniel RW, Shire AH, Sangwa BMM. Immediate postpartum long-acting reversible contraception: A comparison across six humanitarian country contexts. Frontiers in Global Women's Health. 2021;**6**(2):613338. DOI: 10.3389/fgwh.2021.613338

[49] World Health Organization. Family Planning: A Global Handbook for Providers. 4th ed. Geneva: World Health Organization; 2022. Department of Sexual and Reproductive Health and Research, Johns Hopkins Bloomberg School of Public Health, Center for Communication Programs, Knowledge for Health Project, United States Agency for International Development, Bureau for Global Health, Office of Population and Reproductive Health

Chapter 2

Interprofessional Collaboration to Enhance Contraceptive Uptake among School-Going Adolescents in South Africa

Thabisa Mabusela, Nomawonga Msutwana and Magnolia Ngcobo-Sithole

Abstract

Sexually active school-going adolescents globally, though receiving some formal education regarding sex and contraceptives, are still lacking the specific knowledge needed for the correct uptake of contraceptives. It is also known that teenage pregnancy is driven by many aspects but mainly limited knowledge and inconsistent contraceptive use, the attitudes of healthcare professionals at Reproductive Health Centres, teenagers having limited options from which to choose and often stigmatisation they receive from being sexually active. There are several efforts that have been implemented to enhance contraceptive uptake among school-going teenagers globally. These efforts often involve collaboration among various stakeholders including government agencies, healthcare professionals, community-based organisations, non-governmental organisations, and educational institutions. This chapter reports on a study that was done in the Eastern Cape, South Africa, which aimed to explore the perceptions and expertise of midwives/nurses, teachers, and psychologists/counsellors regarding a collaboration that will enhance and improve contraceptive uptake by sexually active school-going adolescents. The interprofessional collaboration envisaged is of crucial importance to facilitate contraceptive use and limit pregnancy in this population group.

Keywords: contraceptive uptake, collaboration, teenage pregnancy, comprehensive sexuality education, school-going adolescents

1. Introduction

Teenage pregnancy is a concerning social issue not only in South Africa but globally. However, there are also indications that from the last decade there have been a drop in pregnancy rates, although these improvements are uneven, with countries in the Sub-Saharan Africa still bearing the highest rates globally [1]. South Africa has seen an increase in teenage pregnancies in the last few years following the Covid-19 pandemic. Between April 2021 and March 2022, 90,000 pregnancies were recorded for girls aged 10–19 years, with over 150,000 young girls being pregnant in the 2022–2023 financial year [2]. The interaction of various factors that contribute to teenage pregnancy has been noted in the literature, including low education, challenges with access to contraceptives, economic status, public school attended (as against private schools), early sexual debut, having many sexual partners, transactional sex with older partners for monetary gain, substance use, peer pressure, and family circumstances [3]. The role of forced sex and gender-based violence has also been implicated within the South African context as another contributing factor [1, 4, 5]. Surely, the wide range of interactional factors that seem to contribute to adolescent pregnancy would require a multifaceted approach, and collaborative approaches are key to delivery of quality health care and services. Hence, this study aimed to explore the perceptions and expertise of midwives/nurses, teachers, and psychologists/counsellors regarding a collaboration that will enhance and improve contraceptive uptake by sexually active school-going adolescents. Health care in general relies on teamwork and the integrated knowledge and effort of many different professionals.

2. Teenage prevention in South Africa: An overview

In 1998, the Department of Basic Education introduced Life Orientation (LO) training in the basic school's curriculum aimed at developing and engaging learners in psychosocial and economic skills so that they can achieve their full potential as responsible citizens [6]. Reproductive health care is one of the skills being developed in the LO programme through its sexuality education component. Although the programme is still presented some improvement in reproductive health care (RHC) is still needed as it is perceived as not effectively serving the course of RHC [7, 8]. The South African government has continued to implement various interventions, including free and easily accessible contraceptives, the distribution of condoms, youth friendly services clinic, as well as the adoption of the 2030 Sustainable Development Goals which, among other things, speak to Sexual and Reproductive Health Rights as well as Children's and Adolescent Health [9, 10]. However, pregnancy among school going teenagers still prevails as a going concern. Sepeng et al. [10] contend that most of the stakeholders are not included in the development of strategies for teen pregnancy prevention, which in his view includes parents, community leaders, healthcare professionals, and the teenagers themselves. In South Africa, there is also no interprofessional collaboration of skills and interventions in the approach to this challenge. It is in this context that the study described in this chapter was conceived.

3. Methodology

The study adopted a mixed methods research design that is concurrent in nature and the qualitative design as the leading design [11]. The target population were the professionals who are working in the Nelson Mandela Bay Health District (NMBHD) as nurses at primary healthcare clinics, teachers who are teaching RHC at secondary schools, and psychologists/counsellors. Selection was through probability, purposive, and criterion-based methods to enhance the richness of the collected data [11]. The sampled nurses were those who work at antenatal, postnatal, mother, and child healthcare clinics for more than 6 months while the selection criteria for psychologists were psychology practitioners in private practice within Nelson Mandela Bay Metro (NMBM). Selection criteria included educational, clinical, counselling psychologists, and registered counsellors.

The setting of the study included 33 comprehensive clinics at NMBM with four midwives/nurses per clinic, and thus, there was a total of 132 possible participants. Teacher participants were chosen from the schools that are within a five-kilometre radius distance from the clinics to facilitate the process of the collaboration if possible. There are eight secondary schools in that space, an average of 30 teachers per school, and an average total of 240 teachers to participate. A selection of this setting permitted the researchers to focus solely on previously disadvantaged participants who are underrepresented in studies of this nature.

3.1 Data collection and analysis

A questionnaire comprising of twenty closed-ended questions on a five Likert scale that was piloted beforehand to ensure reliability was distributed. The Likert scale measures attitudes and perceptions by providing a range of responses to which the respondent had to choose one that most aligns with them [12]. The questionnaire covered the quantitative aspect of the study and was divided into three sections: demographic information, knowledge and awareness questions, and attitudinal and perception-based questions. The questionnaires were distributed and completed successfully under the direct and indirect supervision of the fieldworkers, but daily routines were not interrupted. A total of 136 teachers and 130 nurses completed the questionnaires. Data were analysed using SPSS version 26.0. Descriptive statistics were used to describe and synthesise the data using frequencies, percentages, charts, means, medians, and standard deviations. Reliability and validity of the questionnaire were assured, and internal consistency thereof was measured through Cronbach's alpha coefficient.

To collect data from the psychologists/counsellors, semi-structured face-to-face interviews were conducted by a fieldworker and captured by means of a digital voice-recorder. Participants were asked to sign an informed consent form for voluntary participation and the use of a digital voice-recorder[19]. The interview sessions were conducted for a minimum of 45 minutes per interview. The interviews were held in the work offices of the participants but outside work hours. The interviews were conducted in English, and the main question to be responded to by all the participants was:

- Tell me how do you feel about you as a psychologist/counsellor having a collaboration with midwives/nurses and teachers to assist teenagers with uptake of contraceptives?

An interview schedule was used to direct the flow of the interview and responses. A pilot study was conducted to test the reliability and feasibility as well as the trustworthiness of the study [13]. The main interviews were conducted and continued until data saturation [14] was confirmed; thus, ten participants were interviewed from the 15 that were approached for participation.

Tesch's method of data analysis [15] was used, and the results were finalised in the presence of an independent coder who was a psychologist and a qualitative research expert. The researchers reviewed the data, organised, and coded it into categories, sub-themes, and themes. Five themes emerged from the data, and these are presented in the next section.

3.2 Trustworthiness, reliability, and validity

The trustworthiness of this study was confirmed using Lincoln and Guba's model of trustworthiness [16]. This model is based on four different criteria: credibility, transferability, dependability, and confirmability. Specific strategies were used to enhance the trustworthiness to ensure the authenticity of the study. To ensure credibility, prolonged engagement with participants was used. Multiple data collection methods were used to preserve triangulation. Transferability and dependability were in the form of a specific selection criteria and use of the services of independent reviewer to evaluate accuracy of data collected to avoid bias. Confirmability and authenticity were achieved by means of a pilot study and using verbatim quotes, respectively.

4. Presentation of findings

Herewith, a presentation of the quantitative data and qualitative data, respectively:

4.1 Quantitative results

4.1.1 Characteristics of the sample

Descriptive statistics of the study population (N = 266) are presented in **Table 1**.

The total occupation of participants were 130 (100%) midwives and 136 (100%) teachers. A total of 77% was females that participated. A total of 33% of participants presented with work experience above 20 years where 22% reported work experience less than 1–4 years. Regarding the education level, 65% of participants completed a degree compared to 33% that completed a diploma. A small number of both teachers and nurses did not indicate their educational level nor years of experience.

Characteristics of study participants (N = 266)						
	Occupation					
Age	**Midwives**		**Teachers**		**Total**	
20–30	30	23%	39	29%	69	26%
31–40	34	26%	31	23%	65	24%
41–50	28	22%	21	15%	49	18%
>51	38	29%	45	33%	83	31%
Total	130	100%	136	100%	266	100%
Chi^2(d.f. = 3, n = 266) = 2.77; p = .429						
Occupation and Gender						
	Occupation					
Gender	Midwives		Teachers		Total	
Female	102	78%	103	76%	205	77%
Male	28	22%	33	24%	61	23%
Total	130	100%	136	100%	266	100%

Characteristics of study participants (N = 266)						
	Occupation					
Age	**Midwives**		**Teachers**		**Total**	
Chi^2(d.f. = 1, n = 266) = 0.28; p = .597						
Occupation and Work Experience						
	Occupation					
Work Experience Category	Midwives		Teachers		Total	
1–4 years	15	14%	37	29%	52	22%
5–19 years	60	56%	47	36%	107	45%
20+ years	33	31%	45	35%	78	33%
Total	108	100%	129	100%	237	100%
Chi^2(d.f. = 2, n = 237) = 10.96; p = .004; V = 0.22 Small						
Occupation and Educational Level						
	Occupation					
Educational Level	Midwives		Teachers		Total	
Diploma	72	56%	14	10%	86	33%
Degree	51	40%	121	90%	172	65%
Other	5	4%	0	0%	5	2%
Total	128	100%	135	100%	263	100%
Chi^2(d.f. = 2, n = 263) = 72.47; p < .0005; V = 0.52 Large						

Table 1.
Characteristics of the sample.

4.1.2 Support/need for collaboration

The need for support or need for collaboration is presented in **Table 2**.

A significant correlation between midwives and teachers presented a need for collaboration at 79%, with 21% of the sample either neutral or negative towards collaboration.

The one-sample t-test conducted in **Tables 3** and **4** presents that the communication systems presented with the highest scores from both the midwives and teachers sampled.

	Occupation					
Support/Need for collaboration	**Midwives**		**Teachers**		**Total**	
Negative: 1.00–2.59	5	4%	30	22%	35	13%
Neutral: 2.60–3.40	5	4%	15	11%	20	8%
Positive: 3.41–5.00	120	92%	91	67%	211	79%
Total	130	100%	136	100%	266	100%
Chi^2(d.f. = 2, n = 267) = 27.60; p < .0005; V = 0.32 Medium						

Table 2.
Support/need for collaboration.

One-sample t-test classification and inferential ranking—Collaboration aspects: Midwives						
	Descriptive statistics			95% CI classification		
					H_1:	$\mu \neq 3.40$
Factors	N	Mean	S.D.	Low	High	Category
8. Communication systems	127	4.06	0.95	3.90	4.23	Positive
2. Teenager centred reproductive care	130	3.60	1.11	3.41	3.79	Neutral to Positive
1. Mutual goals	130	3.55	1.11	3.36	3.75	Neutral to Positive
9. Assist the teenagers	130	3.51	1.08	3.32	3.70	Neutral to Positive
3. Shared knowledge	130	3.49	1.08	3.30	3.68	Neutral to Positive
6. Collective management	130	3.47	1.05	3.29	3.65	Neutral to Positive
4. Confidence levels of care	130	3.38	1.07	3.20	3.57	Neutral to Positive

Table 3.
T-test classification and inferential ranking: Collaboration aspects: Midwives/Nurses.

One-sample t-test classification and inferential ranking—Collaboration Aspects; Occupation = Teachers						
	Descriptive statistics		One-sample t-test classification			
Factors	N	Mean	d.f.	t-value	Cohen's d	Category
	S.D.		H1	p-value		
8. Communication systems	137	3.43	136	0.26	n/a	Neutral to Positive
	1.39		$\mu \neq 3.40$	.796		
9. Assist the teenagers	136	3.10	135	−2.41	0.21	Neutral
	1.47		$\mu \neq 3.40$	.017		
1. Mutual goals	137	2.92	136	2.82	0.24	Neutral
	1.33		$\mu \neq 2.60$	.006		
6. Collective management	137	2.77	136	1.47	n/a	Negative to Neutral
	1.32		$\mu \neq 2.60$	.144		
4. Confidence levels of care	137	2.72	136	0.97	n/a	Negative to Neutral
	1.39		$\mu \neq 2.60$	.332		
5. Policy/ strategies in different levels of care	137	2.68	136	0.70	n/a	Negative to Neutral
	1.32		$\mu \neq 2.60$	.485		
3. Shared knowledge	137	2.67	136	0.62	n/a	Negative to Neutral
	1.34		$\mu \neq 2.60$	.533		
2. Teenager centred reproductive care	136	2.64	135	0.33	n/a	Negative to Neutral
	1.39		$\mu \neq 2.60$	.740		

Table 4.
T-test classification and inferential ranking: Collaboration aspects: Teachers.

The questionnaire developed yielded good to excellent reliability as Cronbach alpha scores of 0.70 and above indicate.

4.2 Qualitative results

4.2.1 Profile of the participants

Table 5 below gives a description of the participants.

The participants were either educational psychologists (7) or counselling psychologists (2), except for one participant who is a registered counsellor. Only one psychologist had a Ph.D. qualification, while the rest had a master's degree in either educational or counselling psychology. The registered counsellor had qualified with a four-year bachelor's degree in psychology. Five of the psychologists, including the registered counsellor, presented with work experience of between 11 and 20 years, while the remaining participants had work experience of between 3 and 6 years.

4.2.2 Results

The qualitative phase was aimed at exploring and describing the experiences of psychologists/counsellors regarding collaborating with nurses and teachers to

Demographic profile of participants interviewed					
Participant no.	**Participant code**	**Age range**	**Gender**	**Qualification**	**Years of experience**
1	EP1	50–55	F	PhD Educational Psychology	20
2	EP2	45–50	F	M. Educational Psychology	18
3	EP3	30–35	F	M. Educational Psychology	6
4	EP4	45–50	F	M. Educational Psychology	13
5	EP5	45–50	F	M. Educational Psychology	18
6	EP6	40–45	F	PGCE & M. Educational Psychology	6
7	EP7	40–45	F	HED & M. Educational Psychology	14
8	CP1	25–30	F	M. Counselling Psychology	3
9	CP2	30–35	M	M. Counselling Psychology	5
10	RC1	35–40	F	BPsych (Registered counsellor)	11

Table 5.
Demographic profile of participants.

enhance the uptake of contraceptives by sexually active school-going adolescents. The proposal for an inter-professional collaboration was acceptable to the participants as it would relieve the burden from one profession and benefit the school-going adolescents. Participants also raised the concern of existing policies that are to be considered, the role of partners in the collaboration, and resources that will be needed for the success of the collaboration.

4.2.2.1 Existing policies on collaboration between teachers and healthcare professionals

The participants noted the policies that might be speaking to the said collaboration, but that they were not explicit on reproductive health prevention. The words of the participants in this regard were as follows:

> *"I think policies [in the Department of Education] do accommodate collaboration, but it may not be specifically saying contraceptive uptake"*—EP2 line 180–181

> *"There's no formal plan or programme that has been driven by the Department [of Education]. As such because it's always been looked upon as it's Department of Health's service okay."*—EP1 line 47–48

The role conflict as displayed on the latter response is a matter that could dampen the motivation for the collaboration in the absence of a clear guide. The participants were insisting on clear roles for the different partners in the collaboration.

4.2.2.2 Determine the roles for each partner in the collaboration

Participants recommended a multi-disciplinary effort, but a careful selection of the drivers to the collaboration. Regarding these matters, participants voiced them as follows:

> *"Then my recommendation will be, psychologists can be approached to be part of the collaboration, but they cannot be the key role players."*—EP1line 242–245

> *"Yes, it's supposed to be a multidisciplinary effort. A social worker, a health promoter, a nurses, a psychologist, a counsellor all of us it's supposed to be a teamwork [hence the need for clear roles of the different partners]."* EP5 line 120–121

Critically, the results in both research designs used revealed a concern about the resources that will be needed for the collaboration as the current needs of the nurse/midwife units will not cope with added responsibilities coming from the inter-professional collaboration.

4.2.2.3 Allocate the needed resources

Budget for the Departments of Health and Basic Education should make provision for the resources needed for the successful collaboration in the uptake of contraceptives by school-going adolescents. One participant had the following to say:

> *"Provide more resources and support to healthcare professionals so that there can be a task team or Department or a section or even a part of a clinic that deals specifically with this"*—CP2 line 142–144

It became apparent that besides the collaboration, there are certain considerations that should be made to enhance contraceptive uptake. Focused education on sexual activity and contraception is also needed.

4.2.2.4 Needed education and appropriate information regarding misconceptions about sexual activity and contraception

The matter of relevant education and sources of information was experienced as needing attention as well. In finding own identity, adolescents do a lot of trials and errors behaviours, consulting social media and Internet to find answers, thus making themselves vulnerable to misinformation. Participants, therefore, expressed a need for a focused education of sexual activity and contraception in schools:

> *The young children they receive wrong information because of the availability of information now like phones like other TV, like other children at schools…* EP5 line 141–144

> *"When I was working in the schools, especially in the high schools, there was a lot of misunderstanding around sexual activity, especially with girls, they hadn't been educated in any way on being sexually active and most especially been educated on contraceptives"*—RC1 line 32–34

4.2.2.5 Leaning towards a holistic approach

Participants also expressed that the education should have more emphasis on safe sex, as contraception and sexual activity are interlinked. Adolescents should be taught about the alternatives if they cannot abstain:

> *"So, I think for teenagers we rather encourage safer sex practices than motivating for contraceptives. .... But if the teenager feels that she cannot, she is unable to manage herself control then contraceptive would be an alternative..."*—EP2 line 82–84 and line 265–267

> *"Yeah! the reality is, not all teenagers will abstain. So that's why then the main focus in schools and in education should be on what contraception .... to use in order to stay safe."*—RC1 line 67–69

The participants were alluding to the comprehensive sexuality education (CSE) that should be intentional in schools, given that early sexual debut is a reality with twenty-first century learners. However, CSE that teaches about alternatives such as the recommended contraceptives among other things is contested as seen in the following aspects.

4.2.2.6 Hindrances by the schools and attitudes unfavourable towards contraception

Access to the clinics and schools was identified as a dominating and a major concern to the goal of contraceptive uptake. Participants raised these experiences as follows:

> *"So, I believe there is still a very big stigma within the health care system, which sort of become a barrier for young girls, for young ladies to go and get contraception or at least enquire about contraception."*—CP line 130–13

> *"... the Department of Education, make it clear that these contraceptives must not be in the schools, they must be in the health care centres, the clinics and so on and so on"*—EP4 line 59–63

> *"One of the problems that the schools are having is that a lot of School Governing Bodies don't want to allow Nurses to come in and to administer it at school."*—EP1 line 28–29

Fear of judgement by the nurses or teachers coupled with prohibitions from the parents (School Governing Bodies) discourage contraceptive uptake by adolescents. Further, matters of concern to access and uptake of contraceptives by the sexually active school-going adolescents are compounded by moral concerns and a lack of training of healthcare professionals.

4.2.2.7 Ethical, legal, and cultural values concerns and lack of training

Moral, cultural, and legal obligations of education practitioners make them reluctant to promote CSE and the implied contraceptive uptake. Responses to this effect were as follows:

> *"I'm in the process of adding the parents' permission to talk about issues of sexuality but it's very sensitive topic with special needs children. If we follow the research we should be more active in terms of protecting the children in my view...."*—EP7 line 144–145

> *"Yeah it comes back to lack of education [and training], let me put it that way from our healthcare professionals ... So I think awareness campaigns and education need to start with the healthcare professionals."*—EP3 line 109–112 and 122–126

These aspects make the collaborators think about what kind of information needs to be shared with the adolescent learners, and who the sources of sexuality knowledge should be.

4.2.2.8 Most appropriate information is needed to be shared with the learners

The important aspect emphasised regarding sharing of appropriate information was the understanding of the information shared. The results from the quantitative data analysis confirmed the need to communicate better within the team and adolescents. Some responses associated with sharing of appropriate information were as follows:

> *"Age-appropriate information and as they grow monitor..."*—EP5 line154–155

> *"Umm, ...we need to be very careful about how the information is given, because if the information is given and the child doesn't always understand it 100% they often make as I said those connections."*—EP6 line 335–337

Parents are seen as the ones who should be the main sources of information about sexual matters including contraceptives. Other sources are school curriculum that is aimed at shaping these adolescents to be worthy citizens when they are older. Young folks are the most users of social media and are at times exposed to incorrect information from media without the knowledge of the parents. The words of the participants associated with these statements were as follows:

> *"... the parents must also be in the position to take [play] role ...]."*—EP4 line 105–108

> *"I think teenagers of today do have information because you would find out now that most of them have cellphones. Most of them have access to media such as television and in schools even the curriculum as a subject there's a lot of information about issues as these. So, I don't think that there's any missing"*—EP3 line 130–133

In spite of all things considered, participants recommended continued support to the school-going adolescents regardless of age and sexuality.

4.2.2.9 Steadfast in support of the school-going adolescent

Some parents are reported as not communicating nor taking the subject of uptake of contraceptives seriously, forcing their children to use these reproductive control measures secretly. Thus, the inconsistent and inappropriate use of these measures may lead to risk of diseases and un-intended pregnancy. The statements of the participants in support of the adolescent are as follows:

> *"...and also, the parents must also be in the position take their part be involved in the education of their learners of their children at a younger age, because it's very difficult to educate them when already they want them."*—RC1 line 105–108

> *"We need to move from 1990s to this new millennium and say things have changed, we have to embrace the changes."*—EP6 line 261

Next, we discuss these findings to make meaning in existing literature and arguing for interprofessional collaboration to enhance contraceptive uptake in school-going adolescents.

5. Discussion of findings

Results revealed that though the possibility of interprofessional collaboration is welcomed and lauded, certain aspects at home and community, in the work environment and education system, are to be addressed for the collaboration to be effective. Platforms and matters regarding sex and sexuality education, especially social media and other influencing issues, are to be considered for the part they play in promoting or demotivating the uptake of contraceptives by sexually active school-going adolescents.

The rising teenage pregnancy reported in South Africa [2, 17] is raising a concern of the future of young girls in terms of education and involvement in the business and economy of the country. In South Africa, aspects that contribute to teenage pregnancy are broad and complex [18]; hence, the cautious attitude demonstrated by the participants in this study. The adolescent health field had broadened from the narrow focus on reduction of risky behaviour in this age group, to a more comprehensive approach to teenage pregnancy prevention [16]. Collaborative partnerships across sectors have been shown to contribute to positive changes in health knowledge, attitudes, and behaviours [19] and supposedly, including collaborations that are aimed at the enhancement of contraceptive intake by school-going adolescents. Findings in this study support the need for collaborative approaches that integrate psychological strengths such as negotiating skills, resilience, and prosocial behaviours in adolescent health prevention programs. In a review of studies, teen pregnancy reduction has been attributed to a range of issues, and efforts are to be aimed at multiple levels and by contributions from individuals across a range of disciplines [20].

Notwithstanding that a need for considering existing policies regarding the proposed collaboration as they were experienced as barriers was raised. Participants acknowledge that there are some policies in the Department of Basic Education that speak onto the collaboration between teachers and healthcare professionals. Even though there are such policies, this does not directly speak into contraceptive uptake by learners at schools. Currently, there is no existing collaboration between teachers, nurses, and psychologists/counsellors regarding facilitating contraception uptake in schools as the Department of Basic Education has always been dependent on the Department of Health for the provision of sexual activity education. In a study conducted by James in NMBHD, teachers who were participants raised a concern about their capacity to teaching RHC as they perceive it as a specialist subject [21].

DOI: http://dx.doi.org/10.5772/intechopen.1008260

They further raised a similar concern that of lack of a collaboration with healthcare professionals.

An interesting finding was that while interprofessional collaboration is an acceptable step towards increasing the rate of uptake of contraceptives by the younger generation at schools, participants warned of the workload that might accompany it. As a result, they are advocating for the allocation of more resources especially in the form of staff. Role conflict was also a concern hence the recommendation for clear roles of each partner in the project. The implications of the findings of this study point towards a holistic approach in which each participating partner has their own role, rather than working as separate entities. As observed by some participants in this study, such collaboration requires awareness about the scope of practice of each discipline, as well as respect and regard for the perspectives and contributions of other disciplines [22].

Misconceptions are to be dealt with and appropriate information shared with the adolescents, but a concern is how to go about this matter. In a study conducted in Indonesia results revealed that social taboos, disgrace, and poor communication between parents and teenagers were some of the reasons that prevented communication about sexuality issues [23]. To address access, education and appropriate information is to be shared. Many studies identify a number of misconceptions regarding the use of contraceptives thus some user default [24]. The sensitivity about communication around the topic of RHC at home and at school is as well associated with religion and cultural values and beliefs of the community [21]. In spite of the importance of culture and beliefs, it is recommended for schools and communities to consider the current times regarding sex and sexuality of the younger generation and learners [25]. Notably, teachers and school principals show interest to sharing appropriate information and involvement but rest the responsibility to the experts who are nurses and midwives for the benefit of accurate and correct information to be shared [21]. Knowledge about RHC has been identified as one of the priorities by all participating groups and is positive of its role to propel the interprofessional collaboration for the benefit of promoting proper uptake of contraceptives by school-going adolescents.

6. Conclusion

This is a first investigation into the collaboration of nurses/midwifes, teachers, and psychologists/counsellors in the Nelson Mandela Bay of South Africa. Authors argue that the pregnancy of school-going adolescents will remain a concern for a long time if steps to resolve it remain isolated from profession to profession. In this regard, the recognition of the benefits of collaborative approaches at government policy level seems imperative. While there may also be a need to review the current content of the Life Orientation programme curriculum in South Africa, relying on single issue strategies does not address the complexities of adolescent sexuality and pregnancy but that those from a holistic perspective are more likely to yield better results.

Acknowledgements

The authors wish to acknowledge the contributions of Professor S. James, Ms. M. Kramer, and Dr. N. Rall in the conception and finalisation of this study.

Conflict of interest

The authors have no conflict of interest to declare.

Author details

Thabisa Mabusela*, Nomawonga Msutwana and Magnolia Ngcobo-Sithole
Nelson Mandela University, Port Elizabeth, South Africa

*Address all correspondence to: thabisa.mabusela@mandela.ac.za

References

[1] WHO. Adolescent Pregnancy. 2024. Available from: https://www.who.int/news-room/fact-sheets/detail/adolescent-pregnancy [Accessed: September 10, 2024]

[2] News24. South Africa's Surge in Teenage Pregnancies: Impacting Mental Health of Young Mothers. 2024. Available from: https://www.news24.com/news24/community-newspaper/noordkaapbulletin [Accessed: September 10, 2024]

[3] Chung H, Kim E, Lee J. Comprehensive understanding of risk and protective factors related to teenage pregnancy in low-and middle-income countries: A systematic review. Journal of Adolescence. 2018;**69**:180-188. DOI: 10.1016/j.adolescence.2018.10.007

[4] Mkwananzi S. Teenage pregnancy in South Africa: Setting a new agenda. South African Review of Sociology. 2017;**1**:42-66. DOI: 10.1080/21528586.2016.1216801

[5] Willan S. A review of teenage pregnancy in South Africa–experiences of schooling, and knowledge and access to sexual and reproductive health services. Partners in Sexual Health. 2013;**8**:1-63

[6] Jacobs A. Life orientation as experienced by learners: A qualitative study in north-West Province. South African Journal of Education. 2011;**31**(2):212-223. DOI: 10.15700/saje.v31n2a481

[7] Francis DA, DePalma R. Teacher perspectives on abstinence and safe sex education in South Africa. Sex Education. 2014;**1**:81-94. DOI: 10.1080/14681811.2013.833091

[8] United Nations Educational, Scientific and Cultural Organization (UNESCO). International Technical Guidance on Sexuality: An Evidence-Informed Approach. Rev. ed. Paris, France: UNESCO; 2018. Available from: https://books.google.co.za/books?hl=en&lr=&id=_w9JDwAAQBAJ&oi=fnd&pg=PA6&dq=International+technical+guidance+on+sexuality:+An+evidence-informed+approach&ots=vIYEsO0FaO&sig=g7jZL-Rv7IELPbXS3HlkaF4nPto#v=onepage&q=International%20technical%20guidance%20on%20sexuality%3A%20An%20evidence-informed%20approach&f=false [Accessed: August 08, 2024]

[9] World Health Organization (WHO). Every Woman Every Child 2015: The Global Strategy for Women's, Children's and Adolescents Health (2016-2030). 2016. Available from: https://platform.who.int/data/maternal-newborn-child-adolescent-ageing/global-strategy-data [Accessed: September 12, 2024]

[10] Sepeng NV, Mulaudzi FM, Mathivha P, Musie MR, Seretlo RJ. Strategies to enhance sexual health education for prevention of teenage pregnancy in Vhembe District, Limpopo Province: Different stakeholders' perspectives, a cooperative inquiry qualitative protocol paper. Reproductive Health. 2023;**20**:1-20. DOI: 10.1186/s12978-023-01669-x

[11] Gerish K, Lathlean J. The Research Process in Nursing. Chichester: Wiley; 2015

[12] Sullivan GM, Artino AP. Analyzing and interpreting data from likert-type scales. Journal of Graduate Medical Education. 2013;**5**(4):541-542. DOI: 10.4300%2FJGME-5-4-18

[13] Grove S, Gray J, Sutherland S. The Practice of Nursing Research. Saunders: Elsevier; 2017

[14] Polit DF, Beck CT. Nursing Research; Generating and Assessing Evidence for Nursing Practice. 10th ed. Philadelphia, Chicago: Walters Kluwer; 2017

[15] Creswell JW, Creswell JD. Qualitative inquiry and research design: Choosing among five approaches. In: Creswell JW, Creswell JD, editors. Research Design: Qualitative and Mixed Methods Approaches. 4th ed. Los Angeles, California: SAGE Publications; 2018, inclusive pages

[16] Brindis CD. A public health success: Understanding policy changes related to teen sexual activity and pregnancy. Annual Review of Public Health. 2006;**27**:277-295. Available from: https://www.annualreviews.org/doi/10.1146/annurev.publhealth.27.021405.102244 [Accessed: July 12, 2024]

[17] Francke R. Shocking Stats SA Report Shows 33 000 Teen Mothers in 2020, 660 of them Younger than 10 Years Old. 2021. Available from: https://www.iol.co.za/news/south-africa/western-cape/shocking-stats-sa-report-shows-33-000-teen-mothers-in-2020-660-of-them-younger-than-10-years-old-ffbceb71-f44a-42c1-936e-0dfee472ed51 [Accessed: July 8, 2024]

[18] Newton-Levinson A, Leichliter JS, Chandra-Mouli V. Sexually transmitted infection services for adolescents and youth in low-and middle-income countries: Perceived and experienced barriers to accessing care. Journal of Adolescent Health. 2016;**59**(1):7-16. DOI: 10.1016/j.jadohealth.2016.03.014

[19] Adelelye OA, Ofili AN. Strengthening intersectoral collaboration for primary health care in developing countries: Can the health sector play broader roles? Journal of Environmental and Public Health. 2010;**1**:1-6. Available from: https://www.researchgate.net/publication/44584715_Strengthening_Intersectoral_Collaboration_for_Primary_Health_Care_in_Developing_Countries_Can_the_Health_Sector_Play_Broader_Roles

[20] Holt MK, Green JG, Tsay-Vogel M, Davidson J, Brown C. Multidisciplinary approaches to research on bullying in adolescence. Adolescent Research. 2017;**Rev. 2**:1-10. Available from: https://www.researchgate.net/publication/308187681_Multidisciplinary_Approaches_to_Research_on_Bullying_in_Adolescence

[21] James S. The impact of the responsibility of teachers regarding reproductive healthcare to teenage learners. African Journal of Reproductive Health. 2022;**26**(4):82-91. DOI: 10.29063/ajrh2022/v26i4.9

[22] Foley S, Wittmann D, Balon RA. Multidisciplinary approach to sexual dysfunction in medical education. Academic Psychiatry. 2010;**34**:386-389. Available from: https://link.springer.com/article/10.1176/appi.ap.34.5.386

[23] Muthmainnah NI, Siswantara P, Rachmayanti RD, Devi YP. Implementation of adolescent health programs at public schools and religion-based schools in Indonesia. Journal of Public Health Research. 2021;**10**(4):1954. DOI: 10.4081/jphr.2021.1954

[24] Mbachu CO, Agu IC, Obayi C, Eze I, Ezumah N, Onwujekwe O. Beliefs and misconceptions about contraception and condom use among adolescents in south-East Nigeria. Reproductive Health. 2021;**18**:7. Available from: https://link.springer.com/article/10.1186/s12978-020-01062-y

[25] Msutwana NV. Meaningful teaching of sexuality education framed by culture: Xhosa secondary school teachers' views. Perspectives in Education. 2021;**39**(2):339-355. DOI: 10.18820/2519593X/pie.v39.i2.23

Section 2

Maternal-Fetal Medicine

Chapter 3

Diet as a Risk Factor for the Development of Gestational Diabetes Mellitus: A Narrative Review

Lucas Almeida das Chagas, Rosângela Maria Lopes de Sousa, Rosiane Mattar, Julio Elito Júnior and Edward Araujo Júnior

Abstract

Based on the understanding of the complexity of gestational diabetes mellitus (GDM) and the various factors associated with the disease's onset, including the type of diet consumed, this chapter aims to assess the relationship between the role of diet and the risk of women developing GDM. GDM is defined as any degree of carbohydrate intolerance of varying severity, diagnosed for the first time during pregnancy, which does not meet the diagnostic criteria for pre-existing diabetes, and which may or may not persist after delivery. The etiology of this condition is not fully understood, but the diagnosis of GDM is fundamental to the prevention of complications for both mother and child. Currently, the gold standard for diagnosing GDM is the oral glucose tolerance test (OGTT), which should be performed between 24 and 28 weeks of pregnancy. Because of the high prevalence of GDM and its associated complications, it is imperative that pregnant women modify their eating habits and engage in regular physical activity to prevent the adverse effects of hyperglycemia. Lifestyle changes combined with dietary interventions such as the inclusion of fruits, vegetables, and complex carbohydrates rich in fiber should be followed to improve glycemic control and prevent the adverse effects of hyperglycemia during pregnancy.

Keywords: pregnancy, gestational diabetes mellitus, diet, lifestyle, maternal and perinatal outcomes

1. Introduction

Pregnancy is considered a period in a woman's life when she undergoes various changes, including physical, biological, and hormonal [1]. It is during this period that there are changes in glucose metabolism to meet the increased need for glucose in view of the development of the fetus, and it is also a time when hormonal changes lead to increased insulin resistance, thus causing a greater risk of developing gestational diabetes mellitus (GDM) [2].

GDM is defined as any degree of carbohydrate intolerance of varying severity that is first diagnosed during pregnancy, does not meet the diagnostic criteria for pre-existing diabetes, and may or may not persist after delivery [3]. The prevalence of GDM is increasing worldwide, in parallel with rates of obesity and unhealthy diets [4–6]. According to the International Diabetes Federation (IDF), the global prevalence of GDM is 14% [7], while in Brazil, according to the criteria proposed by the International Association for Diabetes Studies (IADSPG), it is 18% [5]. This wide variation is due to differences in the characteristics of the participants studied (such as age and obesity) and the use of different diagnostic methods and criteria [4, 8].

Hyperglycemia during pregnancy can cause health problems for women and their unborn babies [9]. Women diagnosed with GDM have a high risk of developing GDM in future pregnancies and an increased risk of developing type 2 diabetes mellitus in the future. There is also evidence in the literature of risks to the fetus, such as higher rates of stillbirth, preterm birth, macrosomia, hyperinsulinemia, and clinical neonatal hypoglycemia [9]. However, timely and appropriate treatment of GDM, including a healthy diet, can reduce the risk of these complications [10].

In recent years, several studies have demonstrated the importance of dietary factors in the control and prevention of GDM [11]. Dietary patterns low in fiber, polyunsaturated fatty acids, and low glycemic index foods, combined with the consumption of fats and sugary beverages, are associated with a higher risk of GDM [12, 13]. On the other hand, a diet rich in fruits, vegetables, vegetable oils, whole grains, and skimmed dairy products is associated with a lower release of pro-inflammatory mediators, which would make it an anti-inflammatory diet and prevent the occurrence of GDM [14, 15].

The increasing prevalence of GDM and the maternal-fetal risks associated with this disease reinforce the importance of studying the effectiveness of healthy food consumption in controlling the disease [16]. The literature highlights the important role of the Mediterranean diet in the prevention of GDM due to the antioxidant and anti-inflammatory properties of this diet, which is rich in fiber and monounsaturated fatty acids [17]. Li et al. [18], in their study of healthy eating patterns and common complications in pregnancy (a longitudinal study), confirmed the association between adherence to the Mediterranean diet during pregnancy and a lower risk of developing GDM [18]. Other studies have also found a positive association between healthy eating patterns before pregnancy and a lower risk of GDM [19, 20].

Given the complexity of GDM and its potential complications for both mother and fetus, there is consensus on the importance of screening these women with treatment interventions by a multidisciplinary team followed by nutritional counseling to prevent adverse perinatal outcomes. Based on the extensive knowledge of the disease and the importance and problems associated with this condition, the aim of this study was to evaluate the relationship between the role of diet and the risk of GDM according to literature reports.

2. Pathophysiology

The mechanisms involved in the pathophysiology of GDM are thought to be complex and multifactorial. The literature shows that some pathogenic genes (TCF7L2, GCK, IRS1, KCNQ1, CDKAL1, IGF2BP2, HNF1α, and MTNR1B) are involved in the development of GDM as a result of insulin resistance, and the vast majority of them negatively affect the function of pancreatic β-cells and, as a consequence, cause the disease in pregnancy [21, 22].

Another important factor promoting increased insulin resistance during pregnancy is increased maternal adiposity, which contributes to facilitated lipolysis at the end of pregnancy, resulting in greater insulin sensitivity [23]. Some literature reports suggest that mechanisms such as low-grade inflammation and excessive release of free fatty acids may also contribute to the glucose intolerance observed in GDM [21, 22]. Other evidence also suggests that the insulin secretory response in women who develop GDM is present from the pre-pregnancy period and increases in early pregnancy [24, 25]. These findings suggest that some women with GDM may have chronic or pre-existing pancreatic β-cell dysfunction, which may be mediated by several hormones, including leptin [25].

There is currently no specific causal factor for the development of GDM; however, there are risk factors that increase the likelihood of women developing this condition during pregnancy. Understanding the mechanisms involved in the pathophysiology of GDM is fundamental to promoting detection and treatment management strategies to prevent adverse outcomes.

3. Diagnosis

The diagnosis of GDM can be made at any point during pregnancy as part of routine gestational screening protocols during prenatal care visits. However, in some countries, screening is only performed following a risk assessment conducted by an obstetrician [21, 26].

GDM diagnosis can be carried out using various methods; however, most countries worldwide rely on two main methods for detecting the condition: Fasting Plasma

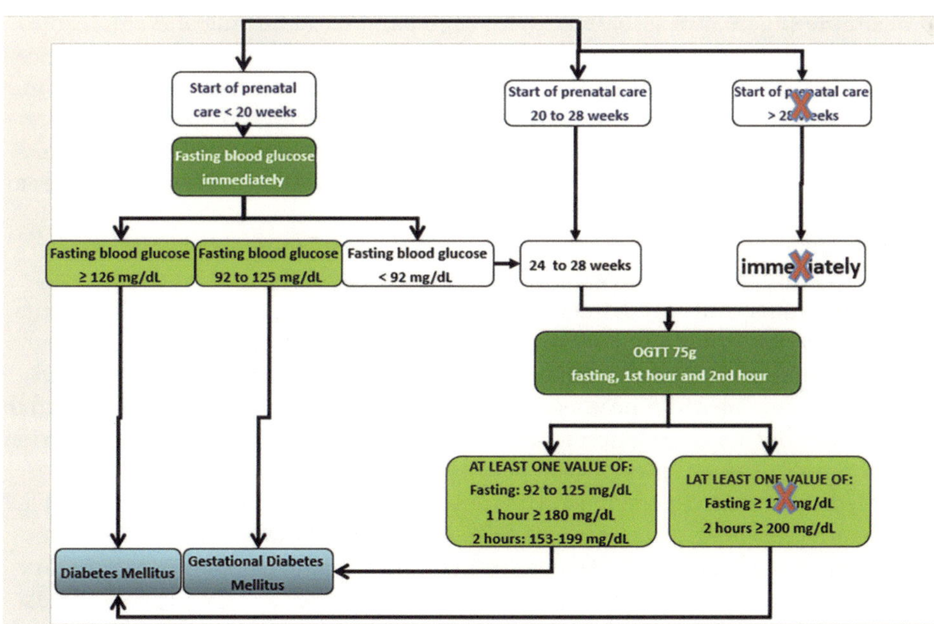

Figure 1.
Flowchart for screening pregnant women suspected of having gestational diabetes mellitus.

Glucose (FPG) and the Oral Glucose Tolerance Test (OGTT). Pregnant women with FPG levels of up to 91 mg/dL at the beginning of pregnancy are considered normal, and it is recommended to repeat testing with OGTT between 24 and 28 weeks to confirm the diagnosis. However, if the pregnant woman has FPG levels between 92 and 125 mg/dL, GDM is diagnosed early in pregnancy, as recommended by the International Association of the Diabetes and Pregnancy Study Groups (IADPSG) and the World Health Organization (WHO) [3, 5, 9, 27].

In Brazil, the Ministry of Health recommends that pregnant women without a diabetes diagnosis by 24 to 28 weeks of gestational age undergo OGTT with a 75-gram glucose load. If one or more of the following values exceed the thresholds suggested by the HAPO study—fasting glucose 92–125 mg/dL, 1-hour ≥180 mg/dL, or 2-hour 153–199 mg/dL [9]—the patient is diagnosed with GDM [1, 27].

Scientific evidence shows that early diagnosis of GDM is associated with favorable pregnancy outcomes. Although there is no global consensus on the diagnostic criteria for GDM, OGTT remains the most widely accepted and is considered the gold standard for diagnosing the condition, as endorsed by WHO and adopted by many countries, including those in Latin America such as Brazil [9]. **Figure 1** shows a flowchart for screening pregnant women suspected of having GDM.

4. Treatment

The increasing prevalence of GDM and the maternal and fetal risks associated with this condition underscore the importance of investigating the efficacy of a healthy diet in conjunction with lifestyle changes, including physical activity, in controlling the disease [28, 29].

Different components of the diet may have positive or negative effects on the glycemic profile of women with GDM. Unhealthy dietary patterns, including diets high in simple sugars, are associated with high pancreatic fatigue and can lead to persistent hyperglycemic peaks, which may result in maternal and fetal complications [30]. In recent years, the importance of elements of the diet that make it more or less inflammatory before and during pregnancy has been reported. A healthy diet during pregnancy is considered an important factor in modifying inflammation and can be considered one of the strategies to optimize perinatal outcomes and glycemic control [31].

Studies suggest a positive association between higher blood concentrations of pro-inflammatory markers and a diet rich in processed foods, full-fat dairy products, refined grains, and soft drinks [12, 13]. On the other hand, a diet rich in fruits, vegetables, vegetable oils, whole grains, and skimmed dairy products is associated with a lower release of pro-inflammatory mediators, which would make it an anti-inflammatory diet [14, 15]. These associations are observed not only in relation to this dietary pattern but also in relation to the composition and quantity of macronutrients and micronutrients in the diet [14].

The Mediterranean dietary pattern is associated with a lower incidence of GDM and fewer adverse perinatal outcomes [17]. Increasing dietary fiber intake through the consumption of fruits, vegetables, and legumes is another important dietary factor in controlling the disease [32]. Fiber is responsible for slowing food digestion and reducing the rate of glucose absorption, thereby altering blood glucose levels and the response to insulin. Fiber also reduces appetite and improves insulin resistance [32].

Adequate protein and fat intake during pregnancy in women with GDM is also associated with improved glycemic control and reduced appetite [33]. Eating a balanced diet is also important for controlling gestational weight gain. International guidelines do not recommend low-calorie diets for pregnant women because of the association of these diets with fetal growth restriction and other complications [33]. In general, diet is considered an important factor in the prevention and management of GDM, as well as in reducing complications associated with this condition.

5. Short- and long-term maternal-fetal complications

Diet is considered an important factor for maternal and fetal health [18]. Maintaining healthy eating patterns with the recommended intake of fruits, vegetables, and proteins, along with the exclusion of fats and simple carbohydrates, is associated with a reduction in gestational complications [11]. However, it is noted that some countries, such as the United States, still lack specific nutritional guidelines for pregnant women [18]. Healthy dietary patterns such as the Mediterranean diet, the alternative healthy eating index, and the Dietary Approaches to Stop Hypertension (DASH) are associated with a reduction in cardiometabolic disorders in the general population. During pregnancy, these dietary patterns are also linked to a reduction in maternal and fetal complications [18]. Several studies have demonstrated the protective role of the Mediterranean diet in preventing GDM and reducing complications for both mother and child. The Mediterranean diet is known for its ability to reduce the inflammatory state in pregnant women with GDM [17, 34, 35].

It is important to emphasize that all pregnant women should follow healthy eating patterns to prevent excessive weight gain [36], which is associated with maternal and fetal complications such as preterm birth, cesarean delivery, macrosomia, perineal lacerations, and uterine rupture resulting from fetal macrosomia and polyhydramnios [24, 36–38].

According to the Hyperglycemia and Adverse Pregnancy Outcome (HAPO) study, women with GDM also have an increased risk of gestational hypertension and preeclampsia. Another potential complication associated with GDM is the possibility that these women may develop GDM in future pregnancies or become type 2 diabetics after delivery or later in life [24]. Therefore, it is crucial that all pregnant women receive guidance on the important role of a healthy and nutrient-balanced diet during pregnancy to prevent these complications.

6. Conclusion

GDM is a silent and challenging disease that affects millions of women during pregnancy and can result in health problems for the woman and her unborn child. Dietary interventions such as the consumption of fruits, vegetables, and fiber-rich complex carbohydrates should be followed to improve glycemic control and prevent the adverse effects of hyperglycemia during pregnancy. Another important lifestyle change for pregnant women is regular physical activity, which has been shown to be an important ally in glycemic control. These lifestyle changes reduce the risk of pregnancy complications for the mother and fetus, as well as the future consequences of hyperglycemia during pregnancy.

Author details

Lucas Almeida das Chagas[1], Rosângela Maria Lopes de Sousa[2], Rosiane Mattar[1], Julio Elito Júnior[1] and Edward Araujo Júnior[1*]

1 Department of Obstetrics, Paulista School of Medicine – São Paulo Federal University (EPM-UNIFESP), São Paulo-SP, Brazil

2 Department of Nutrition, Ceuma University, São Luiz-MA, Brazil

*Address all correspondence to: araujojred@terra.com.br

References

[1] ElSayed NA, Aleppo G, Aroda VR, Bannuru RR, Brown FM, Bruemmer D, et al. Classification and diagnosis of diabetes: Standards of care in diabetes-2023. Diabetes Care. 2023;**46**:S19-S40

[2] Nunes RD, Flôres ME, Seemann M, Traebert E, Traebert J. Two criteria of oral glucose tolerance test to diagnose gestational diabetes mellitus. Revista da Associação Médica Brasileira. 2020;**66**:139-145

[3] World Health Organization. Diagnostic criteria and classification of hyperglycaemia first detected in pregnancy: A World Health Organization guideline. Diabetes Research and Clinical Practice. 2014;**103**:341-363

[4] Guariguata L, Linnenkamp U, Beagley J, Whiting DR, Cho NH. Global estimates of the prevalence of hyperglycaemia in pregnancy. Diabetes Research and Clinical Practice. 2014;**103**:176-185

[5] Trujillo J, Vigo A, Duncan BB, Falavigna M, Wendland EM, Campos MA, et al. Impact of the International Association of Diabetes and Pregnancy Study Groups criteria for gestational diabetes. Diabetes Research and Clinical Practice. 2015;**108**:288-295

[6] Shah NS, Wang MC, Freaney PM, Perak AM, Carnethon MR, Kandula NR, et al. Trends in gestational diabetes at first live birth by race and ethnicity in the US. 2011-2019. Journal of the American Medical Association. 2021;**326**:660-669

[7] Wang H, Li N, Chivese T, Werfalli M, Sun H, Yuen L, et al. IDF diabetes atlas: Estimation of global and regional gestational diabetes mellitus prevalence for 2021 by International Association of Diabetes in pregnancy study group's criteria. Diabetes Research and Clinical Practice. 2022;**183**:109050

[8] Magliano DJ, Boyko EJ. IDF Diabetes Atlas 10th Edition Scientific Committee. IDF Diabetes Atlas. 10th ed. Brussels, Belgium: International Diabetes Federation; 2021. ISBN 978-2-930229-98-0

[9] Zajdenverg L, Façanha CFS, Dualib PM, Golbert A, Moisés ECD, Calderon IMP, et al. Rastreamento e diagnóstico da hiperglicemia na gestação. Sociedade Brasileira de Diabetes; 2022. [updated 2021-12-02] Available from: https://diretriz.diabetes.org.br/rastreamento-e-diagnostico-da-hiperglicemia-na-gestacao [Accessed: July 26, 2022]

[10] Plejemann A. Maternal diabetes and perinatal programming. Early Human Development. 2011;**87**:743-747

[11] Deepa R, Lewis MG, Van Schayck OCP, Babu GR. Food habits in pregnancy and its association with gestational diabetes mellitus: Results from a prospective cohort study in public hospitals of urban India. BMC Nutrition. 2020;**6**:63

[12] Lopez-Garcia E, Schulze MB, Fung TT, Meigs JB, Rifai N, Manson JE, et al. Major dietary patterns are related to plasma concentrations of markers of inflammation and endothelial dysfunction. The American Journal of Clinical Nutrition. 2004;**80**:1029-1035

[13] Neustadt J. Western diet and inflammation. Integrative Medicine. 2006;**5**:14-18

[14] Estruch R. Anti-inflammatory effects of the Mediterranean diet: The

experience of the PREDIMED study. The Proceedings of the Nutrition Society. 2010;**69**:333-340

[15] Urpi-Sarda M, Casas R, Chiva-Blanch G, Romero-Mamani ES, Valderas-Martínez P, Arranz S, et al. Virgin olive oil and nuts as key foods of the Mediterranean diet effects on inflammatory biomakers related to atherosclerosis. Pharmacological Research. 2012;**65**:577-583

[16] Hu J, Oken E, Aris IM, Lin PD, Ma Y, Ding N, et al. Dietary patterns during pregnancy are associated with the risk of gestational diabetes mellitus: Evidence from a Chinese prospective birth cohort study. Nutrients. 2019;**11**:405

[17] Jafari Nasab S, Ghanavati M, C T Clark C, Nasirian M. Adherence to Mediterranean dietary pattern and the risk of gestational diabetes mellitus: A systematic review and meta-analysis of observational studies. Nutrition & Diabetes. 2024;**14**:55

[18] Li M, Grewal J, Hinkle SN, Yisahak SF, Grobman WA, Newman RB, et al. Healthy dietary patterns and common pregnancy complications: A prospective and longitudinal study. The American Journal of Clinical Nutrition. 2021;**114**:1229-1237

[19] Tobias DK, Zhang C, Chavarro J, Bowers K, Rich-Edwards J, Rosner B, et al. Prepregnancy adherence to dietary patterns and lower risk of gestational diabetes mellitus. The American Journal of Clinical Nutrition. 2012;**96**:289-295

[20] Schoenaker DA, Soedamah-Muthu SS, Callaway LK, Mishra GD. Pre-pregnancy dietary patterns and risk of gestational diabetes mellitus: Results from an Australian population-based prospective cohort study. Diabetologia. 2015;**58**:2726-2735

[21] Alejandro EU, Mamerto TP, Chung G, Villavieja A, Gaus NL, Morgan E, et al. Gestational diabetes mellitus: A harbinger of the vicious cycle of diabetes. International Journal of Molecular Sciences. 2020;**21**:5003

[22] Plows JF, Stanley JL, Baker PN, Reynolds CM, Vickers MH. The pathophysiology of gestational diabetes mellitus. International Journal of Molecular Sciences. 2018;**19**:3342

[23] Barbour LA, McCurdy CE, Hernandez TL, Kirwan JP, Catalano PM, Friedman JE. Cellular mechanisms for insulin resistance in normal pregnancy and gestational diabetes. Diabetes Care. 2007;**30**:S112-S119

[24] Sweeting A, Wong J, Murphy HR, Ross GP. A clinical update on gestational diabetes mellitus. Endocrine Reviews. 2022;**43**:763-793

[25] Powe CE, Huston Presley LP, Locascio JJ, Catalano PM. Augmented insulin secretory response in early pregnancy. Diabetologia. 2019;**62**:1445-1452

[26] Bhattacharya S, Nagendra L, Krishnamurthy A, Lakhani OJ, Kapoor N, Kalra B, et al. Early gestational diabetes mellitus: Diagnostic strategies and clinical implications. Medical Sciences (Basel). 2021;**9**:59

[27] Pereira BG, Fernandes CE, Saunders C, Nascimento DJ, Moisés ECD, Calderon IMP, et al. Organização Pan-Americana da Saúde. Ministério da Saúde. Federação Brasileira das Associações de Ginecologia e Obstetrícia. Sociedade Brasileira de Diabetes. Tratamento do diabetes mellitus gestacional no Brasil. Brasília, DF: OPAS; 2019. 57 p.: il. ISBN: 978-85-94091-12-3

[28] Duarte-Gardea MO, Gonzales-Pacheco DM, Reader DM, Homas AM,

Wang SR, Gregory RP, et al. Academy of nutrition and dietetics gestational diabetes evidence-based nutrition practice guideline. Journal of the Academy of Nutrition and Dietetics. 2018;**118**:1719-1742

[29] Mijatovic-Vukas J, Capling L, Cheng S, Stamatakis E, Louie J, Cheung NW, et al. Associations of diet and physical activity with risk for gestational diabetes mellitus: A systematic review and meta-analysis. Nutrients. 2018;**10**:698

[30] Yamamoto JM, Kellett JE, Balsells M, García-Patterson A, Hadar E, Solà I, et al. Gestational diabetes mellitus and diet: A systematic review and meta-analysis of randomized controlled trials examining the impact of modified dietary interventions on maternal glucose control and neonatal birth weight. Diabetes Care. 2018;**41**:1346-1361

[31] Phillips CM, Chen L, Heude B, Bernard JY, Harvey NC, Duijts L, et al. Dietary inflammatory index and non-communicable disease risk: A narrative review. Nutrients. 2019;**11**:1873

[32] Zhang Z, Li J, Hu T, Xu C, Xie N, Chen D. Interventional effect of dietary fiber on blood glucose and pregnancy outcomes in patients with gestational diabetes mellitus. Zhejiang Da Xue Xue Bao. Yi Xue Ban. 2021;**50**(3):305-312

[33] Griffith RJ, Alsweiler J, Moore AE, Brown S, Middleton P, Shepherd E, et al. Interventions to prevent women from developing gestational diabetes mellitus: An overview of cochrane reviews. Cochrane Database of Systematic Reviews. 2020;**6**:CD012394

[34] HAW B, Dodds J, Placzek A, Beresford L, Spyreli E, Moore A, et al. Mediterranean-style diet in pregnant women with metabolic risk factors (ESTEEM): A pragmatic multicentre randomised trial. PLoS Medicine 2019; 16:e1002857

[35] Karamanos B, Thanopoulou A, Anastasiou E, Assaad-Khalil S, Albache N, Bachaoui M, et al. Relation of the Mediterranean diet with the incidence of gestational diabetes. European Journal of Clinical Nutrition. 2014;**68**:8-13

[36] Augustin H, Winkvist A, Bärebring L. Poor dietary quality is associated with low adherence to gestational weight gain recommendations among women in Sweden. Nutrients. 2020;**12**:317

[37] Englund-Ögge L, Brantsæter AL, Sengpiel V, Haugen M, Birgisdottir BE, Myhre R, et al. Maternal dietary patterns and preterm delivery: Results from large prospective cohort study. BMJ. 2014;**348**:g1446

[38] Jastrow N, Roberge S, Gauthier RJ, Laroche L, Duperron L, Brassard N, et al. Effect of birth weight on adverse obstetric outcomes in vaginal birth after cesarean delivery. Obstetrics and Gynecology. 2010;**115**:338-343

Chapter 4

Normal Prolonged Labor: Do Calcium and Thyroid Have a Role?

Yuditiya Purwosunu, Amanda Rumondang and Nathalia Isabella Muskitta

Abstract

Prolonged labor is a common finding in labor wards. One known cause is that the smooth muscle of the uterus did not contract well enough, so the cervical opening and head position failed to follow the progress line in the partograph. Few detailed data exist regarding this because we usually directly give patients more contraction agents, such as oxytocin and amniotomy, rather than look for the cause. Tapping into a mother's natural strength is a gentler and just as practical approach. Calcium is known to affect smooth muscle contraction. Thyroid hormone is also known to affect the calcium level in the body. This chapter ponders the question, "How do calcium and thyroid hormone solve prolonged labor problems?" We consider prepared antenatal care with normal calcium and FT4 levels supplementation worth a trial to have the chance of normal prolonged labor without augmentation.

Keywords: prolong labor, labor, calcium, thyroid, uterine contraction

1. Introduction

Prolonged labor is common during obstetric practice and is consequently the most common intrapartum indication for cesarean section [1, 2]. Cesarean section is known to have higher postoperative complications than vaginal delivery. Meanwhile, vaginal delivery with a prolonged course itself also has maternal and fetal side effects, such as trauma, low Apgar score, and puerperal infection [3–5]. Both bring a dilemma to practicians as to where or when prolonged labor should be allowed to avoid the expense of postoperative complications of cesarean section [3, 5, 6].

This condition is very challenging to diagnose and manage [6, 7]. Sometimes, many practitioners cannot estimate the speed of physiological labor. Therefore, they cannot decide to do specific management. Friedman [8] established a standard baseline to evaluate labor progress. It helps to form prolonged labor management protocols. Philpott [9] also designed a partograph to help monitor the labor progress based on Friedman's curves. The prolonged first stage of labor is often defined as crossing the action line of the partograph or labor progress curve in the first stage of labor, after the latent phase, and before reaching full dilatation of the cervix [9].

The American College of Obstetricians and Gynecologists (ACOG)/Society for Maternal-Fetal Medicine criteria for diagnosis of labor arrest are: (1) the dilatation of the cervix is 6 cm or more; (2) ruptured of the membrane found; and (3) cervical changes after at least 4 hours with adequate contraction or at least 6 hours of oxytocin administration with inadequate uterine activity are not found. Indeed, prolonged labor can be judged only in retrospect [10].

Most of the time, inadequate uterine contraction is the first reason to be suspected when prolonged labor occurs other than cephalo-pelvic disproportion (CPD). Since CPD is a per-exclusion diagnosis that is established in the presence of adequate uterine contractions, many practitioners directly and quickly augment contraction [11, 12]. The ACOG also made clinical practice guidelines for amniotomy, oxytocin, and other interventions to manage prolonged labor [10]. All these actions are intended to make labor adhere more to the partograph, and an intervention to expedite birth is taken rather than to look at the cause in more detail.

By this clinical decision, some women with slower progress of dilation (even though it is normal) are prone to have an intervention with its consequences (fetal distress or infection). With the recent advanced methods of fetal monitoring during labor (such as continuous CTG), a longer duration of labor than a partograph should be more feasible.

However, the pathogenesis of prolonged labor is poorly described, primarily due to the lack of research in this area [6]. There is still limited discussion about preventing prolonged labor or better preparation during antenatal care. Our perinatal statistics demonstrate that prolonged labor is possible as long as standard fetal monitoring is maintained during labor. This chapter will discuss the role of calcium and thyroid in prolonged labor.

2. Prolonged second stage of labor

The prolonged second stage of labor differs from the prolonged first stage. The typical second stage of labor varies in duration from minutes to many hours, but the optimal limit on the duration of the second stage is unknown [5]. A more prolonged second stage of labor brings a significant increase in the risk of fistula, vaginal injury, and postpartum hemorrhage (PPH) [5]. Second-stage cesarean birth is also more challenging to do and brings more maternal operative complications, as with an impacted head of the fetus in the pelvis [13]. However, clinicians should outweigh the risks and benefits of cesarean section in the prolonged second stage of labor compared to vaginal birth.

The National Institute for Health and Care Excellence (NICE) advises intervention after three hours of active second stage for women giving birth for the first time (nulliparous) and two hours for multiparous [14]. However, a systematic review found no consistent evidence connecting the duration of the second stage with adverse outcomes [15]. The study was affected by confounding data and the broad categorization of the second stage duration. However, after adjusting or confounding factors, the odds of NICU admission reduced with increasing duration of the second stage [15].

3. Active management of labor

Active management of labor was first intended to reduce the rate of prolonged labor by making sure all women adhere to partograph or faster [16, 17]. This would make obstetricians make fewer decisions based on inadequate uterine contractions or slower dilatation of the cervix [16, 18–20]. Three large randomized controlled trials compared a policy of active management of nulliparous labor with routine management [19]. In these studies, active management included precisely diagnosing labor, performing early amniotomy, conducting vaginal examinations frequently, and administering high-dose oxytocin to augment slow labor progress characterized by less than 1 cm of cervical dilatation per hour [19, 21]. All three studies have reported a reduction in the duration of labor, and two found reduced maternal infectious morbidity [19, 21, 22]. Therefore, the issue of whether a policy of active management of nulliparous labor can reduce cesarean section rates is still unresolved [19, 23, 24]. One study found a reduced cesarean section rate with active labor management, but only after controlling for confounding factors [19, 23].

The criticism of active labor management is related to more interventions during labor rather than understanding the diversity of labor progress in every patient possible [19, 23]. This resulted in a more medicalized birth process rather than looking into the cause over which women have less control [19, 23, 24]. Meta-analyses have concluded that neither of these single interventions effectively reduced cesarean section rates [19, 23]. The expected rate of increase (1 cm per hour) in all labor is standardization and has not proven to be applicable in all first labors, nor does standardize the 12-hour time allocation in partograph [19, 24].

4. MRI and other methods to predict prolonged labor

Vaginal delivery remains needs fetus–pelvis fit proportion. Previous studies have demonstrated that MRI can be reliable in evaluating labor outcomes [25–27]. Fox et al. [28] have attempted to validate MRI pelvimetry in women with previous cesarean sections. The obstetric conjugate is the most significant predictive pelvic measurement among all MRI pelvimetry parameters, as it shows a strong positive correlation with vaginal delivery [29].

Klemt et al. [30] used an obstetric conjugate of 12 cm to represent a sufficient pelvic inlet for the trial of labor. Meanwhile, Joyce et al. [31] reported that a 3400-g weight fetus requires minimal obstetric conjugate of 10 cm to pass through the birth canal. However, the applicability of these findings is limited by racial differences. A higher body mass index (BMI) may significantly affect soft-tissue pelvic volume, which is closely associated with prolonged labor [29]. Li et al. [32] wrote that women with lower BMIs as well as larger interspinous distance (ISD) and intertuberous distance (ITD) were more likely to have a successful vaginal delivery. The ISD represents the mid-pelvis is particularly important, as its narrowing can obstruct the fetus' internal rotation, hindering the descent of the head [33]. Women with lower BMIs, smaller fetal biparietal diameter (BPD), and AC should be allowed to continue trying labor under close monitoring. MRI pelvimetry could be a valuable tool for selecting nulliparous women who can undergo a trial of labor [32].

5. Uterine muscle contractility, oxytocin, and calcium

Figure 1 describes the mechanism of uterine contraction. Uterine contraction starts by activating a second messenger of prostaglandin and oxytocin, which are G protein-coupled receptors (GPCR) on the cell membrane [35]. GPCR then triggers a

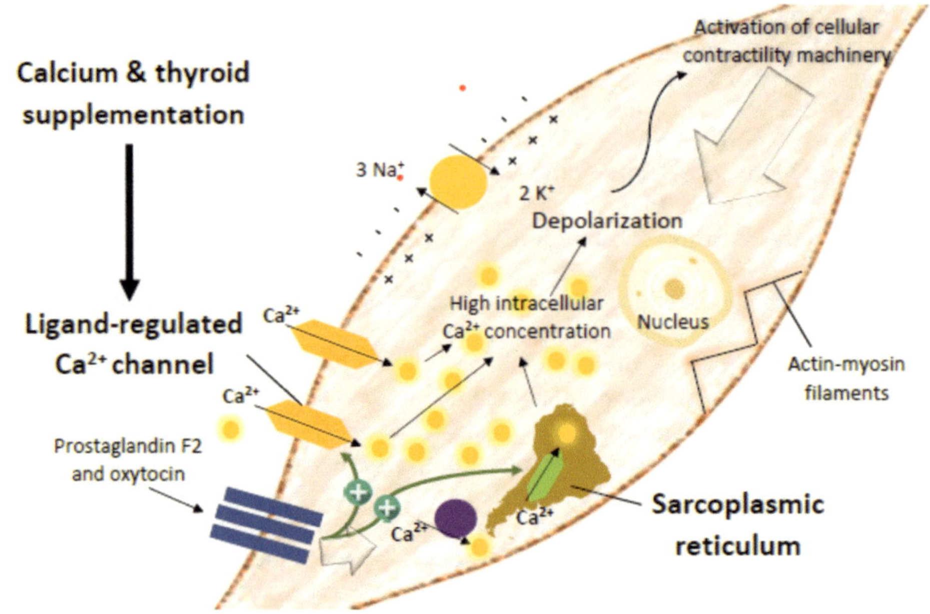

Figure 1.
The mechanism of uterine contraction [34].

cascade of events that release calcium mostly from the sarcoplasmic reticulum [35]. The intrinsic ionic change also triggers ligand-specific calcium channels. It causes more calcium influx, so thereby strengthening the uterine contractions [35].

Pehlivanoğlu et al. [35] concluded that calcium released from the sarcoplasmic reticulum is rapidly depleted compared to the extracellular calcium from calcium channels. Loftus et al. [36] demonstrated that calcium influx by ligand-type channel significantly contributes to the depolarization-excitatory phase of the uterine myocyte. Increased intracellular calcium and extracellular Cl^- concentration also activate Ca^{2+}-activated chloride (Cl^-) channels (CaCCs) [27]. The CaCCs then depolarize the myometrial membrane and activate L-type calcium channels [37]. Enhancing uterine contractility by calcium through various pathways offers a physiological basis for using calcium supplementation to improve uterine contractions and reduce the risk of labor dystocia [38].

The frequent use of oxytocin aims to induce or augment labor. A decrease in uterine contraction, even with oxytocin augmentation, may be due to relative calcium insufficiency [39]. Mcalpine et al. [6] reported that exposure to synthetic oxytocin may contribute to oxytocin receptor desensitization, reducing endogenous oxytocin secretion and decreasing uterine contractions.

6. Muscle and lactic acid

Lactic acid can accumulate as metabolism shifts from aerobic to anaerobic during uterine contractions, leading to contraction fatigue. This lactic acid is found in the myometrium as amniotic fluid lactic (AFL). Elevated levels of AFL are linked to labor dystocia and may increase the chance of requiring cesarean section [40]. These findings led to an intervention of administering bicarbonate, a base that alkalinizes the amniotic fluid, reducing AFL levels and restoring the uterine pH for adequate myometrium contractility [41]. Wiberg-Itzel et al. [42] concluded that sodium bicarbonate intervention significantly reduced AFL levels and increased the spontaneous vaginal delivery rate in the group of 200 randomized patients.

Seyedi et al. [41] found that patients receiving sodium bicarbonate and oxytocin had higher rates of spontaneous delivery in cases of prolonged labor. The intervention group had fewer cesarean births and second stages of labor than the control group [41].

7. Normal calcium and labor

Total calcium serum typically ranged at 2.2–2.5 mmol/L, roughly half of this being ionized calcium (average 1.1 and 1.5 mmol/L) [43]. However, it may not accurately reflect the ionized calcium level. The calcium level in the serum might increase the reserve and the influx of extracellular calcium into the intracellular, contributing to better contractions. Therefore, it is hypothesized that increased serum calcium during labor may promote more effective contractions [44].

Calcium homeostasis in the non-pregnant individual is relatively simple [45]. Pregnant women have lower maternal serum levels due to increased fetal demand, estrogen, hemodilution, and uteroplacental calcium transport mechanisms [45–47]. This results in fetal hypercalcemia but hypocalcemia in maternal serum calcium, mainly during the third trimester. Hyperventilation during labor might cause respiratory alkalosis and a shift in the acid-base balance [48, 49]. This results in calcium ions binding with albumin and creating fewer acid compounds [48]. Further, alkalosis inhibits tissue response to parathyroid hormone and reduces serum calcium concentration [48].

A study measured the calcium levels of two groups who had scheduled cesarean and had no labor signs at 38 weeks gestation [50]. Levels of serum calcium were higher in pregnant women who delivered vaginally than those who had scheduled cesarean delivery. The calcium levels in the umbilical vein of the newborns born after spontaneous labor were higher than those after a cesarean section [50].

8. Calcium administration during labor

Danforth and Ivy et al. showed that postpartum uterine contractions do not occur in dogs and rabbits when calcium levels are low [51]. Dystocia in the parturient bitch is also resolved by slow intravenous administration of calcium gluconate [48, 51, 52]. Calcium plays an essential part in preventing uterine dystocia by its quieting effect on the sympathetic nervous system and producing regular uterine contractions [35].

Two mid-twentieth-century studies reported that pregnant women with normal calcium levels experienced shorter labor and lower morbidity than a comparable control group [53, 54]. It concludes that an increase in ionized calcium is essential for spontaneous onset of labor. The changes in the ionized to non-ionized calcium ratio may have contributed to the stronger uterine contractility [54]. Intravenous calcium gluconate was a significant factor in promoting regular and effective uterine contractions [54].

Two dated but significant studies verified labor enhancement through calcium therapy [53, 54]. In 1947, Grier [53] concluded that patients who were given calcium gluconate and intramuscular oxytocin experienced shorter labor than the average labor. 1954, Whyte [54] determined that combining calcium gluconate and oxytocin is a safe and effective approach for labor induction. In that study, the 200 participants who received that combination experienced a shorter duration of labor compared to the standard protocol [54]. No maternal mortality or neonatal deaths attributable to induction were recorded in either study [53, 54].

9. Calcium as a potential intervention to prevent postpartum hemorrhage

Postpartum hemorrhage (PPH) frequently happens following exogenous oxytocin augmentation and its consequence of receptor desensitization to oxytocin. Oxytocin receptor sensitivity is dependent on free-ionized calcium. Optimizing serum calcium can minimize the effects of receptor desensitization to oxytocin and enhance uterine contraction, especially in augmented prolonged labor, which is a risk factor for PPH [55]

For instance, patients with PPH who did not respond to oxytocin were found to have improved uterine contractions and less bleeding after receiving calcium gluconate intravenously. Wang and Lu [56] reported that women with low serum calcium levels were at a higher risk of PPH within 2 hours postpartum than normal serum calcium patients, suggesting that calcium could help prevent uterine atony. Qin and Gou [57] showed that administration of 10 ml of 10% calcium gluconate at the time of labor, especially near full cervical dilatation, had increased mean serum calcium at the time of fetal head crowning. It leads to fewer cases of primary PPH. They also found that the risk of PPH was increased when the antepartum calcium levels in serum were below 1.05 mmol/L. These findings align with the results of the present study, where patients with primary PPH due to uterine atony had a mean serum ionized calcium level of 2.8 ± 0.35 mg/dL, which is lower than this critical value [57].

10. Thyroid and calcium

Thyroid hormones are essential for normal reproductive function and labor course. Hypothyroidism during pregnancy is highly associated with miscarriage, preterm labor and delivery, intrauterine growth restriction (IUGR), and neonatal death [58]. In animal studies, hypothyroidism is associated with dysfunction in the pituitary-ovarian axis and impaired follicular maturation. The endometrium, myometrium, and uterine weight volumes are lower in hypothyroid rats [58].

The catabolic effect of thyroid hormone to increase bone mineral resorption and calcium loss regulates calcium homeostasis [59, 60]. The synchronized function of the parathyroid hormone, vitamin D, and calcitonin also regulate calcium serum [59, 60]. Thyroid hormone inversely inhibits parathyroid hormone secretion, increases the osteoclast activity, and decreases the calcium excretion [59, 61]. Patients with hyperthyroidism tend to have low levels of PTH with an inverse effect on serum calcium levels [59–62]. Thyroid hormone also influences uterine muscle contractility because thyroid receptors are found in the uterine smooth muscle nuclei. The thyroid also acts directly on the smooth vascular muscle as a vasodilator that influences the peripheral vascular system. Thyroid hormone treatment can rapidly reverse higher systemic vascular resistance in pregnant women with hypothyroidism [58].

Free thyroxine (FT4) and thyroid stimulating hormone (TSH) have a role in releasing oxytocin in the labor course. In the third trimester, pregnant women with elevated TSH and Thyroid Peroxidase Antibody (TPOAb) followed by low FT4 are associated with a prolonged duration at the first stage of labor [59]. TPOAb has a role in catalyzing tyrosine iodization and its coupling with iodotyrosyl residues. Cambell et al. wrote that forming free triiodothyronine and FT4 will regulate the release of oxytocin [59, 61].

11. Jakarta experience

Considering these observations, prepared antenatal care aimed at normal calcium and FT4 levels was considered worth a trial. This study aimed to determine whether the women with calcium and levothyroxine supplementation in antenatal care would have normal prolonged labor with no increased risk of maternal and fetal complications. This would allow some women to have more natural progress in labor with optimal outcomes.

12. Material and methods

This retrospective study was conducted in the Department of Obstetrics, Cipto Mangunkusumo Central National Hospital, Jakarta, and Hermina Hospital, Bekasi, between January 2020 and September 2024. It was noted that most of this study's patients were private booked patients. Therefore, they wished to have a vaginal delivery with less or no intervention. All subjects had free thyroxine and ionized calcium measured in the first trimester using a Roche 9180 electrolyte analyzer and Cobas Immunoassay. Regardless of the calcium level and preeclampsia risk screening, they all had at least 1500 mg of calcium daily intake during the second and third trimester of pregnancy until labor started. Levothyroxine 100 mg supplemented daily was only given if the pregnant woman had a free thyroxine level of less than 1.1 ng/dL, regardless of the TSH level or sign of subclinical hypothyroidism. Supplementation of levothyroxine 100 mg was stopped when the free thyroxine level was more than 1.4 ng/dL (just below the normal range of our population). We measured potassium levels only at early labor. There was no modification in diet, and the patients continued to take the vitamin and mineral tablets as usual or had previously been prescribed. Patient with a history of previous cesarean section is also included. We measured femur length and head circumference using ultrasound and presented them in the percentile using the Intergrowth chart.

Cervical dilatation found during labor assessments is plotted on the partograph. Labor progressed steadily at varying rates and intensities. A prolonged first stage of labor is defined as the point at which the action line on the partograph is crossed, occurring between the latent phase and full cervical dilatation. The latent phase refers to the period before active labor begins, typically when the cervix dilatation is less than 4 cm. Augmentation in our study is taken only to exclude the diagnosis of CPD when the head station is less than 2/5. The other reason for augmentation is the patient's request. Five IU of oxytocin and 1 g of calcium gluconate are diluted in 0.9% normal saline, whereby the drop rate can be titrated to achieve regular contractions. Since this study focuses on the prolonged first stage of labor, women with a prolonged second stage were excluded.

In this study, postpartum hemorrhage is defined as total blood loss of 1000 mL or more within 24 hours after the delivery. Meanwhile, puerperal sepsis is defined as a genital tract infection occurring any time between membrane rupture until 42 days postpartum. It is characterized by the presence of at least two of the following signs: pelvic pain, fever, abnormal vaginal discharge, or delayed uterine involution.

13. Results

A total of 2672 of all patients who wished vaginal delivery were included in the study, as shown in **Figure 2**. Among them, 461 consecutive cases of prolonged labor have been retrospectively reviewed. The incidence of prolonged labor in this study group was 17%. It was noted that 92% of the patients (n = 424) with prolonged labor were private booked patients with consent to refuse augmentation of labor to allow more natural labor progress. This group consisted of patients with allowed slower labor progress, and 28% of them were primipara (n = 129).

In this study, 77% of the women had a normal vaginal birth (n = 324) with no augmentation or amniotomy. Augmentation was decided lastly to be given to 93 women to deliver the baby (22%). Most of the labor characteristics in all groups were weak contractions (62%), relative cephalopelvic disproportion (18%) with fetal weight >3400 g, and the occipital posterior position (8%).

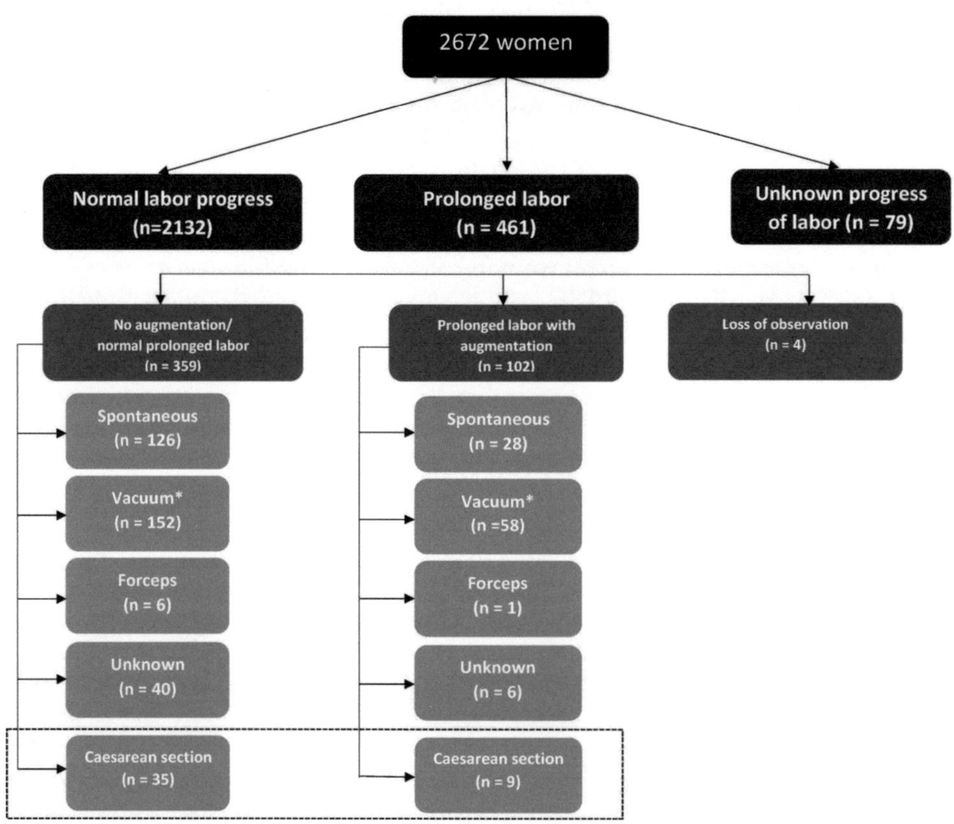

Figure 2.
The flow diagram of the study participants.

The normal prolonged labor group (without augmentation) delivered spontaneously in 39%, using a vacuum in 47%, and forceps in 2%. Regarding the delivery method, there were significant differences in the delivery using a vacuum between the normal prolonged labor group and the prolonged labor with augmentation group ($p < 0.011$).

This study had no maternal and perinatal mortality (**Table 1**). Febrile morbidity after parturition was seen in 19 patients, which correlated to the duration of labor. Perinatal morbidity occurred in 19% of the newborns. Maternal morbidities like PPH, UTI, puerperal sepsis, and wound infection were 19%, 7%, 1%, and 1%, respectively, in the normal prolonged labor group. PPH is more frequent in normal prolonged labor without any augmentation. The patients with PPH in all groups had a mean serum ionized calcium level of 2.8 ± 0.35 mg/dL. Although this study did not assess statistical differences in maternal morbidity, patients with the administration of augmentation agents had significantly lower morbidity in percentage terms.

No neonatal mortality was found in either group. There was no sufficient neonatal morbidity data collected in both group and normal labor progress group for comparison (our limitation). Femur length in the prolonged labor with augmentation group was shorter than that of the normal prolonged group (percentile 32–18%).

Average calcium and free thyroid levels in the normal prolonged labor group (4.6 mg/dL and 1.01 ng/dL, consecutively) were higher than those of prolonged labor with the augmentation group (3.9 mg/dL and 0.89 ng/dL, consecutively). The prevalence rate of hypocalcemia in this study population was relatively high, at 87%. The mean serum calcium levels were significantly lower in the third trimester than in the second trimester.

	Normal prolonged labor (n = 324)	Prolonged labor with augmentation (n = 93)	p-value
Ionized calcium (mg/dL)	4.6 (+1.6)	3.9 (+1.9)	0.03
Free thyroxine (ng/dL)	0.97 (+0.2)	0.89 (+0.4)	NS
Ultrasonography parameters (in percentile)			
Femur length (FL)	32% (+9)	18% (+10)	0.06
Head circumference (HC)	56% (+11)	61% (+8)	NS
Method of delivery			
Spontaneous	126 (35%)	28 (27%)	NS
Vacuum	152 (42%)	58 (57%)	0.009*
Forceps	6 (2%)	1 (1%)	NS
Unknown	40 (11%)	6 (6%)	NS
Caesarean section	35 (10%)	9 (9%)	NS
Maternal morbidity			
Postpartum hemorrhage	62 (19%)	9 (10%)	NS
Urinary tract infection	23 (7%)	5 (5%)	NS
Puerperal sepsis	3 (1%)	1 (1%)	NS
Wound infection	32 (10%)	0 (0%)	0.03

**p-value significant at < 0.05.*

Table 1.
The demographic characteristics of the study participants.

The limitation of this study is the progress of labor in all the patients taking increased supplementary calcium was not compared with that in control antenatal cases.

14. Discussion

In most cases of regular course of labor, a shorter duration of labor is preferred. There was no possibility of having prolonged labor without an intervention to expedite birth if the partograph table crossed. This study would answer whether pregnant women would have normal prolonged labor if calcium and thyroid factors were well prepared at antenatal care.

In this study, without augmentation, normal prolonged labor is possible. With the incidence of prolonged labor of 17%, measuring and preparing calcium and thyroid at antenatal care is a feasible effort to have an optimal contraction in labor rather than rupturing her membranes or administering oxytocin at labor. One positive side of augmentation in the prolonged labor group is that the vacuum is less applied. The high prevalence of low calcium levels in both groups of this study might cause a shorter femur length than the average growth curve.

This study might embrace diversity in the duration of labor, which might not happen if we applied all laboring women with the same partograph. Moreover, to our knowledge, the present idea in this study is relatively new: allowing some women with slower progress of dilation to have "gentle" birth.

15. Conclusion

Prolonged labor is still challenging for many obstetricians. We believe measuring and supplementing calcium (and thyroid) in everyday labor problems is essential rather than generalizing action to augment contraction when the labor is prolonged. Tapping into a mother's natural strength and enhancing her labor environment is a gentler and just as effective (if not more so) approach compared to rupturing her membranes or administering oxytocin.

Calcium is a simple, low-cost treatment that could bring more spontaneous vaginal birth by preventing labor dysfunction and its interventions, thereby preventing cesarean section and its morbid complications. Meanwhile, the thyroid hormone influences uterine muscle contraction by acting in smooth muscle cells.

In summary, the roles of calcium and thyroid hormones are critical in shaping the course of labor. A holistic approach to prenatal care that includes calcium and thyroid supplementation can reduce the incidence of prolonged labor or prevent postpartum hemorrhage.

Acknowledgements

Thank you to all colleagues in the Obstetrics Gynecology Department of Cipto Mangunkusumo General Hospital, Faculty of Medicine, Universitas Indonesia.

Conflict of interest

The authors declare no conflict of interest.

Author details

Yuditiya Purwosunu*, Amanda Rumondang and Nathalia Isabella Muskitta
Fetomaternal Division, Faculty of Medicine, Universitas Indonesia, DKI Jakarta, Indonesia

*Address all correspondence to: yuditiya@icloud.com

References

[1] Wei S, Wo BL, Qi HP, Xu H, Luo ZC, Roy C. Early amniotomy and early oxytocin for prevention of, or therapy for, delay in first stage spontaneous labour compared with routine care. Cochrane Database of Systematic Reviews. 2013;**8**:3

[2] Nelson J. Indications and appropriateness of caesarean sections performed in a tertiary referral Centre in Uganda: A retrospective descriptive study. The Pan African Medical. 2017;**2017**(26):64

[3] Bakker W, van Dorp E, Kazembe M, Nkotola A, van Roosmalen J, van den Akker T. Management of prolonged first stage of labour in a low-resource setting: Lessons learnt from rural Malawi. BMC Pregnancy and Childbirth. 2021;**21**(1):398. DOI: 10.1186/s12884-021-03856-9

[4] Stephansson O, Sandstrom A, Petersson G, Wikstrom AK, Cnattingius S. Prolonged second stage of labour, maternal infectious disease, urinary retention and other complications in the early postpartum period. BJOG. 2016;**123**(4):608-616. DOI: 10.1111/1471-0528.13287. Epub 2015/01/21

[5] Young C, Bhattacharya S, Woolner A, Ingram A, Smith N, Raja EA, et al. Maternal and perinatal outcomes of prolonged second stage of labour: A historical cohort study of over 51,000 women. BMC Pregnancy and Childbirth. 2023;**23**(1):467. DOI: 10.1186/s12884-023-05733-z. Epub 2023/06/23

[6] Mcalpine JM, Vanderlelie JJ, Perkins AV. First do no harm: Intrapartum calcium loading during oxytocic induction of labor. Journal of Womens Health Issues and Care. 2015;**4**(4):1-5

[7] Maghoma J, Buchmann EJ. Maternal and fetal risks associated with prolonged latent phase of labour. Journal of Obstetrics and Gynaecology. 2002;**22**(1):16-19. Epub 2003/01/11. DOI: 10.1080/01443610120101637

[8] Friedman. Primigravid labor a graphicostatistical analysis. Obstetrics and Gynecology. 1955;**6**:567-589

[9] Philpott RH. Graphic records in labour. British Medical Journal. 1972;**21**(4):163-165

[10] American College of Obstetrics and Gynecology SoM-FM. Obstetric care consensus No 1: Safe prevention of the primary cesarean delivery. Obstetrics and Gynecology. 2014;**123**:693-711

[11] Souza JP, Oladapo O, Fawole B, Mugerwa K, Reis R, Barbosa-Junior F, et al. Cervical dilatation over time is a poor predictor of severe adverse birth outcomes: A diagnostic accuracy study. BJOG : An International Journal of Obstetrics and Gynaecology. 2018;**125**:991-1000

[12] Mandiwa C, Zamawe C. Documentation of the partograph in assessnig the progress of labour by health care providers in Malawi's south-west zone. Reproductive Health. 2017;**14**(1):1-7

[13] Fasubaa OB, Ezechi OC, Orji EO, Ogunniyi SO, Akindele ST, Loto OM, et al. Delivery of the impacted head of the fetus at caesarean section after prolonged obstructed labour: A randomised comparative study of two methods. Journal

of Obstetrics and Gynaecology. 2002;**22**(4):375-378. Epub 2003/01/11. DOI: 10.1080/01443610220141290

[14] Guidance N. Intrapartum Care for Healthy Women and Babies. United Kingdom: NICE; 2014

[15] Altman MR, Lydon-Rochelle MT. Prolonged second stage of labor and risk of adverse maternal and perinatal outcomes: A systematic review. Birth. 2006;**33**(4):315-322

[16] O'Driscoll K, Stronge JM. Active management of labor. British Medical Journal. 1973;**3**(5880):590. DOI: 10.1136/bmj.3.5880.590. Epub 1973/09/15

[17] O'Driscoll K, Jackson RJ, Gallagher JT. Active management of labour and cephalopelvic disproportion. The Journal of Obstetrics and Gynaecology of the British Commonwealth. 1970;**77**(5):385-389. Epub 1970/05/01. DOI: 10.1111/j.1471-0528.1970.tb03539.x

[18] Angeby K, Sandin-Bojo AK, Persenius M, Wilde-Larsson B. Women's labour experiences and quality of care in relation to a prolonged latent phase of labour. Midwifery. 2019;**77**:155-164. Epub 2019/08/02. DOI: 10.1016/j.midw.2019.07.006

[19] Sadler LC, Davison T, McCowan LM. A randomised controlled trial and meta-analysis of active management of labour. BJOG : An International Journal of Obstetrics and Gynaecology. 2000;**107**(7):909-915. Epub 2000/07/20. DOI: 10.1111/j.1471-0528.2000.tb11091.x

[20] Sturrock J, Brown R. Prolonged first stage of labour. The Journal of Obstetrics and Gynaecology of the British Empire. 1956;**63**(1):83-86. Epub 1956/02/01. DOI: 10.1111/j.1471-0528.1956.tb05437.x

[21] Frigoletto FD Jr, Lieberman E, Lang JM, Cohen A, Barss V, Ringer S, et al. A clinical trial of active management of labor. The New England Journal of Medicine. 1995;**333**(12):745-750. Epub 1995/09/21. DOI: 10.1056/NEJM199509213331201

[22] Lopez-Zeno JA, Peaceman AM, Adashek JA, Socol ML. A controlled trial of a program for the active management of labor. The New England Journal of Medicine. 1992;**326**(7):450-454. Epub 1992/02/13. DOI: 10.1056/NEJM199202133260705

[23] Dencker A, Berg M, Bergqvist L, Ladfors L, Thorsen LS, Lilja H. Early versus delayed oxytocin augmentation in nulliparous women with prolonged labour--a randomised controlled trial. BJOG : An International Journal of Obstetrics and Gynaecology. 2009;**116**(4):530-536. Epub 2009/03/03. DOI: 10.1111/j.1471-0528.2008.01962.x

[24] AIMS. Common criticisms of active management of labour. AIMS Journal. 1996;**10**(2):1-10

[25] Franz M, Von Bismarck A, Delius M, Ertl-Wagner B, Deppe C, Mahner S, et al. MR pelvimetry: Prognosis for successful vaginal delivery in patients with suspected fetopelvic disporpotions or breech presentation at term. Archives of Gynecology and Obstetrics. 2017;**295**:351-359

[26] Pattinson RC, Cuthbert A, Vannevel V. Pelvimetry for fetal cephalic presentations at or near term for deciding on mode of delivery. Cochrane Database of Systematic Reviews. 2017;**2017**(5):CD000161

[27] Van Loon AJ, Mantingh A, Serlier EK, Mooyaart EL, Huisjes HJ. Randomised controlled trial of magnnetic resonance pelvimetry in

breech presentation at term. Lancet. 1997;**350**:1799-1804

[28] Fox LK, Huerta-Enochian GS, Hamlin JA, Katz VL. The magnetic resonance imaging-based fetal-pelvic index: A pilot study in the community hospital. American Journal of Obstetrics and Gynecology. 2004;**190**:1679-1685

[29] Zaretsky MV, Alexander JM, Mcintire DD, Hatab MR, Twickler DM, Leveno KJ. Magnetic resonance imaging pelvimetry and the prediction of labor dystocia. Obstetrics and Gynecology. 2005;**106**:919-926

[30] Klemt AS, Schulze S, Bruggmann D, Louwen F. MRI-based pelvimetric measurements as predictors for a successful vaginal breech delivery in the Frankfurt Breech at term cohort (FRABAT). European Journal of Obstetrics & Gynecology Reproductive. 2019;**232**:10-17

[31] Joyce DN, Giwa-Osagie F, Stevenson GW. Role of pelvimetry in active management of labour. British Medical Journal. 1975;**4**:505-507

[32] Li J, Lou Y, Chen C, Zheng W, Chen Y, Dong T, et al. Predictive value of MRI pelvimetry in vaginal delivery and its practicability in prolonged labour - a prospective cohort study. Journal of Clinical Medicine. 2023;**12**:442

[33] Gleason RL, Yigeremu M, Debebe T, Teklu S, Zewdeneh D, Weiler M, et al. A safe, low-cost, easy-to-use 3D camera platform to assess the risk of obstruced labor due to cephalopelvic disproportion. PLoS One. 2018;**13**:e0203865

[34] Smith R. Parturition. The New England Journal of Medicine. 2007;**356**(3):271-283. DOI: 10.1056/NEJMra061360. Epub 2007/01/19

[35] Pehlivanoglu B, Bayrak S, Dogan M. A close look at the contraction and relaxation of myometrium: The role of calcium. Journal of the Turkish-German Gynecological Association. 2013;**14**:230-234

[36] Loftus FC, Richardson M, Shmygol A. Single-cell mechanics and calcium signalling in organotypic slices of human myometrium. Journal of Biomechanics. 2015;**48**:1620-1624

[37] Jones K, Shmygol A, Kupittayanant S, Wray S. Electrophysiological characterization and functional importance of calcium-activated chloride channel in rat uterine myocytes. Pflügers Archiv. 2004;**448**:36-43

[38] Raees S, Forgie M, Mitchell R, Malloy E. Calcium carbonate as a potential intervention to prevent labor dystocia: Narrative review of the literature. Journal of Patient Centered Research and Reviews. 2023;**10**(3):128-135. DOI: 10.17294/2330-0698.2010. Epub 2023/07/24

[39] Arrowsmith S, Kendrick A, Wrays S. Drugs acting on the pregnant uterus. Obstetrics Gynecology & Reproductive Medicine. 2010;**20**:241-247

[40] Murphy M, Butler M, Coughlan B, Brennan D, O'Herlihy C, Robson M. Elevated amniotic fluid lactate predicts labor disorders and cesarean delivery in nulliparous women at term. American Journal of Obstetrics and Gynecology. 2015;**213**(673):e1-e8

[41] Seyedi M, Ghorashi Z, Darijani TS. Randomized controlled trial of oral bicarbonate treatment for labor stagnation. The Journal of Obstetrics and Gynaecology Research. 2021;**47**: 114-118

[42] Wiberg-Itzel E, Wray S, Akerud H. A randomized controlled trial of a new treatment for labor dystocia. The Journal Maternal Fetal & Neonatal Medicine. 2018;**31**:2237-2244

[43] Talati Chiraag, Ramchandran N, Carvalho JCA, Kingdom J, Balki M. The effect of extracellular calcium on oxytocin-induced contractility in naive and oxytocin-pretreated human myometrium in vitro. Anesthesia and Analgesia. 2018;**122**(5):1498-1507

[44] Bansal T, Hooda S. Hyperventilation causing symptomatic hypocalcemia during labour in a parturient. Egyptian Journal of Anasthesia. 2013;**29**:333-335

[45] Olausson H, Goldberg G, Laskey MA, Schoenmakers I, Jarjou LM, et al. Calcium economy in human pregnancy and lactation. Nutrition Research Reviews. 2012;**25**:40-67

[46] Malas NO, Shurideh Z. Does serum calcium in preeclampsia and normal pregnancy differ? Saudi Medical Journal. 2001;**22**:868-871

[47] Danforth DN, Ivy A. A consideration of the cause of the onset of labour. Journal of the American College of Surgeons. 1939;**69**:351-360

[48] Hollinshead FK, Hanlon D, Gilbert RO, Vergestren JP, Krekeler N, et al. Calcium, parathyroid hormone, oxytocin, and pH profiles in the whelping bitch. Theriogenology. 2010;**73**:1276-1283

[49] Toonkel RL, Sharma S. Respiratory alkalosis. New York: Springer; 2013

[50] Papandreou L, Chasiotis G, Seferiadis K. Calcium levels during the initiation of labor. Eurpeon Journal of Obstetrics & Gynecology and Reproductive. 2004;**115**:17-22

[51] Danforth DN, Ivy A. Effect of calcium upon uterine activity and reactivity. Experimental Biology and Medicine. 1939;**38**(4):550-551

[52] Pretzer S. Medical management of canine and feline dystocia. Theriogenology. 2008;**70**:332-336

[53] Grier R. Elective induction of labor. American Journal of Obstetrics and Gynecology. 1947;**54**:511-516

[54] Whyte J. Calcium gluconate in the inductoion of labour. Canadian Medical Association Journal. 1954;**70**: 261-262

[55] Lockwood CJ, Krikun G, Schatz F. The decidua regulates hemostasis in human endometrium. Seminars in Reproductive Endocrinology. 1999;**17**(1):45-51. DOI: 10.1055/s-2007-1016211. Epub 1999/07/16

[56] Wang XCX, Lu Y. The exploration of relationship between serum calcium and postpartum hemorrhage. Chinese Journal of Hemorheology. 2002;**2**

[57] Qin LDF, Gou W. A study on prediction by detection of serum calcium ion concentration and prevention from postpartum hemorrhage by 10% of calcium gluconate injection. Foreign Medical Sciences Section of Maternal and Child Health. 2005;**2**

[58] Wei H, Guan Q, Yu Q, Chen T, Wang X, Xia Y. Assessing maternal thyroid function and its relationship to duration of the first stage of labor. European Thyroid Journal. 2022;**11**(2):e210071. Epub 2022/02/16. DOI: 10.1530/ETJ-21-0071

[59] Dhanwal DK. Thyroid disorders and bone mineral metabolism. Indian Journal of Endocrinology and

Metabolism. 2011;**15**(Suppl. 2): S107-S112. DOI: 10.4103/2230-8210.83339. Epub 2011/10/04

[60] Anuj, Modi NS. Effect of thyroid hormones on serum calcium and phosphorous. International Journal of Clinical Biochemistry and Research. 2018;**5**(4):570-573

[61] Campbell I. Thyroid and parathyroid hormones and calcium homeostasis. Anaesthesia and Intensive Care Medicine. 2005;**6**(10):333-336

[62] Begic-Karup S, Wagner B, Raber W, Schneider B, Hamwi A, Waldhausl W, et al. Serum calcium in thyroid disease. Wiener Klinische Wochenschrift. 2001;**113**(1-2):65-68. Epub 2001/03/10

Chapter 5

Oral Health Status among Pregnant and Breastfeeding Women

Medha Wadhwa, Pulkit Kalyan, Anshula Deshpande and Neeraj Deshpande

Abstract

Pregnancy, lasting about 41 weeks, causes significant physiological, biochemical, and physical changes in a woman's body, including the oral cavity. Hormonal shifts, particularly in estrogen and progesterone, increase tissue sensitivity, leading to oral issues like gingivitis, periodontitis, tooth erosion, and dental caries. Changes in saliva pH, dietary imbalances, and poor hygiene further contribute to these problems, including lesions like granulomas. Post-pregnancy, the loss of bone calcification for milk production adds to oral health concerns. Poor oral health during pregnancy has been linked to adverse outcomes like preterm birth and gestational diabetes. Thus, healthcare providers must educate pregnant and breastfeeding women on oral health risks. Collaboration between obstetricians and dentists is essential in minimizing these risks through education and prevention.

Keywords: oral health, pregnancy, breastfeeding, adverse pregnancy outcomes, periodontitis

1. Introduction

Pregnancy is a period of around 41 weeks where women carry the fetus which develops in her womb. These 9 months are critical in the life of a woman and brings diversified changes in the female's body [1]. These changes are not only physical but also physiological and biochemical in nature. The summary of these changes is depicted in **Figure 1** [2]. The different changes in the female body are also reflected in the oral cavity. Oral cavity is closely related to systemic health. The impact of different physiologic changes can be witnessed through the changes in oral cavity. Some of the major changes happening during pregnancy in oral cavity includes gingivitis, oral lesions, tooth mobility and erosion, dental caries, and periodontitis [3].

The pregnancy induced gingivitis is inflammation of gingiva because of dental plaque accumulation, which may worsen to periodontitis. The changes in musculoskeletal aspect of the female body also lead to increased tooth mobility and erosion. The increased prevalence of dental caries during pregnancy has been seen because of increased pH of saliva, intake of junk foods due to pregnancy cravings, and poor awareness toward oral health. Oral lesions like granulomas or pregnancy epulis are common in the anterior gingiva because of increased inflammatory response [4].

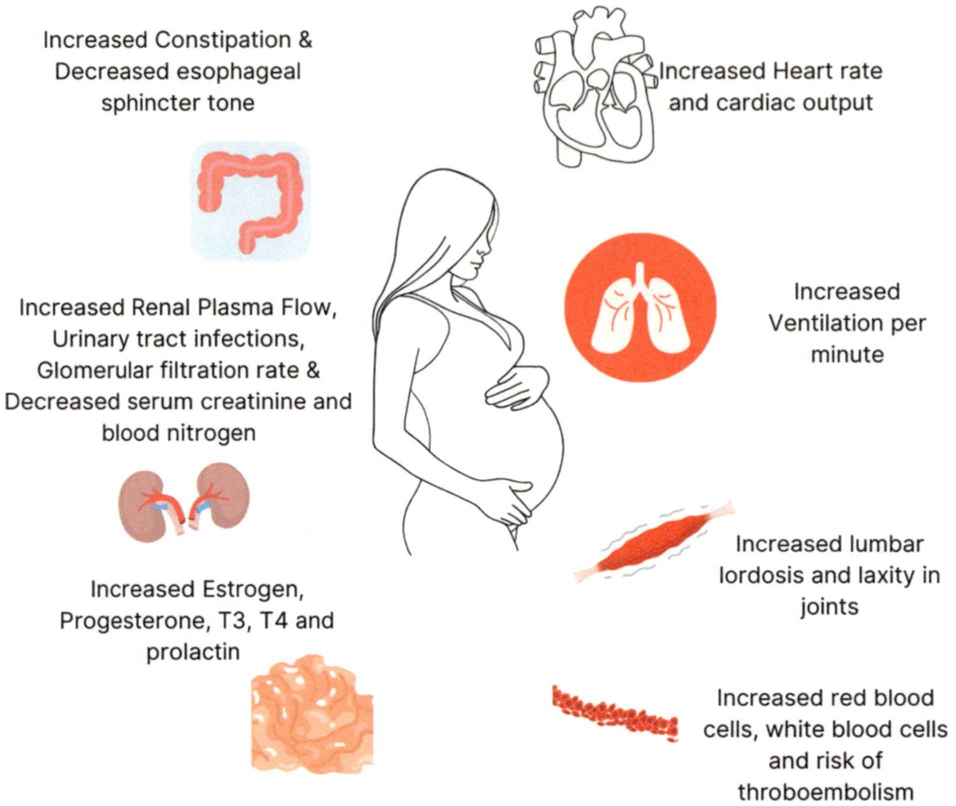

Figure 1.
Changes in females' body during pregnancy.

Further, women who breastfeed are also prone to risk of dental caries and gingivitis. There is evidence that suggest that during breastfeeding, females lose 5% of bone mass as the calcium from bones goes into the feeding milk. This makes them vulnerable to caries and gingival inflammation [5]. It is imperative to advise the women against these expected changes in the oral cavity for proper management.

2. Changes in oral cavity during pregnancy

Increased level of estrogen and progesterone during pregnancy leads to increased sensitivity of tissues. In oral cavity, gingiva becomes more sensitive to irritations. In addition, the increased prevalence of epulis gravidarum during pregnancy leads to an increased risk of bleeding from gums, that is, gingivitis. These changes are due to increased vascular permeability because of increased progesterone. In addition, lower level of vitamin C also leads to the bleeding gums problem. Changes in color of gingiva to red color of strawberry is a major change due to gingivitis. These can worsen to pregnancy-induced periodontitis [3]. The different studies in previous years have reported the prevalence of pregnancy gingivitis in 40% of pregnant women. Further, the poor oral health is also a reflection of systemic changes or gestational complications [6–10]. In addition the teeth undergo changes in terms of tooth decay and erosion. It is believed that the requirement of calcium for fetal growth is fulfilled

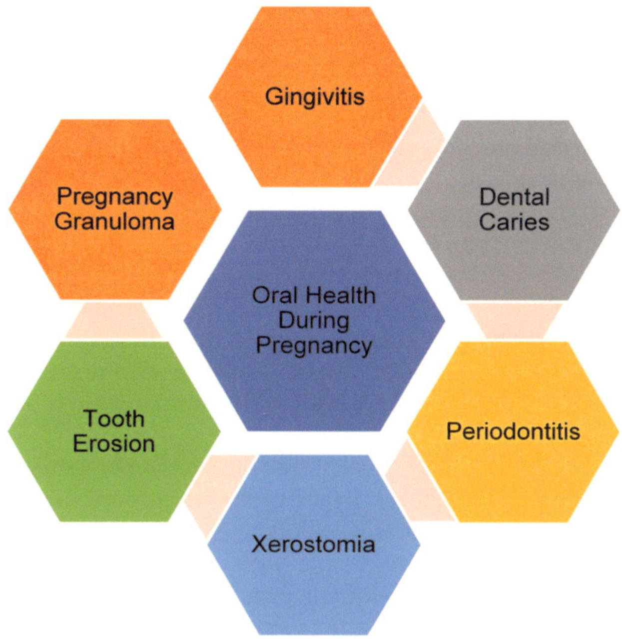

Figure 2.
Summarizing of oral health problems faced by women during pregnancy.

through teeth. Apart from this, the decrease in salivary flow, increased consumption of carbohydrates, and increased formation of plaque worsens the condition of teeth in oral cavity [3]. The changes in oral cavity during pregnancy are represented in **Figure 2**.

3. Impact on pregnancy outcomes

There have been evidence that suggest that poor oral health like periodontitis is associated with adverse pregnancy outcomes (pre-term birth, pre-eclampsia, gestational diabetes, etc.). A systematic review and meta-analysis suggested twice the odds of gestational diabetes mellitus among women who have periodontitis [11]. Earlier studies have also established the presence of periodontal microbial translocation into the peripheral bloodstream by breaking gingival epithelial barrier [12, 13]. In addition, as known from the pathophysiology of periodontitis, it is a host immunoinflammatory response due to a dysbiotic shift in oral microbiota. A similar response is also elicited in case of genitourinary tract infection, and similar antibodies can be seen as an early identifier in oral cavity, thus preventing low birthweight or abortions [14]. Thus, oral cavity can be an early identifier, and proper preventive strategies can help in reducing the prevalence of adverse pregnancy outcomes.

4. Oral health assessment and role of counseling

Pregnancy could be the right moment to create awareness on the importance of oral health as pregnant women are concerned about the health of the developing baby.

The need for counseling and creating awareness arises through the statistics presented in previous literature which highlights that around 56% of pregnant women do not utilize the service of dentist during pregnancy. The same study also highlights that 60% of pregnant women have not utilized dental services for teeth cleaning during pregnancy [15]. The past study has also shown that oral health care during pregnancy improves with counseling [16].

The role of obstetricians is crucial in developing the need for dental care during pregnancy. It is surprising to note that a previous study have highlighted 80% of obstetricians do not have questions pertaining to oral health in the prenatal visit, and around 90% of them do not recommend pregnant women to a dentist for counseling or treatment [17]. During breastfeeding, ignorance toward maintaining oral health can be harmful as *Streptococcus mutans* can be transmitted to the infants [18]. Focused training programs for obstetricians must be conducted to increase the awareness and uptake of dental care services [19].

Simple questions like whether pregnant female is facing bleeding gums, pain in gums, or swollen gums can be helpful. In addition, insight into the previous visit and the time since the last visit can help understand the inclination of the pregnant women toward oral care. This can be further used to develop a mechanism to have dental check-ups done for pregnant woman. Role of counseling thus plays a role in breaking these barriers. Understanding the complexities that may arise when the pregnant or breastfeeding female avoids dental treatment is important. The treatment of root canal, tooth extraction, and restoration are not complex. These treatments along with radiological examination with proper shielding and anesthetic administration does not yield any complexities [20]. Midwives and other prenatal care providers have a unique opportunity to offer preventive oral health services, including assessments, education, and referrals [21]. Integrating oral health into prenatal care, particularly among ethnic and racial minority groups, can be beneficial for maternal and infant health [16]. There is a clear need for improved oral health assessment and counseling during pregnancy. Implementing preventive strategies, such as including oral health education in antenatal visits and involving prenatal care workers in disseminating oral health awareness, can significantly benefit the dental health of both women and children [21, 22].

5. Oral health knowledge and awareness

Oral health knowledge, attitude, and awareness among pregnant and breastfeeding women are generally poor, with significant implications for both maternal and child health. Studies across various regions show that pregnant women often lack adequate knowledge about oral health and its importance during pregnancy. In India, a systematic review found that pregnant women had poor knowledge and awareness regarding oral health, with very few subjects (17.1% and 37.5%) feeling the need to visit a dentist during pregnancy [23]. Similarly, a study in Chennai revealed that the majority (72%) of school-educated pregnant women had never visited a dentist [24].

Interestingly, while some studies report poor knowledge, others indicate a more positive attitude toward oral health. For instance, a study in Hyderabad found that the majority of women showed good knowledge and attitude regarding oral hygiene and its relation to pregnancy. However, the same study noted poor compliance with recommended oral hygiene protocols [25]. This contradiction between knowledge/attitude and practice is also observed in a Nepalese study, where 98.2% of respondents had a positive attitude, but 92.1% had insufficient oral hygiene practices during pregnancy [26].

While awareness and attitudes toward oral health during pregnancy vary, there is a consistent gap between knowledge and practice. Factors such as education level, urban/rural residence, and working status significantly influence oral health awareness and practices [27]. The lack of referrals from gynecologists for dental check-ups during pregnancy (only 6.2% in one study) further compounds the issue [24]. These findings underscore the need for targeted oral health education and intervention programs for pregnant women, as well as better integration of oral health care into prenatal services.

6. Integrated services system for better oral health

The obstetrician holds a key role in care giving to pregnant woman. It is essential to utilize change to positive prenatal behavior, a major attributable factor in success of pregnancy. A holistic approach is a better way of ensuring desirable pregnancy outcomes. The integrated service system depicted in **Figure 3** is a proposed mechanism toward a better oral health of pregnant and breastfeeding women.

The proposed framework includes the questions related to oral health in the examination sheet of the obstetrician. In addition, referral linkage with a dentist can strengthen the oral health of the pregnant and breastfeeding women. The obstetrician can arrange for the counseling sessions through multi-disciplinary team comprising of obstetrician, dentist, nutritionist and physiotherapist. This will ensure the holistic care delivery to the pregnant women.

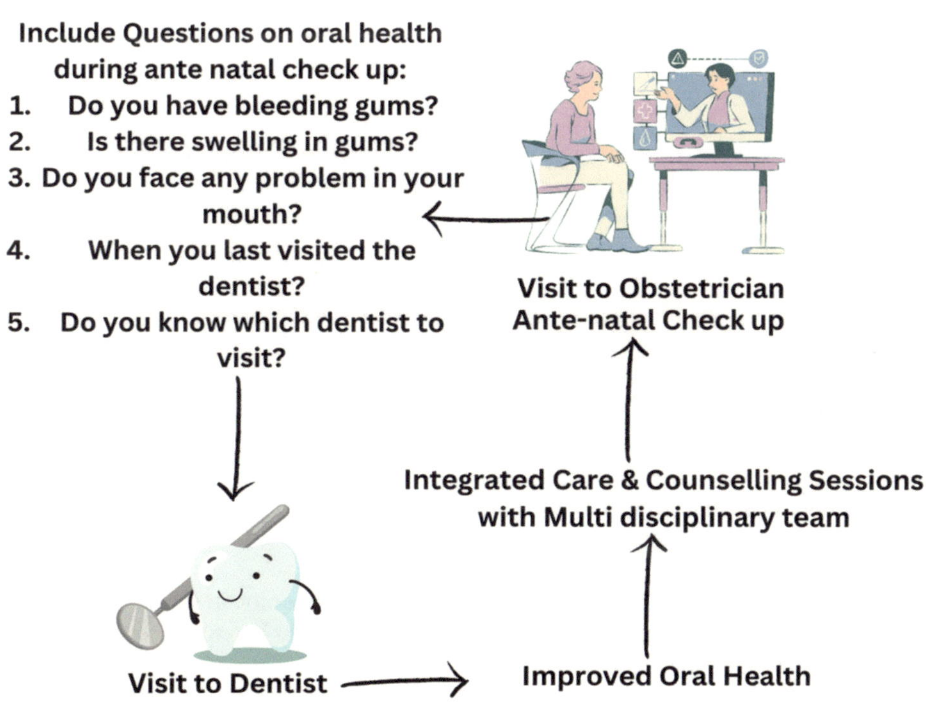

Figure 3.
Integrated services system (healthy mouth, healthy baby).

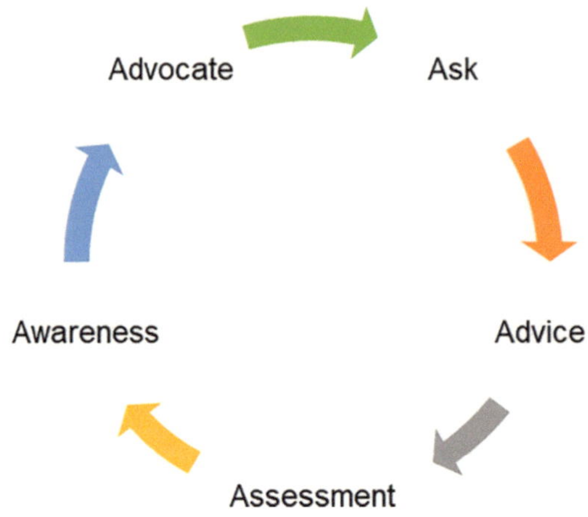

Figure 4.
5A's approach for integrating oral health with regular ante natal checkup.

Ask	Ask the questions pertaining to oral health in each ante natal visit.
Advice	Advice visiting the known dentist or refer to the dentist by obstetrician.
Assessment	Oral Health Assessment should be carried out, and appropriate preventive, diagnostic, and curative measures should be taken for pregnant women.
Awareness	Create awareness of oral health and its association with adverse pregnancy outcomes.
Advocate	Obstetricians should be the advocates for healthy mouth. Ensuring oral health insurance coverage can act like advocacy for healthy mouth.

Table 1.
Description of 5A approach.

The obstetricians can use 5A's approach to sensitize the patients toward importance of oral health. The 5A's approach is depicted in **Figure 4**.

The 5A's approach comprises of the following as shown in **Table 1**.

7. Recommendations for improved oral health during pregnancy and breastfeeding

The obstetricians, community members, family members, and women can keep the following points in mind for better oral health [20, 28]:

1. Obstetrician should discuss oral health with each women during pregnancy and after the birth of infant.

2. Awareness on the importance of oral health as a precursor in impacting the systemic health and also the risk of transfer of potentially harmful caries-causing bacteria from mother to infant.

3. Regular oral health assessment is essential.

DOI: http://dx.doi.org/10.5772/intechopen.1008144

4. Reassuring patients that diagnosis, treatment, and preventive care for healthy mouth is safe. (List of safe procedures are listed in **Table 2**.)

5. Dental care may be covered in state's Medicaid plan. Appropriate referral linkage with dentist can help in advocating importance of healthy mouth.

6. Establishing healthy linkage mechanism between obstetrics and dentists can help.

7. Advocating for better oral health of women before, during, and after pregnancy.

8. Reinforcing healthy oral habits like proper brushing of teeth, flossing, limiting high sugary foods and visit to dentist twice a year will help.

First trimester	• Routine examination • Creating awareness • Periodontal prophylaxis and emergency treatment • Avoid using radiographs. However, if unavoidable, use proper protective devices like lead aprons, thyroid collars, etc.
Second trimester	• Most comfortable time for elective procedures • Educating about oral hygiene
Third trimester	• Avoid elective procedures in second half of third trimester • Avoid using radiographs
Safe medications	Antibiotics safe to be used in pregnancy and lactation • Amoxicillin • Metronidazole • Erythromycin • Penicillin • Cephalosporins • Gentamycin • Clindamycin Analgesics safe to be used in pregnancy and lactation • Acetaminophen • Morphine • Meperidine * Fetal bradycardia with mepivacaine and bupivacaine, hence not to be used in pregnancy but can be used for lactating mothers Sedatives safe to be used in lactation • Nitrous oxide * Risk of spontaneous abortions with nitrous oxide in pregnant women Risk of cleft lip/palate with benzodiazepines in pregnant and lactating women

Table 2.
Safe medications and care during pregnancy and lactation.

8. Conclusion

The chapter highlights the significance of oral health during pregnancy and breastfeeding, emphasizing the physiological changes that occur during this period and their impact on oral health. Pregnant women experience changes in estrogen and progesterone levels, which increase tissue sensitivity, leading to issues like gingivitis, periodontitis, and oral lesions. The hormonal fluctuations, coupled with lifestyle changes, can increase the prevalence of dental caries and tooth erosion due to increased cravings for sugary foods, reduced oral hygiene practices, and altered salivary pH. It is important to understand the critical role of healthcare providers, particularly obstetricians, in promoting oral health through regular assessments, referrals, and counseling. Ignoring oral health can have adverse effects on pregnancy outcomes, such as preterm birth and gestational diabetes, as poor oral hygiene may lead to the translocation of oral bacteria into the bloodstream, affecting systemic health. Thus, by integrating oral health into prenatal care by educating and advocating for regular dental check-ups, providing safe treatments during pregnancy, and establishing collaborative efforts between obstetricians and dentists.

Conflict of interest

The authors declare no conflict of interest.

Author details

Medha Wadhwa[1*], Pulkit Kalyan[2], Anshula Deshpande[3] and Neeraj Deshpande[3]

1 Indian Institute of Public Health, Gandhinagar, India

2 Narsinhbhai Patel Dental College and Hospital, Sankalchand Patel University, Visnagar, India

3 KM Shah Dental College and Hospital, Sumandeep Vidyapeeth, Vadodara, India

*Address all correspondence to: mwadhwa@iiphg.org

References

[1] Flickr F us on. Eunice Kennedy Shriver National Institute of Child Health and Human Development—NICHD [Internet]. 2024. Available from: https://www.nichd.nih.gov/health/topics/factsheets/pregnancy

[2] Kim EG, Park SK, Nho J-H. Factors related to maternal oral health status: Focus on pregnant and breastfeeding women. Healthcare (Basel) [Internet]. 2021;**9**(6):708. DOI: 10.3390/healthcare9060708

[3] Yenen Z, Ataçağ T. Oral care in pregnancy. Journal of the Turkish-German Gynecological Association [Internet]. 2019;**20**(4):264-268. DOI: 10.4274/jtgga.galenos.2018.2018.0139

[4] Oral health care during pregnancy and through the lifespan [Internet]. Acog.org. Available from: https://www.acog.org/clinical/clinical-guidance/committee-opinion/articles/2013/08/oral-health-care-during-pregnancy-and-through-the-lifespan

[5] Digital Resource. Pregnancy, Breastfeeding, and Mother's Dental Health [Internet]. KidShine. 2021. Available from: https://kidshinehawaii.com/pregnancy-breastfeeding-and-mothers-dental-health/

[6] Pinto GDS, Costa FDS, Machado TV, Hartwig A, Pinheiro RT, Goettems ML, et al. Early-life events and developmental defects of enamel in the primary dentition. Community Dentistry and Oral Epidemiology [Internet]. 2018;**46**(5):511-517. DOI: 10.1111/cdoe.12408

[7] George A, Dahlen HG, Reath J, Ajwani S, Bhole S, Korda A, et al. What do antenatal care providers understand and do about oral health care during pregnancy: A cross-sectional survey in New South Wales, Australia. BMC Pregnancy Childbirth [Internet]. 2016;**16**(1). DOI: 10.1186/s12884-016-1163-x

[8] Haber J, Dolce MC, Hartnett E, Altman S, Silk H. Improving oral health during pregnancy: A call to action. Journal of Midwifery & Women's Health [Internet]. 2022;**67**(2):166-169. DOI: 10.1111/jmwh.13357

[9] Guideline on perinatal and infant oral health care. Pediatric Dentistry. 2016;**38**(5):54-58

[10] Sharma A, Mathur VP, Sardana D. Effective management of a pregnancy tumour using a soft tissue diode laser: A case report. Laser Therapy [Internet]. 2014;**23**(4):279-282. DOI: 10.5978/islsm.14-CR-02

[11] Abariga SA, Whitcomb BW. Periodontitis and gestational diabetes mellitus: A systematic review and meta-analysis of observational studies. BMC Pregnancy Childbirth [Internet]. 2016;**16**(1):344. DOI: 10.1186/s12884-016-1145-z

[12] Collins JG, Windley HW 3rd, Arnold RR, Offenbacher S. Effects of a *Porphyromonas gingivalis* infection on inflammatory mediator response and pregnancy outcome in hamsters. Infection and Immunity [Internet]. 1994;**62**(10):4356-4361. DOI: 10.1128/iai.62.10.4356-4361.1994

[13] Kennedy KM. Questioning the fetal microbiome illustrates pitfalls of low-biomass microbial studies. Nature. 2023;**613**:639-649. DOI: 10.52843/cassyni.1d0zcc

[14] Ebersole JL, Novak MJ, Michalowicz BS, Hodges JS, Steffen MJ, Ferguson JE, et al. Systemic immune responses in pregnancy and periodontitis: Relationship to pregnancy outcomes in the Obstetrics and Periodontal Therapy (OPT) study. Journal of Periodontology [Internet]. 2009;**80**(6):953-960. DOI: 10.1902/jop.2009.080464

[15] Hwang SS, Smith VC, McCormick MC, Barfield WD. The association between maternal oral health experiences and risk of preterm birth in 10 states, Pregnancy Risk Assessment Monitoring System, 2004-2006. Maternal and Child Health Journal [Internet]. 2012;**16**(8):1688-1695. DOI: 10.1007/s10995-011-0870-1

[16] Thompson T-A, Cheng D, Strobino D. Dental cleaning before and during pregnancy among Maryland mothers. Maternal and Child Health Journal [Internet]. 2013;**17**(1):110-118. DOI: 10.1007/s10995-012-0954-6

[17] Strafford KE, Shellhaas C, Hade EM. Provider and patient perceptions about dental care during pregnancy. The Journal of Maternal-Fetal and Neonatal Medicine [Internet]. 2008;**21**(1):63-71. DOI: 10.1080/14767050701796681

[18] Köhler B, Andréen I, Jonsson B, Hultqvist E. Effect of caries preventive measures on *Streptococcus mutans* and lactobacilli in selected mothers. European Journal of Oral Sciences [Internet]. 1982;**90**(2):102-108. DOI: 10.1111/j.1600-0722.1982.tb01531.x

[19] Morgan MA, Crall J, Goldenberg RL, Schulkin J. Oral health during pregnancy. The Journal of Maternal-Fetal and Neonatal Medicine [Internet]. 2009;**22**(9):733-739. DOI: 10.1080/14767050902926954

[20] Oral Health Care during Pregnancy: A National Consensus Statement. Washington, DC; 2012

[21] George A, Johnson M, Blinkhorn A, Ellis S, Bhole S, Ajwani S. Promoting oral health during pregnancy: Current evidence and implications for Australian midwives. Journal of Clinical Nursing [Internet]. 2010;**19**(23-24):3324-3333. DOI: 10.1111/j.1365-2702.2010.03426.x

[22] Bansal K, Kharbanda OP, Sharma JB, Sood M, Priya H, Kriplani A. Effectiveness of an integrated perinatal oral health assessment and promotion program on the knowledge in Indian pregnant women. Journal of Indian Society of Pedodontics and Preventive Dentistry [Internet]. 2019;**37**(4):383-391. DOI: 10.4103/JISPPD.JISPPD_201_19

[23] Gambhir RS, Nirola A, Gupta T, Sekhon TS, Anand S. Oral health knowledge and awareness among pregnant women in India: A systematic review. Journal of Indian Society of Periodontology [Internet]. 2015;**19**(6):612-617. DOI: 10.4103/0972-124X.162196

[24] Somasheker G, Lakshmi SP, Vishwanath N, Rao SH, Thirugnanasambandam G. Oral hygiene awareness among pregnant women in Chennai: A cross-sectional study. Indian Journal of Dental Sciences [Internet]. 2021;**13**(3):169-174. DOI: 10.4103/ijds.ijds_56_20

[25] Ahmed Javali M, Abullais Saquib S, Asiri E, Ahmed Kanji M, Abdul Khader M, Yahya Alshahrani A, et al. Oral health knowledge, attitude, and practice of pregnant women in Deccan, South India: A cross-sectional prenatal survey. Journal of Medicine and Life. 2022;**15**(3):420-424. DOI: 10.25122/jml-2019-0095

[26] Awasthi MS, Awasthi KR, Saud B, Adhikari B, Koirala SKR, Datheputhe P, et al. Oral and dental care practices and attitude of pregnant women in Lalitpur, Nepal. International Journal of Nursing and Health Sciences [Internet]. 2020;**2**(1):10-15. DOI: 10.33545/26649187.2020.v2.i1a.16

[27] Khalaf SA, Osman SR, Abbas AM, Ismail TA-AM. Knowledge, attitude and practice of oral healthcare among pregnant women in Assiut, Egypt. International Journal of Community Medicine and Public Health [Internet]. 2018;**5**(3):890. DOI: 10.18203/2394-6040.ijcmph20180743

[28] Kurien S, Kattimani VS, Sriram RR, Sriram SK, Rao VKP, Bhupathi A, et al. Management of pregnant patient in dentistry. International Journal of Oral Health. 2013;**5**(1):88-97

Chapter 6

Pregnancy: A Comprehensive Review

Junna Ye, Jiaxin Li, Yizhu Lin, Yujuan Wang, Jingyi Wu and Zhuochao Zhou

Abstract

Health during pregnancy is a key determinant of population health, with approximately 85% of women worldwide experiencing pregnancy in their lifetime. However, due to different living conditions (local policies, living habits, etc.), medical conditions (genetic testing, medication, etc.), and previous pregnancy experiences (number of previous miscarriages, etc.), pregnant women suffer from a wide range of complications at the time of conception, which will increase the likelihood of adverse pregnancy outcomes, such as miscarriages, stillbirth, preterm labor, and birth defects. These factors also contribute to the physical health of the fetus after birth. In addition, there are some areas where proper contraceptive knowledge has not been disseminated to women of childbearing age, which has led to a number of unwanted pregnancies. Doctors and the government should pay more attention to pregnant women with illnesses and provide them with appropriate support to have a smooth pregnancy and delivery.

Keywords: pregnancy, fetus, physical and mental health, living conditions, contraception

1. Introduction

Pregnancy is the process of growth and development of the embryo and fetus in the mother's body and is divided into three stages: 1–12 weeks, 12–28 weeks and 28–40 weeks. In turn, health during pregnancy is a key determinant of population health, with approximately 85% of women worldwide experiencing pregnancy [1]. However, most pregnant women suffer from comorbidities (e.g., coronary heart disease, obesity, and anxiety) (**Figure 1**) at the time of conception, combined with different living conditions (e.g., smoking, alcohol consumption, etc.), medical conditions (e.g., manner of intervening in the miscarriage, postnatal care, etc.), and previous pregnancy experiences, all of which lead to an increased likelihood of adverse pregnancy outcomes, including miscarriage, stillbirth, preterm labor (extraordinarily preterm, very preterm, moderate to late preterm), birth defects, etc. [2–5]. Worldwide, 20 million women have pregnancies with high risks, and over 800 die from perinatal conditions every day [6]. At the same time, more and more women are experiencing pregnancy complications during pregnancy and after delivery.

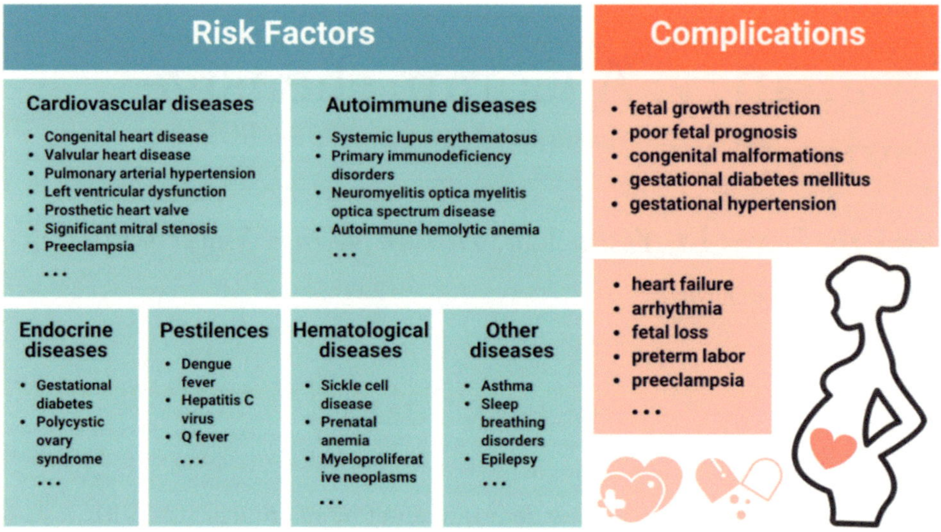

Figure 1.
Risk factors and associated complications for pregnant women.

The postnatal and fetal status is also affected, and the quality of their health is greatly reduced. In addition, women conceive a life due to a lack of knowledge about contraception in some areas. Therefore, the health of pregnant women and fetuses deserves our attention.

This chapter summarizes the relevant literature on pregnancy, describes the effects of maternal physical health, mental health, living conditions, and the number of previous pregnancies on pregnancy outcomes and postnatal neonatal conditions, and discusses the specific roles of these factors to mitigate the likelihood of adverse pregnancy outcomes and unfavorable neonatal conditions through medical care, government support, and other methods.

1.1 Cardiovascular diseases

Cardiovascular diseases are a group of heart and blood vessel disorders, mainly including congenital heart disease, rheumatic heart disease, and hypertension. It is a serious threat to human beings, especially to pregnant women, and is characterized by high prevalence, disability, and mortality.

Maternal deaths due to heart disease are currently on the rise and have become the most important cause of death in Western countries. In a subgroup of 5739 pregnant patients with prevalent diagnoses of congenital heart disease (57%) and valvular heart disease (29%), the highest mortality rate was in the pulmonary arterial hypertension (PAH) group (9%), with heart failure occurring in 11% and arrhythmia in 2% patients [7]. Another study also showed that women with congenital heart disease had a significantly higher frequency of stroke, heart failure, and arrhythmia during pregnancy. Neonatal mortality was significantly higher in the adult congenital heart disease group compared with the non-adult congenital heart disease group (0.83% vs. 0.22%; $p = 0.001$), and newborns of congenital heart disease pregnant women had low/very low or extremely immature birth weight ($p < 0.001$) or required more resuscitation and mechanical ventilation (both $p < 0.001$) [8]. The Norwegian

Health Registry likewise registered all pregnant women in the country and studied whether chronic diseases were associated with miscarriage, and it found that women with cardiometabolic diseases had an increased risk of miscarriage (OR 1.25, 95% CI: 1.20–1.31; $P < 0.001$). And the risk was elevated for all diseases included in cardiometabolic diseases: atherosclerosis (OR 2.22; 95% CI: 1.42–3.49; $p < 0.001$), hypertensive disorders (OR 1.19; 95% CI: 1.13–1.26; $p < 0.001$), and type 2 diabetes mellitus (OR 1.38; 95% CI: 1.26–1.51; $p < 0.001$). In other categories, diseases such as hypoparathyroidism (OR 2.58; 95% CI: 1.35–4.92; $p = 0.004$), and Cushing's syndrome (OR 1.97; 95% CI: 1.06–3.65; $p = 0.03$) had elevated risk [9].

Heart disease is a threat to the health of pregnant women in regions other than the West. At Madras Medical College in India, heart disease (HD) was diagnosed for the first time in 60.5% of pregnant women, with rheumatic HD being the most common (42%). The primary outcomes in pregnant women with heart disease were maternal mortality and maternal combined cardiac events (CE) (15.2%). The highest maternal mortality was in patients with prosthetic heart valves (PHV) (8.6%). The most common maternal combined cardiac event was heart failure (66.0%). So women with heart disease have a high mortality rate, the highest of which are PHV, pulmonary hypertension (PH), and left ventricular systolic dysfunction (LVSD) [10] (**Table 1**). Therefore, pregnant women with heart disease need intensive specialized care and preconception counseling, and women at high risk are advised not to become pregnant.

Another high prevalence of cardiovascular disease is hypertension. A specific group of hypertensive disorders of pregnancy is idiopathic noncirrhotic portal hypertension (INCPH). A study of 24 pregnancies in 16 patients with INCPH found that the overall prognosis for mothers and infants was favorable, despite complications associated with portal hypertension (e.g., miscarriage and preterm labor). Most fetuses at 20 weeks of gestation were healthy, and mothers were asymptomatic at a median follow-up of 27 months postpartum [11]. To minimize hypertensive disorders of pregnancy (HDP) complications, prompt identification and treatment including regular blood pressure monitoring and self-monitoring, combined with equity identification strategies and quality improvement measures, should be used to prevent serious complications and death.

Preeclampsia (PE) is a syndrome of hypertensive disorders of pregnancy that occurs most often after 20 weeks of gestation and is defined as new onset persistent hypertension with proteinuria or systemic involvement [12]. By comparing pregnant women in Sweden and China, a study found that the overall prevalence

	Adverse maternal outcome predictors				
	Pulmonary hypertension	**Prosthetic heart valve**	**Left ventricular dysfunction**	**Significant mitral stenosis**	**Significant aortic stenosis**
Maternal cardiac events	32.5%	34.3%	90.5%	23.4%	13.3%
Maternal death	4.8%	8.6%	7.9%	1.4%	8.6%

Note: all $p < 0.05$ (data from Pregnancy outcomes in women with heart disease: the Madras Medical College Pregnancy and Cardiac (M-PAC) Registry from India [10]).

Table 1.
Impact of various types of heart disease on pregnancy outcomes.

of preeclampsia was similar in both countries, with 16,068 (2.9%) and 1803 (2.3%) cases, but in terms of severity, there were 5222 (32.5%) cases in Sweden and 1228 (68.1%) cases in China. A higher risk factor for preeclampsia in China compared with Sweden was obesity (China: OR 5.12; 95% CI: 3.82–6.86; Sweden: OR 3.49; 95% CI: 3.31–3.67). In contrast, a higher risk factor for preeclampsia in Sweden compared with China was childlessness (Sweden: OR 3.91; 95% CI: 3.65–4.18; China: OR 1.65; 95% CI: 1.20–2.25) (**Table 2**). These suggest an association between obesity and childlessness and preeclampsia [13]. The impact of obesity on pregnancy complications in pregnant women with heart disease was further analyzed in a study, and it showed that pregnant women with a higher body mass index (BMI) (30 kg/m^2 and above) had a higher risk of experiencing an adverse CE in 790 pregnancies (23% vs. 14%; p = 0.006). In multivariate models, obesity (OR 1.7; 95% CI: 1.0–2.7) and higher Canadian Cardiac Disease in Pregnancy risk index (CARPREG II) (OR 1.7; 95% CI: 1.5–1.9) predicted CE. Preeclampsia was more common in obese women compared to normal weight women (8% vs. 2%; p = 0.001). Therefore, obesity is a modifiable risk factor that should be focused on during preconception counseling [14]. These results support the association of increased PE risk with factors such as obesity and childlessness.

	Sweden	China
Variable		
Maternal age: ≥35 vs. <35		
Mild preeclampsia OR (95% CI)	1.31 (1.24–1.38) (p<0.001)	2.15 (1.50–3.08) (p<0.001)
Severe preeclampsia OR (95% CI)	1.50 (1.39–1.62) (p<0.001)	1.87 (1.44–2.43) (p<0.001)
BMI: underweight vs. normal		
Mild preeclampsia OR (95% CI)	0.73 (0.61–0.87) (p<0.001)	0.41 (0.18–0.91) (p<0.001)
Severe preeclampsia OR (95% CI)	0.75 (0.59–0.96) (p = 0.03)	0.68 (0.46–0.99) (p = 0.05)
BMI: overweight vs. normal		
Mild preeclampsia OR (95% CI)	1.81 (1.72–1.90) (p<0.001)	3.20 (2.02–5.06) (p<0.001)
Severe preeclampsia OR (95% CI)	1.44 (1.35–1.55) (p<0.001)	2.12 (1.49–3.03) (p<0.001)
BMI: obesity vs. normal		
Mild preeclampsia OR (95% CI)	3.49 (3.31–3.67) (p<0.001)	5.12 (3.82–6.86) (p<0.001)
Severe preeclampsia OR (95% CI)	2.31 (2.13–2.50) (p<0.001)	4.01 (2.96–5.43) (p<0.001)

Data from preeclampsia prevalence, risk factors, and pregnancy outcomes in Sweden and China [13].

Table 2.
Adjusted odds ratios for risk factors associated with mild preeclampsia and severe preeclampsia from multivariable logistic regression for Sweden and weighted logistic regression for China.

1.2 Pestilences

Dengue infection during pregnancy almost doubles fetal death rate (OR 1.9, 95% CI: 1.6–2.2). Severe dengue infection increases the risk of fetal death approximately fivefold (OR 4.9, 95% CI: 2.3–10.2) [15]. Although the mechanism by which dengue infection leads to stillbirth is not clear, there are three main hypotheses: the symptoms of dengue infection in the mother have a direct effect on the fetus (severe dengue); dengue infection causes changes affecting the placenta, and the dengue virus has a direct effect on the fetus [16].

Pregnant women infected with hepatitis C virus (HCV) had higher odds of adverse perinatal outcomes (preterm labor, fetal dysplasia, fetal distress), but there were no differences in gestational diabetes, preeclampsia, eclampsia, or stillbirth. It is worthwhile to take precautions in advance, as pregnant women are recommended to be screened for HCV during pregnancy since they are still at risk for HCV infection during pregnancy [17].

Other infectious diseases, such as Q fever, also deserve public attention. The effect of Q fever (caused by Coxsackie bodies) on pregnancy is unknown, but available data suggest that it may increase the risk of early miscarriage, late preterm labor, or intrauterine fetal death. In addition, Q fever infection during pregnancy may increase the maternal risk of developing chronic Q fever. And Q fever is usually asymptomatic, so screening and treatment are recommended in high-endemic areas [18].

1.3 Autoimmune diseases

Autoimmune diseases are diseases in which an organism develops an immune response to its own antigens that results in damage to its own tissues. Pregnant women with autoimmune diseases such as systemic lupus erythematosus (SLE) and primary immunodeficiency disorders (PID) are at higher risk for obstetric complications and adverse pregnancy outcomes, including fetal loss, preterm labor, fetal growth restriction, and preeclampsia, and the women are at risk for recurrence and exacerbation of pre-existing autoimmune diseases during pregnancy.

SLE increases the risk of pregnancy complications such as preeclampsia and poor fetal prognosis. A previous study using blood transcriptome analysis and multicolor flow cytometry found that immune markers such as interferon and plasma cells were downregulated in healthy pregnancies, whereas these markers were significantly elevated in preeclampsia and lupus pregnancies with fetal complications [19].

In addition, neuromyelitis optica myelitis optica spectrum disease (NMOSD) is particularly common in women of childbearing age. Pregnancy may exacerbate NMOSD and affect the outcome of the pregnancy, and some treatments carry risks to the fetus [20]. A systematic review and meta-analysis examined 15 studies involving 443 patients with NMOSD. Immunosuppressive therapy during pregnancy and older age at conception was found to be associated with a lower risk of pregnancy-related seizures. The recurrence rate was highest in the first postpartum trimester, while Expanded Disability Status Scale scores worsened significantly during pregnancy and the postpartum period. This suggests that immunosuppressive therapy may help to reduce the risk of pregnancy-related seizures, but the increased risk of recurrence in the postpartum period needs to be further validated [21].

Autoimmune hemolytic anemia (AIHA), on the other hand, may flare up during pregnancy. Between 1997 and 2022, a study evaluated 33 women for recurrence or new onset of autoimmune hemolytic anemia (AIHA) in 45 pregnancies. Of the 20 women diagnosed with AIHA before pregnancy, 10 had recurrences, and 13 had new episodes of AIHA during pregnancy or in the puerperium (2 had recurrences during a second pregnancy). All these hemolytic events were severe and required treatment (e.g., steroids, intravenous human immunoglobulin, and blood transfusions), with complete remission in 65% of cases, maternal complications in 15% of cases, and adverse fetal events in 22% of cases. Despite the high risk of AIHA, a healthy pregnancy can be achieved with close monitoring and prompt treatment [22].

1.4 Endocrine diseases

During pregnancy, the endocrine system undergoes a series of physiologic changes to adapt to and support fetal development. Patients with endocrine disorders will also experience corresponding changes in their underlying diseases during pregnancy. Even some severe endocrine diseases can lead to infertility in patients.

Gestational diabetes (GD) is the most common endocrine disorder during pregnancy, and women with diabetes are at a higher risk of developing complications during pregnancy compared to those without. Hyperglycemia increases the prevalence of congenital malformations in infants before 8–10 weeks of gestation, when the fetus is forming its organs [23]. In addition, a retrospective cohort study investigated the association of history of spontaneous abortion (SAB) and induced abortion with the risk of GD in subsequent pregnancies. The study covered 102,259 pregnant women and showed that a history of SAB was significantly associated with the risk of GD and that this risk increased with the number of SABs.

Polycystic ovary syndrome (PCOS), which causes a range of symptoms in patients, has a prevalence of 5–13% in women [24]. It has been reported that women with PCOS have higher BMI after conception, greater weight gain during pregnancy, and higher chances of having adverse pregnancy outcomes such as miscarriage, gestational diabetes mellitus, gestational hypertension, preeclampsia, and cesarean delivery. Therefore, pregnant women should be screened for PCOS during prenatal checkups [25].

1.5 Hematologic diseases

The hematologic system is one of the most important systems and ensures the normal function of all kinds of blood cells in order to guarantee the health of the organism.

Sickle cell disease (SCD) is a classic inherited blood disorder. The use of hydroxyurea during pregnancy in pregnant women with SCD increases the likelihood of miscarriage and stillbirth due to the association of hydroxyurea with live births of full-term infants with a birth weight of <5.5 pounds for full-term infants in live births, but not with preterm births or serious medical problems at the time of the baby's birth [26]. Meanwhile, a study analyzed the impact of SCD and prenatal anemia on severe maternal morbidity (SMM) and other adverse pregnancy outcomes (APOs) during pregnancy. The study found that the incidence of SMM was significantly higher in patients with SCD than in anemic patients and controls, especially in complications related to thrombosis or SCD-specific pathology. The results suggest that prenatal anemia may play a mediating role in pregnancy risk and that pregnancy risk associated with SCD is similar across many APOs [27].

In addition, a chronic hematologic malignancy, myeloproliferative neoplasms (MPNs), often cause true erythrocytosis, essential thrombocythemia (ET), primary myelofibrosis (PMF), and unclassifiable MPN (MPN-U) [28]. The live birth rate for pregnant women with MPN has been reported to be 65% in polycythemia vera (PV) and 70% in ET [29–32]. In the study, there was a significant increase in preterm labor in MPN group pregnancies, 14% compared to 4% in control group pregnancies ($p < 0.001$). Correspondingly, low birth weight (<2500 g) was significantly increased in MPN pregnancies ($p = 0.042$). Maternal thrombotic complications occurred in three (1%) pregnancies in patients with MPN compared to none in controls. Pregnancy-related bleeding affected 14% of pregnancies in MPN compared with 9% in the control group ($p < 0.110$). Cesarean delivery was more common in MPN pregnancies. The incidence was 12.2 per 100,000 pregnancies. In conclusion, preterm labor is an important complication of MPN pregnancy, and maternal complications are less common than previously reported. Pregnant women with true erythrocytosis are at increased risk of fetal loss, and their high incidence of late miscarriage is associated with the presence of the JAK2v617F mutation, and therapeutically antithrombotic therapy appears to reduce the risk [4].

2. Mental health of pregnant women

Women of childbearing age have a high prevalence of mental illness, mood and anxiety disorders, with at least 15% of women of childbearing age using psychotropic medications—antidepressants, and this percentage is even higher when other mood stabilizers and antipsychotics are added to the equation [33].

More seriously, this may be exacerbated by the disproportionate burden resulting from low and middle incomes. Several studies have therefore investigated the probability of perinatal depression and anxiety among women living in different income countries. Low- and middle-income countries had the highest prevalence, with a combined prevalence of 25.5% (95% CI: 23.8%-27.1%; 197 studies from 23 countries, including 212,103 individuals). The combined prevalence in high- and middle-income countries was 24.7% (95% CI: 23.6% ~ 25.9%; 344 studies from 21 countries, including 364,103 individuals), and in low-income countries it was 20.7% (95% CI: 18.4% ~ 23.0%; 50 studies from seven countries, including 40,502 individuals) [34]. Another study determined the prevalence of six anxiety and related disorders among perinatal women in low- and middle-income countries through a systematic evaluation and meta-analysis. In 203 studies with 212,318 women, one in five pregnant and postpartum women living in low- and middle-income countries suffered from generalized anxiety disorder. In addition, 8.3 percent of women suffered from post-traumatic stress disorder [35]. Overall, depression and anxiety disorders are common in low- and middle-income countries. Therefore, accurate estimates of the prevalence of perinatal depression and anxiety disorders and the treatment of interventions for these disorders in low- and middle-income countries are essential for policy development, allocation of scarce resources and further improvement of the prognosis for women, infants and families.

3. Living conditions of pregnant women

External factors related to living conditions, such as smoking and alcohol consumption, social environment, economic development, ethnicity, regional location, etc., have a great impact on the health of pregnant women and their newborns.

The first is the lifestyle habits of pregnant women. Poor habits during pregnancy such as smoking and drinking increase the risk of pregnancy complications and adverse infant outcomes such as preterm labor, fetal growth restriction, and infant death [36]. In a cohort study, it was found that the risk of late stillbirth in pregnant women with dual exposure to alcohol and smoking after early pregnancy was 2.78 times higher than that of pregnant women with no exposure in early pregnancy or who had quit smoking by the end of early pregnancy [37]. Analysis of data from the Pregnancy Risk Assessment Surveillance System (PRAS) 2021 found that the prevalence of smoking was 12.1% pre-pregnancy, 5.4% during pregnancy, and 7.2% postpartum; 56.1% of women who smoked pre-pregnancy quit during pregnancy. The prevalence of smoking women who quit during pregnancy was 56.1% [36], with the majority of women choosing to actively quit in order to protect the fetus. In addition, external means such as alcohol screening and brief interventions (ASBI) have been shown to prevent or reduce alcohol use during pregnancy; after the intervention, the proportion of pregnant women reporting abstinence increased (OR 2.26; 95% CI: 1.43–3.56) [3].

Second, policies implemented for pregnant women in the country and city where they live can directly affect pregnancy. From 2015 to 2017, China implemented a comprehensive preconception-pregnancy management program for women with type 1 diabetes (T1D) in 11 centers from eight cities. Pregnant women in the original prospective cohort with serious pregnancy outcomes were compared with two control groups after implementation of the program, and the incidence of serious adverse pregnancy outcomes was lower in the prospective cohort (6.02%) than in the retrospective cohort (18.30%; corrected odds ratio 0.31; 95% CI: 0.13–0.74) [38]. On the other hand, in 2015, a publicly funded fertility program was introduced in Ontario, Canada to increase access to fertility treatment. For *in vitro* fertilization (IVF), the program provided for a selective single embryo transfer (eSET) policy. Statistically, comparing the pre-introduction and post-introduction of selective single embryo transfer (eSET), it was found that the rate of multiple pregnancies after Ovulation Promotion/Artificial Insemination (AI) decreased from 12.9% to 9.1%. After IVF, the rate of multiple pregnancies decreased from 29.4% to 7.1%. Therefore, the policy significantly reduced the multiple pregnancy rate [39]. The uniform management of the policy and the technical support provided a better and easier solution to the problems of pregnant women during pregnancy.

4. Medical care of diseases during pregnancy

For pregnant women suffering from various diseases during pregnancy, medical centers should take appropriate measures to monitor the development of the diseases in a timely manner, and to alleviate the pain caused by the diseases to the pregnant woman and her family through medication, surgery, and other means, and increase the likelihood of a good outcome of the pregnancy.

4.1 Drug delivery

One of the major challenges in the treatment of diseases during pregnancy is the transit of small molecule drugs through the placenta and their toxicity to the developing fetus. The placenta is responsible only for providing nutrients, removing waste products, and protecting the fetus from toxic substances in the maternal circulation.

Thus, the placenta is a biological barrier between the mother and the fetus for drug delivery. The latest research in nanoparticle technology offers the opportunity for safe drug delivery during pregnancy by controlling the interaction of therapeutic drugs with placenta [40].

4.1.1 Diabetes mellitus

For patients with diabetes mellitus, there is currently no commercially available customized hybrid closed-loop insulin delivery system to achieve specific glycemic targets during pregnancy. A study was designed to evaluate the feasibility and performance of a customized closed-loop insulin delivery system (CLC-P) based on a regional model predictive controller for use at home by patients with gestational combined type 1 diabetes. Ten pregnant women with type 1 diabetes using insulin pumps in mid- or late-gestation (HbA1c 5.8 ± 0.6%) and with a mean gestational week on the system of 23.7 ± 3.5 weeks participated in the experiment. Compared with the break-in period (break-in 64.5 ± 16.3% vs. CLC-P 78.6 ± 9.2%; p = 0.002), the mean percentage of intervals increased by 14.1 percentage points, equivalent to 3.4 hours per day. Time above 140 mg/dL (p = 0.033) and time below 63 mg/dL and 54 mg/dL (both p = 0.037) were significantly reduced during CLC-P use (**Table 3**). Nine subjects exceeded the consensus goal of 70% or more of the time range during CLC-P use. The results suggest that extended use of CLC-P at home until delivery is feasible (**Figure 2**). This finding is helpful for pregnant women with diabetes, but larger randomized studies are needed to further evaluate systemic efficacy and pregnancy outcomes [41].

Furthermore, regarding medications for the treatment of type 2 diabetes mellitus (T2DM) in pregnant women, it has been suggested that women with T2DM who are treated with oral hypoglycemic agents, such as metformin and sulfonylureas, should be switched to insulin prior to conception or, at the latest, after the diagnosis of pregnancy. However, it needs to be noted that metformin crosses the placenta and interacts with fetal environmental factors to adversely affect the fetus [42] (**Figure 3**).

Variable	Run-in	CLC-P	Absolute difference (95% CI)	P value
Primary outcome				
Time in 63–140 mg/dL, %	64.5 ± 16.3	78.6 ± 9.2	14.1 (6.6 to 21.7)	0.002
Secondary outcomes				
Time < 63 mg/dL, % [IQR]	3.7 [1.5 to 6.4]	1.6 [1.4 to 2.1]	−2.8 (−8.3 to −0.3)	0.037
Time < 54 mg/dL, % [IQR]	1.0 [0.3 to 2.2]	0.4 [0.3 to 0.4]	−0.9 (−3.7 to −0.02)	0.037
Time > 140 mg/dL, %	29.8 ± 19.5	19.7 ± 9.5	−10.1 (−19.2 to −1.0)	0.033
Mean glucose, mg/dL	123.1 ± 24.1	115.1 ± 10.6	−8.0 (−19.1 to 3.1)	0.139

Note: all p < 0.05 (data from At-Home Use of a Pregnancy-Specific Zone-MPC Closed-Loop System for Pregnancies Complicated by Type 1 Diabetes: A Single-Arm, Observational Multicenter Study. Diabetes Care [41].)

Table 3.
Continuous glucose monitoring outcomes for run-in versus CLC-P use.

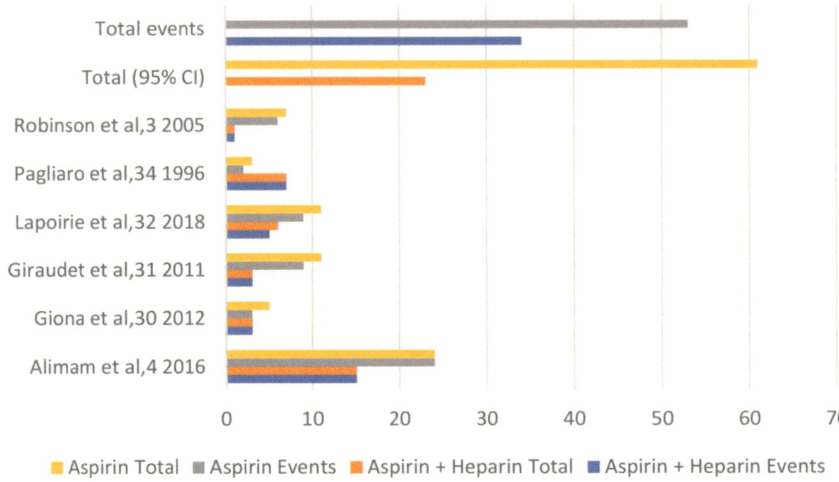

Figure 2.
Continuous glucose monitoring outcomes for run-in versus CLC-P use.

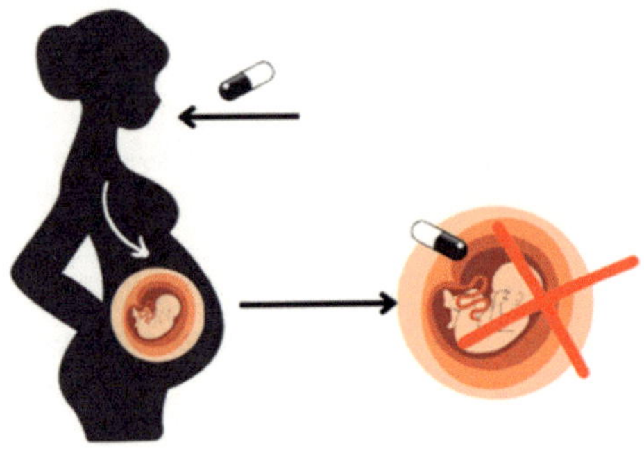

Figure 3.
Drugs taken during pregnancy can adversely affect the fetus.

4.1.2 Eclampsia

Regarding eclampsia, low-dose aspirin (LDA) is an effective measure to prevent preeclampsia. A study analyzed risk factors for preeclampsia and their incidence using 2019 birth data from the United States. The results showed that the majority of pregnant women met the criteria for high- or moderate-risk factors in the 2021 LDA Recommended Guidelines, with multiple pregnancies and low socioeconomic status being the main risk factors. These data support the current guidelines and suggest that LDA should also be recommended for pregnant women with a single moderate risk factor to further reduce the incidence of pregnancy-related hypertension [43].

4.1.3 Myeloproliferative neoplasms (MPNs)

MPNs are increasingly being detected in women of childbearing age. Pregnancy in women with MPNs has been associated with maternal thrombosis, hemorrhage, and placental dysfunction, leading to fetal growth restriction or loss. A total of 22 studies including 1210 pregnancies were included. The live birth rate was 71.3%

(95% CI: 65.1% ~ 77.6%). The use of aspirin (11 studies, 227 patients; uncorrected ratio, 8.6; 95% CI: 4.0 ~ 18.1) and interferon (6 studies, 90 patients; uncorrected ratio 9.7; 95% CI: 2.3 ~ 41.0) was associated with a higher live birth rate. The addition of heparin to aspirin was not associated with an increased risk of live birth (6 studies, 96 patients; unadjusted odds ratio 2.1; 95% CI: 0.5 ~ 9). The most common maternal adverse event was preeclampsia, with an incidence of 3.1% (95% CI: 1.7% ~ 4.5%). Evidence suggested that aspirin or interferon therapy was associated with a higher rate of live births in patients with myeloproliferative tumor pregnancies [44].

4.1.4 Depression

In addition to insomnia, it is not uncommon for stress and physical discomforts of pregnancy to lead to depression during pregnancy. Pregnancy is physically and mentally more difficult for women who already suffer from depressive symptoms. About half of women treated for affective disorders discontinue antidepressants during pregnancy, but discontinuation may lead to postpartum relapse. A cohort study used a Danish and Norwegian sample consisting of 41,475 live-born singleton pregnant women in Denmark (1997–2016) and 16,459 women in Norway (2009–2018) who had been prescribed antidepressants at least once in the 6 months before pregnancy. Based on mixed data from Denmark and Norway, those who discontinued medication late (prior stabilization) were found to have a slightly elevated probability of developing psychiatric disorders compared to those who discontinued medication continuously. These findings suggest that women with severe mental illness who are currently receiving stable treatment may benefit from continued antidepressant treatment and individualized therapeutic counseling during pregnancy [45].

Therefore, when prescribing medication, doctors should take into account factors such as the stage of the pregnancy and whether or not the medication will pass through the placenta. In addition, drug researchers are supposed to consider developing drugs and materials that protect pregnant women and fetuses.

4.2 Genetic testing

Trisomy 21 is a group of chromosomal disorders that have an enormous impact on newborns and families, and many regions are now taking steps to prevent the occurrence of trisomy 21 in the early stages of pregnancy. Offering free deoxyribonucleic acid (cfDNA) testing in the first trimester of pregnancy to women at high risk for trisomy 21 may reduce invasive fetal karyotyping and the number of miscarriages. However, a randomized analysis of 2051 eligible women found that offering cfDNA screening but still requiring invasive testing in the event of a positive test did not significantly reduce the rate of miscarriage compared with invasive testing alone [46].

4.3 Complementary therapy

It is estimated that one in seven heterosexual couples are affected by infertility and therefore require the help of assisted reproductive therapy (ART) to conceive [47]. Interventions that may reduce the risk of miscarriage or increase the chances of a live birth include intrauterine injection of hCG at the time of embryo transfer at the stage of embryonic division, use of dehydroepiandrosterone and embryo culture media high in hyaluronic acid in women, and use of antioxidant therapy in men. Interventions that increase the potential risk of miscarriage or decrease the chance of live birth include the use of PGT-A fluorescence *in situ* hybridization and injection of embryo culture supernatant prior to embryo transfer in frozen cycles. When choosing an intervention, it is important to seek the advice of a medical professional and select the most appropriate one [48].

5. Adverse pregnancy outcomes

Adverse pregnancy outcomes are undesirable outcomes of pregnancy that may pose a threat to health and life of the mother and child, including miscarriage, stillbirth, and preterm labor.

5.1 Miscarriage

Research shows that parental age affects the risk of miscarriage. The risk of miscarriage is low (10%) for women aged 25–29 years, which rising rapidly after the age of 30 years, and as high as 53% for those aged 45 years and over [49]. For fathers, men aged 25–29 years had the lowest risk of miscarriage, which then increased with age, e.g., 1.04 (95% CI: 0.90–1.21) in the 30–34 year old group versus the 25–29 year old group [50]. So the optimal age for both parents to have children is 25–29 years, after which the risk of miscarriage increases with age.

Moreover, most pregnant women choose to conceive again after a miscarriage, but the timing and number of intervals between pregnancies is also critical. Most mothers between the ages of 25 and 34 choose to have another child after an interval of six months. Pregnancy intervals of more than 24 months were more common among women who smoked and had lower levels of education. However, the length of the interval between pregnancies was not found to be associated with subsequent risk of miscarriage, preterm labor, or birth of a small-for-gestational-age child [51]. At the same time, if another miscarriage occurred after a second pregnancy, the higher the number of miscarriages, the higher the risk of recurrence, with age-adjusted ratio of 1.54 (95% CI: 1.48–1.60) after one miscarriage, 2.21 (95% CI: 2.03 to 2.41) after two miscarriages, and 3.97 (95% CI: 3.29 to 4.78) after three consecutive miscarriages [49].

5.2 Stillbirth

In full-term pregnancies (37–42 weeks), the risk of stillbirth increases with gestational age. The perinatal risk is lowest at 39 weeks of gestation, while delivery before or after this time increases the risk of adverse outcomes [52]. Besides, at 41 weeks, the risk of labor and stillbirth increased significantly, and neonatal mortality did not decrease compared to the previous period. And the risk of stillbirth increased even more markedly when labor was resumed after 41 weeks [53].

In addition, the lifestyle habits of pregnant women are also associated with stillbirth. The relative risk of late stillbirth in pregnant women with prenatal exposure to alcohol, smoking, or both was 2.22, 1.60, and 2.78, respectively, compared to pregnant women with no exposure to alcohol or smoking [37]. Adverse lifestyle habits significantly increase the risk of stillbirth.

5.3 Prematurity

Live birth at less than 37 weeks of gestation is called preterm labor, where the extremely preterm (<28 weeks) and very preterm (28–32 weeks) are accompanied by a high prevalence of neurologic and respiratory complications in the newborn [5]. There are three factors that contribute to preterm labor, the first of which is maternal age. Pregnant women aged 20–34 years have an increased risk of adverse fetal outcomes and an increased risk of spontaneous preterm labor compared to pregnant women aged 35 years and older. And for women of any age, the shorter the interval between pregnancies, the greater the likelihood of adverse outcomes [54].

Besides, the environment in which a pregnant woman lives can also affect pregnancy outcomes; for example, air pollutants (nitrogen oxides, particulate matter, and polycyclic aromatic hydrocarbons) have been associated with the risk of preterm labor and congenital malformations [55–58].

6. Neonatal status

During pregnancy, the state of the pregnant woman (e.g., pregnancy complications, drug delivery, and immune system) can affect fetal development, damage organs, and ultimately affect the health of the fetus after birth. The effects on the state of the fetus will be described next in terms of both the immune system and drug delivery.

Pregnant women sometimes take medications during pregnancy, and some of these medications can reach the fetus through the placenta and affect fetal health. For example, prenatal exposure to opioids is associated with an increased risk of asthma, dermatitis, infections, and eczema, but not autoimmune diseases or allergies [59]. Whereas the use of exogenous opioids during pregnancy has been found through rodent models, exposing the fetus to opioids during a critical period in the development of the immune system leads to an overreaction of the immune system, which in turn causes immune activation [60, 61]. One solution to minimize adverse fetal effects and improve therapeutic safety is to prevent placental-specific drug delivery through placental channels.

7. Contraception

Women can choose whether or not to have children. In some cases, women do not want children, and they need to learn contraception, deliberately preventing pregnancy through devices or drugs (**Figure 4**). However, in 2017, the teenage pregnancy rate in Brazil was 68.4/1000 (higher than the global (46/1000) and Latin American average (65.5/1000)). In addition, 66% of adolescent pregnancies are unwanted, and about 75% of adolescent mothers do not attend school. Although nearly 250 million women globally would like to delay or avoid pregnancy, about half of all pregnancies each year are unintended. This requires multifaceted preventive measures and emphasizes quality, comprehensive sexuality education from an early age [63].

In addition, although the contraceptive pill has been approved for more than 60 years, product gaps and unmet needs remain, and women who think about

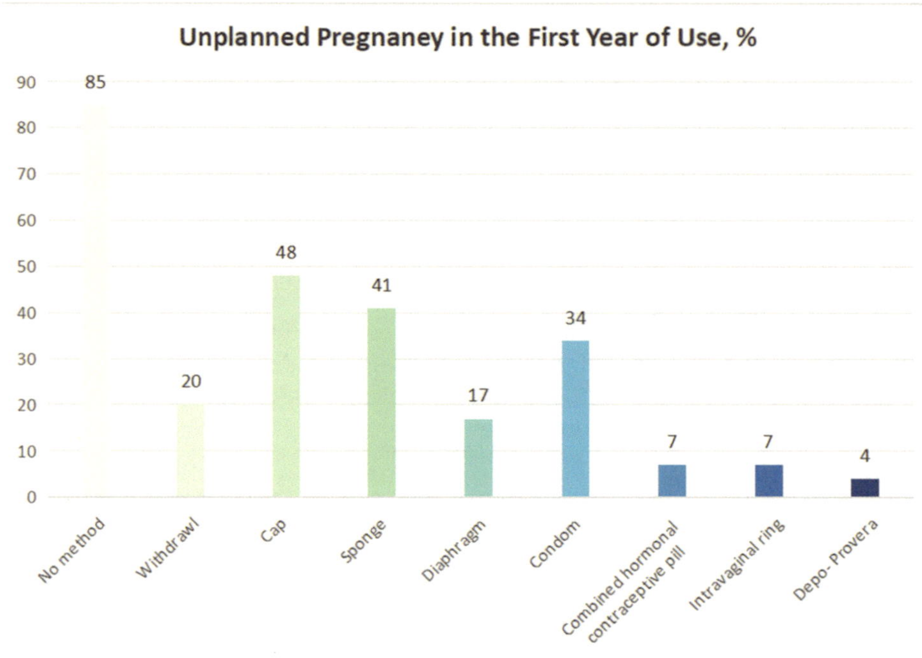

Figure 4.
Contraception efficacy rates (data from contraception [62] and figure made by Chiplot).

contraception are unable to use it for fear of side effects on their bodies. And the primary mechanism for male contraception—the condom—has remained unchanged for 100 years [64].

In summary, increasing the choice and use of contraceptives, popularizing sex education can contribute to the development of healthy families and slow population growth that places a disproportionate burden on the environment.

8. Conclusion

A pregnant woman's own illness is the main factor that primarily affects her pregnancy status and the status of her fetus. Therefore, pregnant women should pay more attention to their pregnancy status and undergo regular checkups. On the other hand, doctors should also pay more attention to pregnant women with illnesses and choose appropriate treatments and medications for them. Local governments should also provide appropriate support to ensure that pregnant women can have a smooth pregnancy and delivery.

DOI: http://dx.doi.org/10.5772/intechopen.1007951

Author details

Junna Ye[1*], Jiaxin Li[2], Yizhu Lin[2], Yujuan Wang[2], Jingyi Wu[1] and Zhuochao Zhou[1]

1 Department of Rheumatology and Immunology, Ruijin Hospital, Shanghai Jiao Tong University School of Medicine, Shanghai, China

2 Shanghai Jiao Tong University School of Medicine, Shanghai, China

*Address all correspondence to: yjn0912@qq.com

IntechOpen

References

[1] Stock SJ, Aiken CE. Barriers to progress in pregnancy research: How can we break through? Science. 2023;**380**(6641):150-153. DOI: 10.1126/science.adf9347

[2] Brown CC, Adams CE, George KE, Moore JE. Associations between comorbidities and severe maternal morbidity. Obstetrics and Gynecology. 2020;**136**(5):892-901. DOI: 10.1097/aog.0000000000004057

[3] Luong J, Board A, Gosdin L, Dunkley J, Thierry JM, Pitasi M, et al. Alcohol use, screening, and brief intervention among pregnant persons—24 U.S. jurisdictions, 2017 and 2019. MMWR. Morbidity and Mortality Weekly Report. 2023;**72**(3):55-62. DOI: 10.15585/mmwr.mm7203a2

[4] Bertozzi I, Rumi E, Cavalloni C, Cazzola M, Fabris F, Randi ML. Pregnancy outcome and management of 25 pregnancies in women with polycythemia vera. American Journal of Hematology. 2018;**93**(9):E234-E2e5. DOI: 10.1002/ajh.25210

[5] Subtil D, Brabant G, Tilloy E, Devos P, Canis F, Fruchart A, et al. Early clindamycin for bacterial vaginosis in pregnancy (PREMEVA): A multicentre, double-blind, randomised controlled trial. Lancet. 2018;**392**(10160):2171-2179. DOI: 10.1016/s0140-6736(18)31617-9

[6] Holness N. High-risk pregnancy. The Nursing Clinics of North America. 2018;**53**(2):241-251. DOI: 10.1016/j.cnur.2018.01.010

[7] Roos-Hesselink J, Baris L, Johnson M, De Backer J, Otto C, Marelli A, et al. Pregnancy outcomes in women with cardiovascular disease: Evolving trends over 10 years in the ESC registry of pregnancy and cardiac disease (ROPAC). European Heart Journal. 2019;**40**(47):3848-3855. DOI: 10.1093/eurheartj/ehz136

[8] Lammers AE, Diller GP, Lober R, Möllers M, Schmidt R, Radke RM, et al. Maternal and neonatal complications in women with congenital heart disease: A nationwide analysis. European Heart Journal. 2021;**42**(41):4252-4260. DOI: 10.1093/eurheartj/ehab571

[9] Magnus MC, Morken NH, Wensaas KA, Wilcox AJ, Håberg SE. Risk of miscarriage in women with chronic diseases in Norway: A registry linkage study. PLoS Medicine. 2021;**18**(5):e1003603. DOI: 10.1371/journal.pmed.1003603

[10] Justin Paul G, Anne Princy S, Anju S, Anita S, Cecily Mary M, Gnanavelu G, et al. Pregnancy outcomes in women with heart disease: The Madras medical college pregnancy and cardiac (M-PAC) registry from India. European Heart Journal. 2023;**44**(17):1530-1540. DOI: 10.1093/eurheartj/ehad003

[11] Andrade F, Shukla A, Bureau C, Senzolo M, D'Alteroche L, Heurgué A, et al. Pregnancy in idiopathic non-cirrhotic portal hypertension: A multicentric study on maternal and fetal management and outcome. Journal of Hepatology. 2018;**69**(6):1242-1249. DOI: 10.1016/j.jhep.2018.08.007

[12] Brown MA, Magee LA, Kenny LC, Karumanchi SA, McCarthy FP, Saito S, et al. The hypertensive disorders of pregnancy: ISSHP classification, diagnosis & management recommendations for international practice. Pregnancy Hypertens. 2018;**13**:291-310. DOI: 10.1016/j.preghy.2018.05.004

[13] Yang Y, Le Ray I, Zhu J, Zhang J, Hua J, Reilly M. Preeclampsia prevalence, risk factors, and pregnancy outcomes in Sweden and China. JAMA Network Open. 2021;**4**(5):e218401. DOI: 10.1001/jamanetworkopen.2021.8401

[14] Pfaller B, Siu SC, D'Souza R, Wichert-Schmitt B, Kumar Nair GK, Haberer K, et al. Impact of obesity on outcomes of pregnancy in women with heart disease. Journal of the American College of Cardiology. 2021;**77**(10):1317-1326. DOI: 10.1016/j.jacc.2021.01.010

[15] Paixão ES, Costa M, Teixeira MG, Harron K, de Almeida MF, Barreto ML, et al. Symptomatic dengue infection during pregnancy and the risk of stillbirth in Brazil, 2006-12: A matched case-control study. The Lancet Infectious Diseases. 2017;**17**(9):957-964. DOI: 10.1016/s1473-3099(17)30366-3

[16] Goldenberg RL, McClure EM, Saleem S, Reddy UM. Infection-related stillbirths. Lancet. 2010;**375**(9724):1482-1490. DOI: 10.1016/s0140-6736(09)61712-8

[17] Chen PH, Johnson L, Limketkai BN, Jusuf E, Sun J, Kim B, et al. Trends in the prevalence of hepatitis C infection during pregnancy and maternal-infant outcomes in the US, 1998 to 2018. JAMA Network Open. 2023;**6**(7):e2324770. DOI: 10.1001/jamanetworkopen.2023.24770

[18] Ghanem-Zoubi N, Paul M. Q fever during pregnancy: A narrative review. Clinical Microbiology and Infection. 2020;**26**(7):864-870. DOI: 10.1016/j.cmi.2019.10.024

[19] Hong S, Banchereau R, Maslow BL, Guerra MM, Cardenas J, Baisch J, et al. Longitudinal profiling of human blood transcriptome in healthy and lupus pregnancy. The Journal of Experimental Medicine. 2019;**216**(5):1154-1169. DOI: 10.1084/jem.20190185

[20] Mao-Draayer Y, Thiel S, Mills EA, Chitnis T, Fabian M, Katz Sand I, et al. Neuromyelitis optica spectrum disorders and pregnancy: Therapeutic considerations. Nature Reviews. Neurology. 2020;**16**(3):154-170. DOI: 10.1038/s41582-020-0313-y

[21] Wang L, Su M, Zhou Z, Zhou L, ZhangBao J, Tan H, et al. Analysis of pregnancy-related attacks in neuromyelitis optica spectrum disorder: A systematic review and meta-analysis. JAMA Network Open. 2022;**5**(8):e2225438. DOI: 10.1001/jamanetworkopen.2022.25438

[22] Fattizzo B, Bortolotti M, Fantini NN, Glenthøj A, Michel M, Napolitano M, et al. Autoimmune hemolytic anemia during pregnancy and puerperium: An international multicenter experience. Blood. 2023;**141**(16):2016-2021. DOI: 10.1182/blood.2022018890

[23] Mills JL, Baker L, Goldman AS. Malformations in infants of diabetic mothers occur before the seventh gestational week. Implications for treatment. Diabetes. 1979;**28**(4):292-293. DOI: 10.2337/diab.28.4.292

[24] Bozdag G, Mumusoglu S, Zengin D, Karabulut E, Yildiz BO. The prevalence and phenotypic features of polycystic ovary syndrome: A systematic review and meta-analysis. Human Reproduction. 2016;**31**(12):2841-2855. DOI: 10.1093/humrep/dew218

[25] Bahri Khomami M, Shorakae S, Hashemi S, Harrison CL, Piltonen TT, Romualdi D, et al. Systematic review and meta-analysis of pregnancy outcomes in women with polycystic ovary syndrome. Nature Communications. 2024;**15**(1):5591. DOI: 10.1038/s41467-024-49749-1

[26] Kroner BL, Hankins JS, Pugh N, Kutlar A, King AA, Shah NR, et al. Pregnancy outcomes with hydroxyurea use in women with sickle cell disease. American Journal of Hematology. 2022;**97**(5):603-612. DOI: 10.1002/ajh.26495

[27] Early ML, Eke AC, Gemmill A, Lanzkron S, Pecker LH. Comparisons of severe maternal morbidity and other adverse pregnancy outcomes in pregnant people with sickle cell disease vs anemia. JAMA Network Open. 2023;**6**(2):e2254545. DOI: 10.1001/jamanetworkopen.2022.54545

[28] Barbui T, Thiele J, Gisslinger H, Finazzi G, Vannucchi AM, Tefferi A. The 2016 revision of WHO classification of myeloproliferative neoplasms: Clinical and molecular advances. Blood Reviews. 2016;**30**(6):453-459. DOI: 10.1016/j.blre.2016.06.001

[29] Griesshammer M, Sadjadian P, Wille K. Contemporary management of patients with BCR-ABL1-negative myeloproliferative neoplasms during pregnancy. Expert Review of Hematology. 2018;**11**(9):697-706. DOI: 10.1080/17474086.2018.1506325

[30] Gangat N, Joshi M, Shah S, Yogarajah M, Patnaik MM, Pardanani A, et al. Pregnancy outcomes in myeloproliferative neoplasms: A Mayo clinic report on 102 pregnancies. American Journal of Hematology. 2020;**95**(5):E114-E1e7. DOI: 10.1002/ajh.25748

[31] Gangat N, Guglielmelli P, Al-Kali A, Wolanskyj-Spinner AP, Camoriano J, Patnaik MM, et al. Pregnancy in patients with myelofibrosis: Mayo-Florence series of 24 pregnancies in 16 women. British Journal of Haematology. 2021;**195**(1):133-137. DOI: 10.1111/bjh.17626

[32] Gangat N, Tefferi A. Myeloproliferative neoplasms and pregnancy: Overview and practice recommendations. American Journal of Hematology. 2021;**96**(3):354-366. DOI: 10.1002/ajh.26067

[33] Yonkers KA. Treatment of psychiatric conditions in pregnancy starts with planning. The American Journal of Psychiatry. 2021;**178**(3):213-214. DOI: 10.1176/appi.ajp.2020.20121791

[34] Roddy Mitchell A, Gordon H, Lindquist A, Walker SP, Homer CSE, Middleton A, et al. Prevalence of perinatal depression in low- and middle-income countries: A systematic review and meta-analysis. JAMA Psychiatry. 2023;**80**(5):425-431. DOI: 10.1001/jamapsychiatry.2023.0069

[35] Roddy Mitchell A, Gordon H, Atkinson J, Lindquist A, Walker SP, Middleton A, et al. Prevalence of perinatal anxiety and related disorders in low- and middle-income countries: A systematic review and meta-analysis. JAMA Network Open. 2023;**6**(11):e2343711. DOI: 10.1001/jamanetworkopen.2023.43711

[36] Kipling L, Bombard J, Wang X, Cox S. Cigarette smoking among pregnant women during the perinatal period: Prevalence and health care provider inquiries—Pregnancy risk assessment monitoring system, United States, 2021. MMWR. Morbidity and Mortality Weekly Report. 2024;**73**(17):393-398. DOI: 10.15585/mmwr.mm7317a2

[37] Odendaal H, Dukes KA, Elliott AJ, Willinger M, Sullivan LM, Tripp T, et al. Association of prenatal exposure to maternal drinking and smoking with the risk of stillbirth. JAMA Network Open. 2021;**4**(8):e2121726. DOI: 10.1001/jamanetworkopen.2021.21726

[38] Zheng X, Yang D, Luo S, Yan J, Guo X, Yang H, et al. Association of Implementation of a comprehensive preconception-to-pregnancy management plan with pregnancy outcomes among Chinese pregnant women with type 1 diabetes: The CARNATION study. Diabetes Care. 2021;**44**(4):883-892. DOI: 10.2337/dc20-2692

[39] Velez MP, Soule A, Gaudet L, Pudwell J, Nguyen P, Ray JG. Multifetal pregnancy after implementation of a publicly funded fertility program. JAMA Network Open. 2024;7(4):e248496. DOI: 10.1001/jamanetworkopen.2024.8496

[40] Figueroa-Espada CG, Hofbauer S, Mitchell MJ, Riley RS. Exploiting the placenta for nanoparticle-mediated drug delivery during pregnancy. Advanced Drug Delivery Reviews. 2020;**160**:244-261. DOI: 10.1016/j.addr.2020.09.006

[41] Levy CJ, Kudva YC, Ozaslan B, Castorino K, O'Malley G, Kaur RJ, et al. At-home use of a pregnancy-specific zone-MPC closed-loop system for pregnancies complicated by type 1 diabetes: A single-arm, observational multicenter study. Diabetes Care. 2023;**46**(7):1425-1431. DOI: 10.2337/dc23-0173

[42] Ringholm L, Damm P, Mathiesen ER. Improving pregnancy outcomes in women with diabetes mellitus: Modern management. Nature Reviews. Endocrinology. 2019;**15**(7):406-416. DOI: 10.1038/s41574-019-0197-3

[43] Wheeler SM, Myers SO, Swamy GK, Myers ER. Estimated prevalence of risk factors for preeclampsia among individuals giving birth in the US in 2019. JAMA Network Open. 2022;**5**(1):e2142343. DOI: 10.1001/jamanetworkopen.2021.42343

[44] Maze D, Kazi S, Gupta V, Malinowski AK, Fazelzad R, Shah PS, et al. Association of Treatments for myeloproliferative neoplasms during pregnancy with birth rates and maternal outcomes: A systematic review and meta-analysis. JAMA Network Open. 2019;**2**(10):e1912666. DOI: 10.1001/jamanetworkopen.2019.12666

[45] Trinh NTH, Munk-Olsen T, Wray NR, Bergink V, Nordeng HME, Lupattelli A, et al. Timing of antidepressant discontinuation during pregnancy and postpartum psychiatric outcomes in Denmark and Norway. JAMA Psychiatry. 2023;**80**(5):441-450. DOI: 10.1001/jamapsychiatry.2023.0041

[46] Malan V, Bussières L, Winer N, Jais JP, Baptiste A, Le Lorc'h M, et al. Effect of cell-free DNA screening vs direct invasive diagnosis on miscarriage rates in women with pregnancies at high risk of trisomy 21: A randomized clinical trial. JAMA. 2018;**320**(6):557-565. DOI: 10.1001/jama.2018.9396

[47] National Collaborating Centre for Ws, Children's H. National Institute for Health and Clinical Excellence: Guidance. Fertility: Assessment and Treatment for People with Fertility Problems. London: Royal College of Obstetricians & Gynaecologists. Copyright © 2013, National Collaborating Centre for Women's and Children's Health; 2013

[48] Holt-Kentwell A, Ghosh J, Devall A, Coomarasamy A, Dhillon-Smith RK. Evaluating interventions and adjuncts to optimize pregnancy outcomes in subfertile women: An overview review. Human Reproduction Update. 2022;**28**(4):583-600. DOI: 10.1093/humupd/dmac001

[49] Magnus MC, Wilcox AJ, Morken NH, Weinberg CR, Håberg SE. Role of

maternal age and pregnancy history in risk of miscarriage: Prospective register based study. BMJ. 2019;**364**:l869. DOI: 10.1136/bmj.l869

[50] du Fossé NA, van der Hoorn MP, van Lith JMM, le Cessie S, Lashley E. Advanced paternal age is associated with an increased risk of spontaneous miscarriage: A systematic review and meta-analysis. Human Reproduction Update. 2020;**26**(5):650-669. DOI: 10.1093/humupd/dmaa010

[51] Regan AK, Gissler M, Magnus MC, Håberg SE, Ball S, Malacova E, et al. Association between interpregnancy interval and adverse birth outcomes in women with a previous stillbirth: An international cohort study. Lancet. 2019;**393**(10180):1527-1535. DOI: 10.1016/s0140-6736(18)32266-9

[52] Hamilton I, Martin N, Liu J, DeFranco E, Rossi R. Gestational age and birth outcomes in term singleton pregnancies conceived with infertility treatment. JAMA Network Open. 2023;**6**(8):e2328335. DOI: 10.1001/jamanetworkopen.2023.28335

[53] Muglu J, Rather H, Arroyo-Manzano D, Bhattacharya S, Balchin I, Khalil A, et al. Risks of stillbirth and neonatal death with advancing gestation at term: A systematic review and meta-analysis of cohort studies of 15 million pregnancies. PLoS Medicine. 2019;**16**(7):e1002838. DOI: 10.1371/journal.pmed.1002838

[54] Schummers L, Hutcheon JA, Hernandez-Diaz S, Williams PL, Hacker MR, VanderWeele TJ, et al. Association of short interpregnancy interval with pregnancy outcomes according to maternal age. JAMA Internal Medicine. 2018;**178**(12):1661-1670. DOI: 10.1001/jamainternmed.2018.4696

[55] Bekkar B, Pacheco S, Basu R, DeNicola N. Association of air pollution and heat exposure with preterm birth, low birth weight, and stillbirth in the US: A systematic review. JAMA Network Open. 2020;**3**(6):e208243. DOI: 10.1001/jamanetworkopen.2020.8243

[56] Ren S, Haynes E, Hall E, Hossain M, Chen A, Muglia L, et al. Periconception exposure to air pollution and risk of congenital malformations. The Journal of Pediatrics. 2018;**193**:76-84.e6. DOI: 10.1016/j.jpeds.2017.09.076

[57] Ghassabian A, Pierotti L, Basterrechea M, Chatzi L, Estarlich M, Fernández-Somoano A, et al. Association of exposure to ambient air pollution with thyroid function during pregnancy. JAMA Network Open. 2019;**2**(10):e1912902. DOI: 10.1001/jamanetworkopen.2019.12902

[58] Wang X, Liu C, Zhang M, Han Y, Aase H, Villanger GD, et al. Evaluation of maternal exposure to PM(2.5) and its components on maternal and neonatal thyroid function and birth weight: A cohort study. Thyroid. 2019;**29**(8):1147-1157. DOI: 10.1089/thy.2018.0780

[59] Kelty E, Rae K, Jantzie LL, Wyrwoll CS, Preen DB. Prenatal opioid exposure and immune-related conditions in children. JAMA Network Open. 2024;**7**(1):e2351933. DOI: 10.1001/jamanetworkopen.2023.51933

[60] Newville J, Maxwell JR, Kitase Y, Robinson S, Jantzie LL. Perinatal opioid exposure primes the peripheral immune system toward hyperreactivity. Frontiers in Pediatrics. 2020;**8**:272. DOI: 10.3389/fped.2020.00272

[61] Rushworth FH, Backos M, Rai R, Chilcott IT, Baxter N, Regan L. Prospective pregnancy outcome in untreated recurrent miscarriers

with thyroid autoantibodies. Human Reproduction. 2000;**15**(7):1637-1639. DOI: 10.1093/humrep/15.7.1637

[62] Woodhams EJ, Gilliam M. Contraception. Annals of Internal Medicine. 2019;**170**(3):Itc18-itc32. DOI: 10.7326/aitc201902050

[63] The L. Preventing teenage pregnancies in Brazil. Lancet. 2020;**395**(10223):468. DOI: 10.1016/s0140-6736(20)30352-4

[64] Anderson DJ, Johnston DS. A brief history and future prospects of contraception. Science. 2023;**380**(6641):154-158. DOI: 10.1126/science.adf9341

Chapter 7

Tunisian Pregnant Women Benefiting from Cervical Ripening in the Third Trimester

Montacer Hafsi, Eya Kristou, Fathi Mraihi and Dalenda Chelli

Abstract

Cervical maturation in the third trimester is crucial to prepare the cervix for childbirth and ensure successful vaginal delivery. This study aimed to describe the profile of patients requiring cervical maturation and evaluate the outcomes of mechanical and chemical methods. A retrospective study was conducted on 100 parturients at the Obstetric Gynecology Department "D" of Tunis maternity and neonatology center (CMNT) between 2020 and 2022. Pregnant women at term with unfavorable Bishop scores and cephalic presentation were included. Exclusions were based on contraindications to vaginal delivery and multiple pregnancies. The primary outcome was the rate of vaginal delivery, with secondary outcomes including labor duration and maternal and neonatal results. The average patient age was 29 years, with 50% being primiparous. Post-term pregnancy was the most common indication for cervical maturation. The Foley catheter was used in 70% of cases, while Misoprostol was used in 30%. Labor lasted 15 hours with Misoprostol and 18 hours with the Foley catheter. Vaginal delivery occurred in 80% of cases, with a 40% cesarean rate for failed inductions. Tachysystole occurred in 6% of cases, and perineal tears were reported in 26.09% (Misoprostol) and 21.06% (Foley catheter) cases. Most newborns had satisfactory Apgar scores, with 5% requiring resuscitation and 10% needing hospitalization. Both methods are effective, but risks require careful management.

Keywords: childbirth, Misoprostol, extra-amniotic balloon, cervical ripening, obstetric labor

1. Introduction

Cervical maturation in the third trimester is a critical step in preparing the cervix for childbirth. It involves essential anatomical and physiological changes such as dilation, effacement, and softening, which are necessary for a smooth and efficient labor process. However, in some women, cervical immaturity can lead to obstetric complications, including prolonged labor, higher cesarean rates, and increased maternal and fetal health risks [1, 2].

In Tunisia, specific epidemiological factors, including limited access to proper care and deteriorating healthcare infrastructure, exacerbate these complications. Despite the importance of cervical maturation, few studies have focused on this issue within the Tunisian population, highlighting a significant gap in the literature [3]. Cervical ripening methods, including mechanical methods such as the Foley catheter and pharmacological agents like Misoprostol, are commonly used [4].

However, the use of Misoprostol for cervical ripening lacks official market authorization (AMM) in some countries, such as Tunisia and France [5, 6].

This study aims to address this gap by describing the epidemiological profile of pregnant women requiring cervical maturation in the third trimester and reporting on the outcomes of mechanical and chemical methods used to facilitate the process.

2. Materials and methods

2.1 Study design

This was a retrospective, descriptive, observational study conducted at a single center, focused on clinical case series.

2.2 Study period and location

The study took place at the Department D of Gynecology and Obstetrics at the Maternity and Neonatology Center of Tunis (CMNT), spanning from January 2020 to December 2022.

2.3 Study population

- *Inclusion criteria*: Women with a single-term pregnancy (>37 weeks), age >18 years, advanced term (≥41 weeks), cephalic presentation, unfavorable Bishop score (<6), and a normal fetal heart rate (FHR) were included. Informed consent was obtained from all participants.

- *Exclusion criteria*: Women with contraindications to vaginal delivery or medical contraindications to the use of Misoprostol or the extra-amniotic catheter were excluded (e.g., severe asthma, known prostaglandin allergy, placenta previa).

- *Exclusion of records*: Patients with incomplete or missing medical records, those lost to follow-up, or those who left against medical advice were excluded.

2.4 Data collection

Data were extracted from patient medical records and delivery logs. A standardized form, developed based on literature, was completed anonymously using this information. Variables were compiled into a comprehensive dataset for analysis.

2.5 Data analyzed

1. *General population description*:

    - Maternal age (<25, 25–35, ≥35 years)

    - BMI categories: underweight (<20), normal (20–25), overweight (25–30), moderate obesity (30–35), severe obesity (≥35)

- Medical and surgical history (e.g., diabetes, hypertension, thyroid dysfunction)
- Gynecological history (e.g., gravidity, parity, previous cesarean sections)
- Pregnancy details: term at admission, prenatal follow-ups, and ultrasound findings
- Fetal data: estimated fetal weight, amniotic fluid volume, and FHR

2. *Labor induction characteristics*:

- Gestational age at induction (categorized: 37–38 + 6 weeks, 39–40 + 6 weeks, ≥41 weeks)
- Primary reasons for induction (e.g., post-term, gestational diabetes, reduced fetal movements)
- Bishop score prior to induction (<3, 4–5, ≥6)
- Methods of cervical ripening (Misoprostol, extra-amniotic catheter, or both)
- Duration of labor phases (latent and active), dosage of Misoprostol, and time to labor onset

3. *Labor and delivery outcomes*:

- Total labor duration, amniotic fluid characteristics (clear, stained, meconium)
- Use of oxytocin, FHR abnormalities (CNGOF classification: green, yellow, orange, red)
- Delivery mode (spontaneous, instrumental, cesarean)
- Episiotomy and indications for instrumental or cesarean delivery

4. *Maternal outcomes*:

- Uterine contractility issues, perineal tears, uterine rupture, postpartum hemorrhage

5. *Neonatal outcomes*:

- Birth weight, Apgar score at 1 and 5 minutes, need for resuscitation, neonatal unit admission

2.6 Cervical maturation

2.6.1 Maturation techniques

- Foley catheter

- Mechanical method used to dilate the cervix by applying controlled pressure through a Foley catheter (18 Fr gauge) filled with 60 ml of saline. The catheter stays in place until it naturally falls out, with a maximum duration of 24 hours.
- Procedure: visual inspection of the cervix using a speculum, antiseptic cleaning with Betadine, catheter insertion, balloon inflation, and traction application.
- Equipment: sterile gloves, speculum, saline, clamps, Foley catheter, etc.

- Misoprostol
  - Synthetic prostaglandin E1 analog, used for its quick action and low cost.
  - Administration methods: oral, sublingual, vaginal (vaginal dosage: 50 µg every 8 hours, up to 3 doses within 24 hours).
  - Fetal heart rate monitoring (FHR) is conducted 1 hour before and after each dose.

2.6.2 Maturation protocols

- After the decision to induce labor, an initial Bishop score is calculated, and FHR is monitored. Following Foley or Misoprostol administration, regular FHR checks are conducted.
- If the Bishop score remains unfavorable post-treatment, oxytocin (Syntocinon®) may be used. Labor induction failure is defined by an inability to achieve a favorable Bishop score after six Misoprostol doses.
- Labor monitoring continues via vaginal exams and contractions. Labor details are documented in the partogram.

2.7 Bibliographic research

- Key databases used: NCBI, Science Direct, ClinicalKey, Cochrane, and medical university databases.
- Keywords: labor induction, Misoprostol, Foley catheter, cervical maturation, obstetric labor

2.8 Statistical analysis

1. Studied variables
   - Epidemiological variables: Age, medical/surgical history, BMI, parity, number of natural deliveries
   - Pregnancy variables: Complications, gestational age, reasons for induction

- Induction protocol: Latency and active labor phases, delivery method, and complications

- Neonatal outcome: APGAR score, birth weight, reasons for NICU admission

- Maternal outcome: Uterine hypertonia, rupture, hemorrhage, and perineal tears

2. Statistical analysis

- Descriptive: Qualitative variables (frequencies) and quantitative variables (means, standard deviation, or medians)

- Analytical: Chi-square tests for qualitative variables, T-test or Mann–Whitney U test for quantitative

2.9 Ethical agreement and data protection

Data was collected after receiving department approval, and all patient information was anonymized to protect privacy. Data integrity and confidentiality were maintained throughout the study.

2.10 Conflict of interest declaration

No conflicts of interest or external funding influenced the study results.

3. Results

3.1 Maternal and obstetric data

3.1.1 Age

The mean age was higher in the extra-amniotic group (30.2 years) compared to the Misoprostol group (28.5 years), with no significant difference (p = 0.84) (**Table 1**).

Age group	Misoprostol (n = 30) (%)	Extra-amniotic (n = 70) (%)	p-Value
20–25	23.34	18.57	0.84
26–30	36.67	40	0.64
31–35	26.67	28.57	0.61
36–40	10	10	0.92
41–45	3	2.85	0.99

Table 1.
Distribution by age group in the two groups.

3.1.2 Weight and height

The mean weight was 72.15 kg in the Misoprostol group and 75.16 kg in the extra-amniotic group. No significant differences in weight (p = 0.45) or height (p = 0.35) were observed.

3.1.3 BMI

The mean BMI in the Misoprostol group was 26.53, while it was 28.66 in the extra-amniotic group, with no significant difference (p = 0.45) (**Table 2**).

3.1.4 Medical history

A total of 21% of patients had chronic conditions such as diabetes, asthma, and hypothyroidism. There was no significant difference between groups (p = 0.44) (**Table 3**).

3.1.5 Surgical history

Totally, 5% of patients had a history of surgery (e.g., appendicectomy, cholecystectomy). There was no significant difference (p = 0.88).

3.1.6 Gestational age

The average gestational age was similar across both groups (Misoprostol: 38 weeks + 5 days; extra-amniotic: 39 weeks + 1 day). No significant difference was found (p = 0.84) (**Table 4**).

3.2 Induction and labor data

3.2.1 Indication for induction

The most common indications were post-term pregnancy and premature rupture of membranes (Misoprostol) or preeclampsia (extra-amniotic group) (**Table 5**).

BMI	Misoprostol	Extra-amniotic	p-Value
Mean	26.53	28.66	0.45
Minimum	17.89	23.15	
Maximum	34.10	40.10	

Table 2.
BMI of patients in our series.

Medical history	Misoprostol (n = 30) (%)	Extra-amniotic (n = 70) (%)	p-Value
Yes	20	21.42	0.44
No	80	78.57	0.44

Table 3.
Medical history of patients in our series.

Gestational age	Misoprostol (n = 30) (%)	Extra-Amniotic (n = 70) (%)	p-Value
37–37 + 6 weeks	6.66	11.42	0.84
38–38 + 6 weeks	33.34	21.42	0.64
39–39 + 6 weeks	23.34	24.28	0.99
40–40 + 6 weeks	10	17.14	0.61
>41 weeks	26.66	25.71	0.92

Table 4.
Distribution of patients by pregnancy term.

Indication	Misoprostol (n = 30) (%)	Extra-amniotic (n = 70) (%)	p-Value
Post-term pregnancy	26.66	25.72	0.80
Preeclampsia	16.66	24.28	0.38
Gestational diabetes	6.66	10	0.70
Double dysgravidy (HTN + GD)	10	17.14	0.70
Premature rupture of membranes >12 h	23.33	0	1.00

Table 5.
Distribution of patients by labor induction indications.

3.2.2 Bishop score

The mean initial Bishop score was 3.4, with no significant difference between groups (p = 0.65) (**Table 6**).

3.2.3 Labor duration

The total labor duration was longer in the extra-amniotic group (18 h 30 m) compared to the Misoprostol group (15 h 20 m) though the difference was not significant (p = 0.15) (**Table 7**).

3.2.4 Amniotic fluid

There was a higher occurrence of stained amniotic fluid in the Misoprostol group (17%) compared to the extra-amniotic group (10%), but this difference was not significant (p = 0.14) (**Table 8**).

Bishop score	Misoprostol (n = 30) (%)	Extra-amniotic (n = 70) (%)	p-Value
≤3	23.34	35.71	0.65
3–4	46.66	40	0.88
5	30	24.28	0.73

Table 6.
Distribution of patients by initial Bishop score.

Labor duration (hours)	Misoprostol (n = 23) (%)	Extra-amniotic (n = 57) (%)	p-Value
<12 h	34.78	26.31	0.15
12–24 h	43.48	61.40	
>24 h	21.74	13.72	

Table 7.
Population distribution by labor induction.

Amniotic fluid	Misoprostol (n = 30) (%)	Extra-amniotic (n = 70) (%)	p-Value
Clear	76.67	82.85	0.84
Stained	16.67	10	0.14
Meconium	6.66	7.15	0.99

Table 8.
Amniotic fluid color by induction method.

3.2.5 Oxytocin use

Oxytocin was administered to 67 patients, with no significant difference between groups ($p = 0.75$) (**Table 9**).

3.2.6 Fetal heart rate (FHR) abnormalities

FHR monitoring showed pathological traces in 40% of parturients. There was no significant difference between groups ($p = 0.66$) (**Table 10**).

3.3 Mode of delivery and complications

3.3.1 Mode of delivery

The cesarean section rate was slightly higher in the Misoprostol group (23.34%) compared to the extra-amniotic group (18.58%), though the difference was not statistically significant ($p = 0.21$) (**Table 11**).

Oxytocin use	Misoprostol (n = 30) (%)	Extra-amniotic (n = 70) (%)	p-Value
Yes	63.33	68.57	0.75
No	36.67	31.43	

Table 9.
Use of oxytocics by induction method.

FHR abnormalities	Misoprostol (n = 30) (%)	Extra-amniotic (n = 70) (%)	p-Value
Pathological Traces	43.33%	38.57%	0.66

Table 10.
FHR abnormalities by induction method.

Delivery mode	Misoprostol (n = 30) (%)	Extra-amniotic (n = 70) (%)	p-Value
Vaginal	66.66	78.57	0.70
Instrumental	10	2.85	0.03*
Cesarean	23.34	18.58	0.21

**Significant p-value for instrumental delivery between groups.*

Table 11.
Delivery rates by induction method.

Indication for cesarean	Misoprostol (n = 7) (%)	Extra-amniotic (n = 13) (%)	p-Value
Failed induction	42.87	38.46	0.88
Fetal distress	28.57	30.78	0.65

Table 12.
Indications for cesarean delivery.

3.3.2 Indications for cesarean

The primary reasons for cesarean were failed induction and fetal distress, with no significant difference between groups (p = 0.88) (**Table 12**).

3.3.3 Complications during labor

Labor complications occurred in 15% of patients in the Misoprostol group and 17% in the extra-amniotic group, with no significant difference (p = 0.3) (**Table 13**).

3.4 Neonatal outcomes

3.4.1 Birth weight

Neonatal birth weights averaged 3483 g in the Misoprostol group and 3560 g in the extra-amniotic group. No significant differences were observed (p = 0.91) (**Table 14**).

Complications	Misoprostol (n = 30) (%)	Extra-amniotic (n = 70) (%)	p-Value
Yes	23.33	25.71	0.30
No	76.67	73.29	

Table 13.
Labor complications.

Birth weight (g)	Misoprostol (n = 30) (%)	Extra-amniotic (n = 70) (%)	p-Value
<2500	13.33	8.57	0.87
2500–4000	80	87.14	0.91
4000–4500	6.66	4.29	0.84

Table 14.
Birth weight in our population.

Apgar score	1 min – misoprostol (%)	1 min - extra-amniotic (%)	5 min – misoprostol (%)	5 min - extra-amniotic (%)	p-Value
7–10	87	92	100	100	0.95

Table 15.
Apgar score at 1 minute and 5 minutes in our population.

NICU admission	Misoprostol (n = 30) (%)	Extra-amniotic (n = 70) (%)	p-Value
Yes	13	10	0.96
No	87	90	

Table 16.
Neonatal unit hospitalizations.

3.4.2 Apgar scores

- Apgar scores at 1 and 5 minutes were similar between groups, with no significant differences (p = 0.95) (**Table 15**).

3.4.3 NICU admission

NICU admission rates were slightly higher in the Misoprostol group (13%) compared to the extra-amniotic group (10%), but the difference was not statistically significant (p = 0.96) (**Table 16**).

4. Discussion

4.1 Summary of results

Induction of labor involves artificially initiating labor before its spontaneous onset with the aim of facilitating childbirth. This procedure has become increasingly common worldwide, including in Tunisia, where it is one of the most frequently performed interventions in obstetric care. Despite the lack of market authorization for Misoprostol in Tunisia and the high authority of health (HAS) in France's guidelines advising against the regular use of the extra-amniotic balloon catheter, both methods are widely used for cervical ripening in clinical practice.

Our study included 100 pregnant women in the third trimester, all of whom underwent cervical ripening with either the extra-amniotic balloon catheter or Misoprostol. The aim was to compare the effectiveness and safety of these methods in terms of labor progression, mode of delivery, and maternal and neonatal outcomes. The average age of the participants was 29 years, with a notable majority presenting with either normal weight or overweight, and 21% classified as obese. The most common indication for induction was post-term pregnancy (45%), followed by other factors like decreased fetal movements, prolonged rupture of membranes (RPM), gestational diabetes, and preeclampsia.

In 70% of cases, the extra-amniotic balloon catheter was used, while the remaining 30% of cases were induced using Misoprostol. Despite the differences in the techniques, both methods were equally effective in inducing labor, with the majority of women delivering vaginally. There were no significant differences in the total duration of labor between the two groups. Importantly, there was no evidence of increased maternal or neonatal morbidity associated with either method of induction.

4.2 Discussion of results

4.2.1 Epidemiological profile of the parturients

4.2.1.1 Age

Maternal age plays a crucial role in determining the mode of delivery, particularly in terms of cesarean rates. Studies have demonstrated that advanced maternal age, typically defined as 35 years and older, is associated with a significantly higher risk of cesarean section due to complications like prolonged labor or fetal distress [7]. Research by the American College of Obstetricians and Gynecologists [7] emphasizes that the likelihood of cesarean delivery increases markedly in women aged 40 and above, with the risks being threefold higher compared to younger women [8].

Our study, however, involved a younger population with an average age of 29 years. This aligns with previous studies where younger maternal age was linked to higher rates of successful vaginal deliveries [1, 9]. The relative youth of our cohort likely contributed to the high success rate of vaginal deliveries observed. However, larger studies that span a wider age range may reveal trends more in line with advanced maternal age and cesarean risk [10, 11].

4.2.1.2 Parity

Parity is another important predictor of labor induction success. Nulliparous women (those giving birth for the first time) are generally more prone to complications during labor induction, with increased rates of cesarean section compared to multiparous women (those who have given birth before) [12, 13].

Our findings are consistent with the literature; multiparous women in our study were more likely to deliver vaginally. This may be due to their more favorable cervical status and uterine muscle responsiveness, as previously noted in studies such as those by Leelarujijaroen et al. [14] and Diaz-Martinez et al. [15–17].

4.2.1.3 Body mass index (BMI)

The relationship between obesity and labor induction failure has been well established. In our study, women with a BMI of 30 or higher had a significantly higher rate of cesarean section compared to women with a BMI below 30, a finding that mirrors previous research [12, 18]. Several studies, including those by Ellis et al. [19], highlight that obesity complicates cervical ripening and prolongs labor, often necessitating higher doses of oxytocin and increasing the chances of cesarean delivery [20].

Further, studies have shown that obese women may have a slower cervical response to prostaglandins, including Misoprostol, due to alterations in hormonal sensitivity or distribution [10]. This suggests that BMI should be considered when choosing an induction method, as certain techniques might be less effective in obese patients [10, 12].

4.3 Evaluation of the effectiveness of ripening methods

4.3.1 Labor progression

Our study found no significant difference in labor progression between the extra-amniotic balloon catheter and Misoprostol groups, a finding consistent with the results of the PROBAAT-II trial [21, 22] and studies by Lanka et al. [23], which reported comparable labor durations for both methods [20, 24]. However, studies such as Levine et al. [25] demonstrated that combining Misoprostol with mechanical methods like the Foley catheter can significantly reduce the induction-to-delivery interval [13, 26].

These differences highlight the importance of tailoring cervical ripening methods to individual patient profiles, as certain combinations may yield faster and more efficient labor progress in specific populations, such as those with higher parity or more advanced maternal age (**Table 17**) [27].

Table 17 illustrates the variation in labor progression between studies. Our findings are comparable with international data, showing that the extra-amniotic balloon catheter led to shorter times to onset of uterine contractions than Misoprostol alone, a pattern also observed in other countries.

4.3.2 Vaginal delivery rates within the first 24 hours

The rate of vaginal delivery within the first 24 hours of induction is a key indicator of the success of labor induction techniques. In our study, 76.66% of women who received Misoprostol delivered vaginally, compared to 81.42% in the extra-amniotic balloon group. These rates align with other studies, such as Aduloju et al. [24], which found similar vaginal delivery rates between mechanical and pharmacological induction methods [17].

While some studies suggest a slight advantage for mechanical methods, others, including the work of Osoti et al. [20], have demonstrated that Misoprostol alone is just as effective when administered under appropriate conditions [28]. This variation highlights the need for clinical flexibility when selecting induction methods, especially in resource-limited settings (**Table 18**) [13, 20].

Study	Year	Country	Misoprostol	Foley catheter	Combined	p-Value
Lanka et al.	2014	Nigeria	27.64 h (15.63)	26.52 h (15.24)	**	0.65
Levine et al.	2016	USA	17.6 h	17.7 h	13.1 h	0.001
PROBAAT-II	2016	Netherlands	29 h	30 h	**	0.97
Gilani et al.	2018	Pakistan	19.26 h	**	16.46 h	0.033
Al-Ibraheemi et al.	2018	USA	19 h	**	15 h	0.001
Osoti et al.	2018	Kenya	18.9 h	**	14.1 h	<0.001
Priyadarshini et al.	2021	India	24.99 h	**	19.65 h	0.002
Inamdar et al.	2020	India	17.9 h	**	14.6 h	<0.0001
Current study	2023	Tunisia	8h + 53 min	15 h + 26 min	15 h + 26 min	0.02

Table 17.
Time between ripening and onset of uterine contractions.

Study	Year	Country	Misoprostol	Foley catheter	Combined	p-Value
Lanka et al.	2014	Nigeria	50.79%	50.79%	**	1.00
Levine et al.	2016	USA	70%	73.2%	87.8%	0.001
PROBAAT-II	2016	Netherlands	39.7%	30.2%	**	<0.001
Gilani et al.	2018	Pakistan	75.0%	**	54.17%	0.033
Al-Ibraheemi et al.	2018	USA	62%	**	70%	0.23
Priyadarshini et al.	2021	India	56.8%	**	76%	0.2
Current study	2023	Tunisia	76.66%	81.42%	81.42%	0.70

Table 18.
Vaginal delivery rates within 24 hours.

Table 18 highlights the variability in vaginal delivery rates across different studies. While our findings show high success rates for both methods, the slight advantage of the extra-amniotic balloon catheter in our study is consistent with the results from other research.

4.3.3 Oxytocin use

Oxytocin is frequently used to augment labor once cervical ripening has been achieved, particularly when labor is slow to progress. In our study, oxytocin was administered in 63.33% of the Misoprostol group and 68.57% of the extra-amniotic balloon group, with no significant differences between the groups. These findings are consistent with studies by Aduloju et al. [24] and PROBAAT-II [22], where oxytocin use was equally common across various induction methods [20, 24].

The similar rates of oxytocin use suggest that both methods are equally effective in achieving adequate uterine contractions. However, obese women and those with unfavorable Bishop scores may require higher doses of oxytocin to reach the same labor progression as other women, as noted by studies on labor induction in obese populations (**Table 19**) [10, 27].

Table 19 summarizes oxytocin usage in different studies. Our findings align with other research, where both methods of cervical ripening necessitate similar levels of oxytocin administration to ensure labor progression.

Study	Year	Country	Misoprostol (%)	Foley catheter (%)	Combined (%)	p-Value
Lanka et al.	2014	India	46.03	**	46.03	0.37
Aduloju et al.	2016	Nigeria	61.4	94.2	31.4	0.001
Levine et al.	2016	USA	68.6	89.9	70.7	<0.001
PROBAAT-II	2016	Netherlands	68.4	80.3	**	<0.001
Current study	2023	Tunisia	63.33	68.57	68.57	0.75

Table 19.
Oxytocin use.

4.4 Evaluation of potential morbidities

4.4.1 Maternal complications

In terms of maternal complications, our study found that uterine tachysystole occurred in 6% of women induced with Misoprostol, a rate comparable to other studies, including those by Aregeb et al. [17] and Kehl et al. [12, 13]. No cases of uterine rupture were reported in our cohort, which is consistent with the findings of Kehl et al. [12], who also reported low rates of uterine rupture with mechanical methods [12].

The low rate of maternal complications in our study aligns with international standards for cervical ripening techniques, particularly when these methods are used in women without prior uterine surgery [13].

4.4.2 Neonatal complications

Neonatal outcomes were similarly favorable in both groups. The rates of neonatal admission to intensive care units (NICU) were low, and there were no significant differences in Apgar scores at 1 and 5 minutes between the groups. This aligns with the findings of studies like those by Carbone et al. [28] and Levine et al. [25], which reported no significant differences in neonatal outcomes based on the method of cervical ripening [27].

In our study, there were no cases of neonatal death, and the few neonates who required NICU admission were primarily from mothers induced with Misoprostol. This pattern, while not statistically significant, mirrors findings in studies like those by Al-Ibraheemi et al. [27], where Misoprostol was associated with slightly higher rates of neonatal distress compared to mechanical methods. However, these differences were minor and did not result in long-term adverse outcomes [20, 25].

4.5 Limitations and strengths of the study

4.5.1 Study limitations

1. *Sample size*: Although our study included 100 patients, this sample size may be insufficient to detect rare outcomes or subtle differences between the two methods. A larger sample size would allow for more robust conclusions, especially regarding rare complications like uterine rupture.

2. *Study design*: This was a retrospective observational study, which limits the ability to establish causality. Randomized controlled trials would provide stronger evidence of the relative efficacy and safety of the two methods.

3. *Methods of ripening*: Our study focused on two specific methods of cervical ripening, namely the extra-amniotic balloon catheter and Misoprostol. Other methods, such as prostaglandin gels or oral Misoprostol, were not evaluated, potentially limiting the generalizability of our findings to other clinical settings.

4.5.2 Study strengths

1. *Recent data*: Our study is based on recent data, reflecting current clinical practices in labor induction. This ensures that our findings are relevant to contemporary obstetric care.

2. *Diversity of methods*: By comparing two commonly used methods of cervical ripening, our study provides valuable insights into their relative effectiveness and safety, helping inform clinical decision-making in everyday practice.

3. *Clinical relevance*: The findings of our study are directly applicable to clinical practice, particularly in resource-limited settings like Tunisia, where cost-effective and efficient labor induction methods are essential.

5. Conclusions

The artificial induction of labor (DAT) is a procedure designed to initiate labor before its natural onset, distinct from cervical ripening, which is often required beforehand. Successful induction typically leads to vaginal delivery, though the time to achieve this can vary. The decision to proceed with induction must be made collaboratively between the patient and healthcare provider, ensuring all available resources are used for a safe delivery.

In Tunisia, Misoprostol is frequently used for cervical ripening despite lacking AMM for third-trimester use. The extra-amniotic balloon catheter is also widely employed, reflecting local practices despite guidelines advising against its use in some countries.

Our study aimed to describe the epidemiological profile of women requiring cervical ripening and to evaluate outcomes using mechanical and chemical methods. The study, conducted with 100 women at a Tunisian maternity center, focused on vaginal delivery rates and other outcomes such as labor duration, maternal, and neonatal complications.

Key findings showed that Misoprostol and the extra-amniotic catheter were effective in cervical ripening, facilitating vaginal deliveries in most cases. However, safety concerns have been raised regarding Misoprostol's use, and the extra-amniotic catheter is not recommended by some health authorities, highlighting the need for cautious administration to prioritize maternal and fetal safety.

Acknowledgements

The authors would like to express their sincere gratitude to the obstetric gynecology department "D" at the Center de Maternité et de Néonatologie de Tunis (CMNT) for their support and assistance during the course of this study. Special thanks to Dr. Dalenda Chelli and the medical team for their invaluable insights and contributions.

Parts of this chapter were previously published in the doctoral thesis by the same author: Montacer Hafsi, Faculty of Medicine of Tunis, University Tunis El Manar. The author acknowledges the use of Grammarly AI for language polishing of the manuscript.

Conflict of interest

The authors declare no conflict of interest.

Notes

The authors extend their appreciation to all the healthcare professionals who participated in the data collection process and to the patients whose cooperation was essential for the completion of this study.

Author details

Montacer Hafsi*, Eya Kristou, Fathi Mraihi and Dalenda Chelli
Department D of Gynecology and Obstetrics, Maternity and Neonatology Center of Tunis, Tunisia

*Address all correspondence to: montacer.hafsi@etudiant-fmt.utm.tn

References

[1] Robinson D, Campbell K, Hobson SR, et al. Guideline no. 432b: Cervical ripening. Journal of Obstetrics and Gynaecology Canada. 2023;**45**(1):56-62

[2] National Institute for Health and Care Excellence. Inducing Labour: NICE Guidance. 2023. Available from: https://www.nice.org.uk/guidance/ng207/history

[3] Haute Autorité de Santé. Synthèses des recommandations professionnelles: Déclenchement artificiel du travail à partir de 37 semaines d'aménorrhée. Revue Sage Femme. 2009;**8**(1):14-18. Available from: https://www.sciencedirect.com/science/article/abs/pii/S1637408808002411

[4] Ducloy Bouthors AS, Keita Meyer H, Bouvet L, et al. Accouchement normal: Accompagnement de la physiologie et interventions médicales. Gynécologie Obstétrique Fertilité & Sénologie. 2020;**48**(12):891-906

[5] Dore S, Ehman W. No. 396: Intrapartum consensus guideline. Journal of Obstetrics and Gynaecology Canada. 2020;**42**(3):316-348

[6] Trabelsi H, Mathlouthi N, Zayen S, et al. Maturation cervicale à terme: Étude prospective randomisée: Misoprostol versus dinoprostone. La Tunisie Médicale. 2011;**90**(5):362-369

[7] American College of Obstetricians and Gynecologists. Obstetric care consensus no. 11: Pregnancy at age 35 years or older. Obstetrics and Gynecology. 2023;**141**(5):1030

[8] Ellis JA, Brown CM, Barger B, et al. Influence of maternal obesity on labor induction: A systematic review. Journal of Midwifery & Women's Health. 2019;**64**(1):55-67

[9] Rydahl E, Declercq E, Juhl M, et al. Cesarean section on the rise: Does advanced maternal age explain the increase? PLoS ONE. 2019;**14**(1)

[10] Roloff K, Peng S, Sanchez Ramos L, et al. Cumulative oxytocin dose during induction of labor according to maternal body mass index. International Journal of Gynaecology and Obstetrics. 2015;**131**(1):54-58

[11] Richards MK, Flanagan MR, Littman AJ, et al. Primary cesarean section and adverse delivery outcomes among women of very advanced maternal age. Journal of Perinatology. 2016;**36**(4):272-277

[12] Kehl S, Weiss C, Rath W. Balloon catheters for induction of labor at term after previous cesarean section: A systematic review. European Journal of Obstetrics, Gynecology, and Reproductive Biology. 2016;**204**:44-50

[13] Gilani S, Ain QT, Hanif M, Mazhar SB, Saeed N. Concurrent use of intracervical Foley's catheter plus vaginal misoprostol versus vaginal misoprostol alone for induction of labour. Journal of the Society of Obstetrics and Gynaecologists of Pakistan. 2018;**8**(3):184-190

[14] Leelarujijaroen C, Pruksanusak N, Geater A, et al. A predictive model for successfully inducing active labor among pregnant women: Combining cervical status and clinical characteristics. European Journal of Obstetrics & Gynecology and Reproductive Biology: X. 2023;**18**:100196

[15] Diaz Martinez A, Monfort Ortiz R, Ye Lin Y, Garcia Casado J, Nieto Tous M, Nieto Del Amor F, et al. Uterine

myoelectrical activity as biomarker of successful induction with dinoprostone: Influence of parity. Biocybernetics and Biomedical Engineering. 2023;**43**(1):142-156

[16] Batinelli L, Serafini A, Nante N, et al. Induction of labor: Clinical predictive factors for success and failure. Journal of Obstetrics and Gynaecology. 2018;**38**(3):352-358

[17] Aregeb ZA, Albromboly W, Abdelhameid AA, Helal KF, Badr MS. Induction of labor using vaginal misoprostol alone or combined with intracervical Foley catheter. Egyptian Journal of Hospital Medicine. 2021;**85**(1):3125-3129

[18] Priyadarshini A, Jaiswar SP, Singh A, Singh S. Comparative outcome of induced labor by intracervical Foley catheter with misoprostol versus misoprostol alone. Journal of Comparative Effectiveness Research. 2019;**8**(1):55-59

[19] Ellis JA, Brown CM, Barger B, Carlson NS. Influence of maternal obesity on labor induction: A systematic review and meta analysis. Journal of Midwifery & Women's Health. 2019;**64**(1):55-67

[20] Osoti A, Kibii DK, Tong TMK, et al. Effect of extra amniotic Foley's catheter and vaginal misoprostol versus vaginal misoprostol alone on cervical ripening and induction of labor in Kenya: A randomized controlled trial. BMC Pregnancy and Childbirth. 2018;**18**(1):300

[21] Ten Eikelder MLG, Neervoort F, Oude Rengerink K, Van Baaren GJ, Jozwiak M, De Leeuw JW, et al. Induction of labour with a Foley catheter or oral misoprostol at term: The PROBAAT-II study, a multicentre randomised controlled trial. BMC Pregnancy and Childbirth. 2013;**13**:67

[22] Ten Eikelder MLG, Oude Rengerink K, Jozwiak M, De Leeuw JW, De Graaf IM, Van Pampus MG, et al. Induction of labour at term with oral misoprostol versus a foley catheter (PROBAAT-II): A multicentre randomised controlled non inferiority trial. Lancet. 2016;**387**(10028):1619-1628

[23] Lanka S, Surapaneni T, Nirmalan PK. Concurrent use of foley catheter and misoprostol for induction of labor: A randomized clinical trial of efficacy and safety: Induction of labor. Journal of Obstetrics and Gynaecology Research. 2014;**40**(6):1527-1533

[24] Aduloju OP, Akintayo AA, Adanikin AI, et al. Combined Foley's catheter with vaginal misoprostol for pre-induction cervical ripening: A randomized controlled trial. The Australian & New Zealand Journal of Obstetrics & Gynaecology. 2016;**56**(6):578-584

[25] Levine LD, Downes KL, Elovitz MA, et al. Mechanical and pharmacologic methods of labor induction: A randomized controlled trial. Obstetrics and Gynecology. 2016;**128**(6):1357-1364

[26] Inamdar S, Toshniwal SM, Sharma SR. Foley's catheter and vaginal misoprostol vs vaginal misoprostol alone for labor induction. Journal of South Asian Federation of Obstetrics and Gynaecology [En ligne]; 14(4):7 p. Consultable à l'URL: https://www.jsafog.com/doi/10.5005/jp-journals-10006-2094 2022 [Consulté le 29 janvier 2023]

[27] Al-Ibraheemi Z, Brustman L, Bimson BE, et al. Misoprostol with Foley bulb compared with misoprostol alone for cervical ripening: A randomized

controlled trial. Obstetrics and Gynecology. 2018;**131**(1):23-29

[28] Carbone JF, Tuuli MG, Fogertey PJ, Roehl KA, Macones GA. Combination of Foley bulb and vaginal misoprostol compared with vaginal misoprostol alone for cervical ripening and labor induction: A randomized controlled trial. Obstetrics and Gynecology. 2013;**121**(2):247-252

Chapter 8

Efficacy and Safety of Metformin Use in Pregestational Insulin Resistance Pregnant Women and in Gestational Diabetes Mellitus in Perinatal Outcome: An Update

Enrique Valdés Rubio

Abstract

Insulin resistance (IR), before and during pregnancy, has long been studied as an etiological and pathophysiological factor in a series of high-risk perinatal pathologies. As a result of those above, the use of metformin (MET) in women with pregestational IR (PIR) or in pregnant women with gestational diabetes mellitus (GDM), before and during pregnancy, has become a prophylactic and therapeutic alternative for a series of pathologies despite not having solid evidence. This chapter aims to evaluate the impact of MET use in pregnant women with PIR and/or in patients with a diagnosis of GDM by evaluating the impact of the use of MET v/s insulin (INS) in high perinatal risk pathologies, for these purposes, an update of the impact of the use of MET during pregnancy was carried out based on an updated review of the literature that meets the highest standards advised by based medicine in the evidence. Thus, the beneficial effects and adverse side effects of the use of MET in the mother-child binomial will be discussed.

Keywords: gestational diabetes mellitus, insulin resistance, metformin, pregnancy, polycystic ovary syndrome

1. Introduction

Insulin resistance (IR) is defined as the decreased cellular response of insulin signaling. Its pathophysiological role is related to a variety of pathologies, such as diabetes mellitus Type 2, metabolic syndrome, polycystic ovary syndrome (PCOS), pre eclampsia (PE), and gestational diabetes mellitus (GDM) [1, 2].

In pregnancy, there are high levels of IR, with its peak being reached in the third trimester. The latter is based on the discovery that IR plays a physiological role that consists of the following: through insulin signaling, free fatty acids (FFA)

are mobilized. These are metabolized by the mother and like hyperglycemia, it is reflected in higher concentrations of glucose that is essential for fetal growth and development [3–5].

During the first trimester of pregnancy, there are a series of changes mediated by IR that are essential for guaranteeing adequate fetal development and growth. Thus, there are a series of hormones that promote and intensify IR such as placental lactogen (the most important in the first trimester), estrogens, progesterone, and cortisol [5]. Therefore, the pregnant woman undergoes a series of metabolic and physiological changes that ensure a euglycemic environment for the mother-child binome. Finally, FFAs are released in large quantities and encourage even higher levels of IR, stimulating a pro-IR mechanism, which creates a virtuous circle that ensures euglycemia for both the mother and the fetus [5, 6].

Higher degrees of insulin resistance and/or alteration in the concentration of its biomarkers (adiponectin [ApN], sex hormone binding globulin (SHBG), leptin, resistin) during pregnancy have been related to high perinatal risk pathologies (GDM, PE, small for gestational age [SGA], macrosomia, GDM, etc.) and therefore, this etiopathogenesis has been studied, obtaining increasingly evident yet controversial results [7–10].

On the other hand, metformin (MET) is a second-generation biguanide whose main action is to be an insulin-sensitizing drug. It improves the sensitivity of tissues to insulin, inhibits glucose synthesis by the liver, increases peripheral glucose consumption, and decreases the concentration of insulin. Its pharmacokinetics highlight that fetal exposure is low, with a placental partition quotient of 36.3% and cord blood concentrations of 0.1–2.9 mg/L during delivery. This, associated with the increase in renal clearance as the term of pregnancy approaches, makes it a safe drug. In fact, it has been classified by the FDA as risk B [11, 12]. MET has been widely studied in perinatology for its eventual benefit in pathologies that affect the mother-child binome. Thus, most of the research that has been carried out seeks to verify its efficacy and safety in the prevention and/or treatment of GDM and its eventual benefit in other pathologies such as PE, PEG, fetal growth restriction (FGR), macrosomia, cesarean section, and its possible early or late adverse effects in their offspring.

This study aims to evaluate the safety and efficacy of the use of MET in pregnant women with pregestational IR (PIR) and/or in those patients with a diagnosis of GDM.

2. Methods

A computerized search was performed in MEDLINE, PubMed, and Cochrane Library Database to identify those studies that presented the following inclusion criteria: Randomized Controlled Trials (RCT), Meta-Analyses, Systematic Reviews, and methodologically correct studies that met the best standards of Evidence-Based Medicine, from 2010 to 2024. These studies researched perinatal outcomes in women with a history of PIR who were treated prophylactically with MET, and/or in women with GDM. The objective of this chapter is to evaluate the safety and efficacy of the use of MET in pregnant women with PIR and/or in those patients with a diagnosis of GDM.

Sixty three articles dealing with this topic were studied, of which 18 met the inclusion criteria requirement.

3. Definitions

Insulin resistance is defined by the presence of any of the following criteria: HOMA test greater than 2.5 and at least one of the following clinical conditions: polycystic ovary syndrome (PCOS), acrochordon, and acanthosis. Parameters are suggested by the American Association of Clinical Endocrinologists and the American College of Endocrinologists [1, 2, 13, 14].

The diagnosis of GDM was defined according to the criteria of the International Association of Diabetes and Pregnancy Study Groups Recommendations on the Diagnosis and Classifications of Hyperglycemia in Pregnancy or any type of carbohydrate intolerance detected during pregnancy. This is diagnosed with a glucose tolerance test (OGTT), with a load of 75 grams, carried out between 24 and 26 weeks of gestation and in high-risk pregnant women at 32 weeks, with fasting blood glucose greater than 92 mg/dl, after 1 hour: 180 hour and after 2 hours: 153 mg/dl [14].

On the other hand, the diagnosis of PE was defined as the presence of arterial hypertension associated with proteinuria in a pregnancy greater than 20 weeks and which is associated with the following findings: blood pressure of 140/90 mmHg or more, repeated on two occasions separated by at least 6 hours, or a single blood pressure of 160/100 mmHg or more, associated with 24-hour proteinuria of 300 mg or more, in the absence of urinary tract infection [15].

Small for gestational age (SGA) was defined as a neonate with a weight less than the 10th percentile for their gestational age based on the local growth charts.

Large for gestational age (LGA) was defined as a neonate with a weight greater than the 90th percentile for its gestational age based on the local growth charts.

Macrosomia is defined as a newborn weighing 4000 grams or more.

The perinatal outcomes that were studied included: first trimester abortion, GDM, PE, fetal growth restriction (FGR), PB, maternal body mass index (BMI), newborn weight (NW), macrosomia, cesarean section (CS), maternal and neonatal hypoglycemia and admission to the intensive care unit (NICU).

4. Outcomes

4.1 Metformin in the prevention of GDM in patients with pregestational insulin resistance (PIR)

There is only one single randomized, double-blind, multicenter study that evaluated the impact of the use of MET in pregnant women with PIR as a risk factor for developing GDM, PE, and SGA [16].

In this study, it was not demonstrated that MET significantly reduced GDM (16/63–25.4) v/s (18.48–37.5) p 0.17, PE (3/57, 5.3) v/s (4/40, 10) (p 0.38) in placebo and MET, respectively. On the other hand, there were no significant differences in FGR (4/58–6.9) v/s (2/434.65) (p 0.6), premature birth, CS, macrosomia, and newborn weight. In this last variable, the group treated with MET had clearly thinner neonates, but the newborn's weight percentile was not significant (57.1 v/s 47.2; p 0.5.) [16].

In this sense, it is important to highlight that all the studies that have been published have evaluated the prophylactic effect of MET on the development of GDM, PB, PE, GRF, and other perinatal pathologies in PCOS patients, but it must be kept in mind that IR It is not always present in this syndrome, being observed in 80% of obese PCOS women and between 30 and 40% of lean women [17–19], therefore there is a bias in the interpretation of the results, since MET is an insulin-sensitizing drug.

4.2 Metformin v/s insulin in patients with GDM

There is evidence that patients with GDM who use MET demonstrate that its effectiveness in maintaining euglycemia is equivalent to and even greater than INS during pregnancy. However, a significant percentage of patients treated with MET were unable to avoid hyperglycemia and had to associate it with INS in order to achieve metabolic goals.

Thus, in the first and most important study published in the New England Journal of Medicine (MiG) [20] in 2008, it was found that 46% of patients treated with MET had to be supplemented with INS. Pregnant women who required supplementation had higher BMI ($p = 0.01$), high fasting blood glucose values ($p = 0.001$), a history of spontaneous abortions ($p = 0.001$), and higher levels of glycosylated hemoglobin ($p = 0.001$) [20]. In subsequent studies, it was necessary to prescribe this supplementation for 20.9–22.94% of pregnant women with GDM. It was identified that the patients who had the lowest risk of combined treatment were those who had a fasting blood glucose level of less than 90 mg/dl [20]. These contradictory results are due to the fact that studies evaluating the effectiveness of MET use a variety of methods to assess blood glucose levels, such as glycosylated hemoglobin and postprandial and fasting blood glucose. However, there is no definition of the ranges that are used to define normality, so the ranges of fasting blood glucose vary between 100 and 110 mg/dl and postprandial blood glucose ranges vary according to the consensus of expert opinions [21] Another very different reality is what is observed in pregnant women with pregestational diabetes (Type 2 DM) where 84.9% of women treated with MET needed supplementation with INS to achieve metabolic objectives [22].

MET (MIG) managed to maintain a postprandial euglycemic profile associated with the consumption of certain foods, fewer episodes of hypoglycemia, less weight gain during pregnancy, lower NB weight, and a lower amount of CS. In those who did not achieve the metabolic objectives, MET succeeded in postponing the indication for insulin therapy, requiring lower doses of this to achieve euglycemia and better adherence to treatment, despite the fact that gastrointestinal intolerance was one of the adverse effects of MET [20]. All the other results of maternal-fetal pathologies did not have a significant difference between the two groups, except in pregnant women with PCOS treated with MET who had a lower rate of spontaneous abortions [20].

On the other hand, the most important evidence that confirms the safety and effectiveness of the use of MET in patients with GDM is a systematic review and meta-analysis of 24 studies that highlight that MET users presented a lower risk of pregnancy-induced hypertension ($p = 0.03$), LGA RN ($p = 0.04$), macrosomia ($p = 0.01$), neonatal hypoglycemia ($p = 0.001$), and NICU admission ($p = 0.01$) [21].

4.3 Effect of MET on neonatal hypoglycemia

Several studies have concluded that MET reduces the risk of neonatal hypoglycemia [19, 20–22, 23] although there are studies that refute this conclusion. What is true is that the ranges to define hypoglycemia are varied and therefore the conclusions vary between studies. On the other hand, it is noteworthy that the incidence of hypoglycemia is greater when MET is associated with INS (MET + INS) 7.8%, INS alone

(30%, p 0.001) [23]. The MiTy study concluded that the neonatal hypoglycemias were similar between the INS + MET group v/s INS + placebo [24].

4.4 Impact of metformin on obesity

Maternal weight gain during pregnancy was lower in the MET group (GDM and PCOS), varying between 0.47 and 1.8 kg, and adherence to treatment was higher in this group. The weight of the newborn was lower in the MET group although not low enough to diagnose FGR, and there is some evidence that preterm birth increases in this group. Obese pregnant women (BMI > 30 kg/m^2) who received MET decreased the incidence of late PE [25]. On the other hand, FGR, macrosomia, cesarean operation, respiratory distress, and ICU admission were similar in both groups.

Finally, a recent RCT study (EMPOWar) evaluated the potential prophylactic effect of MET in obese women (BMI = 30–39 KG/Mtr2 v/s BMI > 40 KG/Mtr2), to prevent high-risk perinatal pathologies, a population in which PIR does not always exist and who did not have Type 2 DM at the time of recruitment. Various biomedical variables were analyzed in the mother and fetus and in all the variables that were studied, no significant difference was found between the MET group and the placebo. The authors conclude that MET is not indicated in obese patients who do not present GDM [26].

4.5 Impact of MET in pregnancy-induced hypertension

Severe insulin resistance and/or its biomarkers (adiponectin, leptin, resistin, and SHBG) during pregnancy have been related to high-risk perinatal pathologies such as PE, a conclusion supported by a meta-analysis based on a small number of publications, which studied the impact of the use of MET in patients with MDG or obesity, concluding that MET could have some effect in reducing hypertensive disorders in patients with GDM, based on the following results: in women with gestational diabetes, metformin use was associated with a reduced risk of pregnancy-induced hypertension when compared with insulin (relative risk [RR], 0.56; 95% CI, 0.37–0.85; $I^2 = 0\%$) and a non-significantly reduced risk of pre-eclampsia (RR, 0.83; 95% CI, 0.60–1.14; $I^2 = 0\%$). In obese women, when compared with placebo, metformin use was associated with a non-significant reduction in risk of pre-eclampsia (RR, 0.74; 95% CI, 0.09–6.28; $I^2 = 86\%$) [27].

Thus, these biomarkers have been studied and increasingly evident controversial results have been obtained.

In the case of adiponectin (ApN), a protein synthesized by adipose tissue, it has been related as a predictor of PE and FGR. PE shares a pathophysiology with IR, since both present endothelial dysfunction, atherosclerosis, and systemic inflammation. Studies supported the fact that maternal serum ApN levels in the first trimester were a predictor of PE and FGR. Other studies evaluating the behavior of ApN concentration in the first trimester did not confirm this finding. However, when ApN concentration was adjusted with BMI, this association was significant as a predictor in the first trimester of FGR [8]. On the other hand, although PIR was related to PE, chronic arterial hypertension, advanced maternal age, and excessive increase in BMI are the variables that significantly proved to be better predictors of PE [8–10].

4.6 Effect of metformin on the incidence of preterm birth

Several studies concluded that the use of MET in patients with GDM had a higher incidence of preterm births compared to the control group, but there are meta-analyses that demonstrate that pregnant women treated with MET did not present significant differences with the control group. Balsells commented that although it is true that in patients treated with MET the effect of prematurity was small (−0.16 weeks), he agreed that PB would increase by 50% (RR 1.50, 95% CCI 1.04ª 2.16, P = 0,03. N 1299 0,51 A 1.50: P = 0.71) [28]. Another study, compared MET with a placebo in patients with PCOS; in this population, there were no significant differences with the control group. Moreover, performed a meta-analysis with the data from this study and concluded that the incidence of PB was lower in the MET group (OR 0.37, 95% CI 0.20–0.68; $p = 0.002$) [29]. A cohort study examined the effects of MET on GDM, Type 2 DM, and PCOS and concluded that pregnant women who received the combination of MET + INS had significantly higher PB. Patients who received only monotherapy (MET or INS) had a similar rate of premature births [25].

Finally, in the study, MiG found that the MET group had a higher incidence of PB (12.1 v/s 7.6%; $p = 0.04$) [20].

4.7 Impact of MET on newborn weight

A meta-analysis compared the birth weight between those patients treated with MET v/s INS and concluded that those with GDM treated with MET had lower weight than the INS users with an average difference of 114.48 (95% CI 37.32–191.64; $p < 0.01$) and 107.69 (95% 182.70–32.68; $p = 0.005$), respectively. In addition, in this study a lower incidence of macrosomia was observed [30].

The MiTy study, It should be taken into account that the effectiveness of MET v/s INS was carried out in pregnant women with Type 2 diabetes mellitus, therefore its results are not comparable with the results obtained in studies where MET v/s INS were performed in GDM reported a decrease in newborn weight, a higher incidence of SGA and a decrease in macrosomia in the group treated with MET + INS v/s INS + placebo ($p = 0.0016$ and $p = 0.026$, $p = 0.046$, respectively). On the other hand, there were no significant differences in LGA between both groups. Finally, this study demonstrated a higher incidence of SGA in patients treated with MET and when this was associated with INS, the risk of presenting LGA significantly increased [24].

4.8 Incidence of cesarean section in pregnant MET users

It is known that GDM patients with poor metabolic control have a high risk of cesarean section [31–33]. Later, studies demonstrated that patients who used MET had a lower incidence of cesarean section. The best evidence was provided by the MiTy study which concluded that pregnant women with a history of Type 2 DM had a lower incidence of cesarean section in those patients treated with MET plus INS v/s INS plus placebo (RR 0.85, 95% CI 0.73–0.99; $p = 0.031$) [24]. Finally, another study that included pregnant women with pregestational Type 2 DM had a lower incidence of cesarean section compared to those who were treated with MEt alone or INS alone (52.2, 81.2, and 82%, respectively; $p < 0.01$) [32].

4.9 Adverse effects in fetuses exposed to metformin

The plasma concentrations of MET in the fetus are similar to those observed in the mother.

No malformations were found and among the early and late effects in the offspring exposed to MET during pregnancy, a possible alteration in fetal programming stands out, causing a greater predisposition to obesity during adolescence and metabolic syndrome in adulthood [34].

In a study in which PCOS pregnant women were treated with MET during pregnancy, the follow-up of the exposed children presented higher fasting blood glucose and systolic blood pressure at 8 years of age [34].

Finally, a study that studied children exposed to MET v/s INS concluded that, although weights were similar until 2 years of age, at 9 years of age BMI was significantly higher in children exposed to MET (MD 0.98.95%; CI 0.23–1.33; p 0.005) [35].

However, a recent systematic review and meta-analysis study evaluated the impact of MET on the neurodevelopment of 7641 children up to 14 years of age, obtaining the following results: metformin use during pregnancy was not associated with neurodevelopmental delay in infancy (relative risk, 1.09; 95% confidence interval, 0.54e2.17; 3 studies; 9668 children) or at ages 3–5 years (relative risk, 0.90; 95% confidence interval, 0.56e1.45; 2 studies; 6118 children). When compared with unexposed peers, metformin use during pregnancy was not associated with altered motor scores (mean difference, 0.30; 95% confidence interval, _1.15 to 1.74; 3 studies; 714 children) or cognitive scores (mean difference, _0.45; 95% confidence interval, _1.45 to 0.55; 4 studies; 734 children), concluding that apparently MET would not affect neurodevelopment in children up to 14 years of age [36].

5. Conclusions

The only RCT that sought to evaluate the impact of MET during pregnancy in PIR pregnant women concluded that MET was not effective in preventing GDM, PE, FGR, premature birth, or macrosomia. On the other hand, comparative studies carried out on pregnant women with GDM, between those treated with MET v/s INS concluded, despite being controversial, that patients with GDM treated with MET presented better metabolic behavior, less maternal weight gain during pregnancy, lower weight of the NB, and higher incidence of premature births. Postprandial glycemia associated with the consumption of certain foods, MET caused fewer episodes of hypoglycemia, less weight gain during pregnancy, and lower weight of the newborn. For those who did not achieve metabolic objectives, MET was able to postpone the indication for insulin therapy, requiring lower doses to achieve euglycemia [21]. Pregnant women had better adherence to treatment, despite the fact that gastrointestinal intolerance was among the adverse effects of MET. All the other results of maternal-fetal pathologies did not have a significant difference between the two groups, except in PCOS pregnant women treated with MET who presented a lower rate of spontaneous abortions and a lower incidence of late PE in obese pregnant women with a body mass index (BMI > 30) Kg/m^2 [24]. Finally, plasma concentrations of MET in the fetus are similar to that of the mother. Pregnancy, an eventual alteration of fetal programming is noteworthy causing a greater predisposition to obesity in adolescence, metabolic syndrome in adulthood, higher 11 > fasting blood glucose and systolic blood pressure in later ages.

Finally, there is a series of maternal antecedents that predict the failure of MET to achieve the metabolic objectives of the GDM and the need to supplement therapy with INS among others; advanced maternal age, obesity, history of GDM, and higher fasting blood glucose levels [37–41].

Solid evidence of the effectiveness and safety of MET during pregnancy is still lacking. On the other hand, there is evidence that exposure to MET in the fetus produces early and late adverse effects in the offspring. It is necessary to continue studying the intrauterine effects before recommending it as a first-line treatment for the treatment of GDM. On the other hand, the dosage of MET has not been established, since it must necessarily be adjusted to an increasing IR as the pregnancy progresses. Finally, MET could only be used in the first semester to avoid spontaneous abortion in PCOS and apparently could be in GDM and in obese pregnant women (BMI >30 kg/m^2) to avoid late-onset PE. On the other hand, there is evidence that in Type 2 diabetes mellitus, the use of MET has a high failure rate. The author has the opinion that this should be combined with insulin therapy, since in early pregnancies, it is necessary to achieve euglycemia quickly to avoid deleterious effects on the embryo and fetus because the effect of MET could take days to achieve the expected effect.

Author contributions

The design, bibliographic search, review, study, interpretation of data, writing, editing and approval of the manuscript fell on the sole author.

Funding sources

This study was not supported by any sponsor or funder.

Conflict of interest

The author has no conflicts of interest to declare.
There are no ethical implications in this study.

Author details

Enrique Valdés Rubio
Department of Obstetrics and Gynecology, Maternal—Fetal Unit, University of Chile, Clinical Hospital, Santiago, Chile

*Address all correspondence to: e.valdes.r63@gmail.com; evaldesr@docente.uss.cl

References

[1] Matthews DR, Hosker JP, Rudenski AS, Naylor BA, Treacher DF, Turner RC. Homeostasis model assessment: Insulin resistance and beta-cell function from fasting plasma glucose and insulin concentrations in man. Diabetologia. 1985;**28**:412-419

[2] Einhorn: American College of Endocrinology Position Statement on the insulin resistance syndrome. Endocrine Practice. 2003;**9**:237-252

[3] Sonagra AD, Biradar SM, Murthy DSJ. Normal pregnancy- a state of insulin resistance. Journal of Clinical and Diagnostic Research. 2014;**8**(11):CC01-CCC3

[4] Tumurbaatar B, Poole AT, Olson G, et al. Adipose tissue insulin resistance in gestational diabetes. Metabolic Syndrome and Related Disorders. 2017;**15**(2):86-92

[5] Moyce B, Dolinsky V. Maternal β-cell adaptations in pregnancy and placental signalling: Implications for gestational diabetes. International Journal of Molecular Sciences. 2018;**19**(11):3467

[6] Plows JF, Stanley JL, Baker PN, Reynolds CM, Vickers MH. The pathophysiology of gestational diabetes mellitus. International Journal of Molecular Sciences. 2018;**19**(11):3342

[7] D'Anna R, Baviera G, Corrado F, Giordano D, De Vivo A, Nicocia G, et al. Adiponectin and insulin resistance in early- and late-onset pre-eclampsia. BJOG. 2006;**113**:1264-1269

[8] Valdés ER, Lattes KA, Muñoz HS, Barja PY, Papapietro KV. First-trimester adiponectin and subsequent development of preeclampsia or fetal growth restriction. Gynecologic and Obstetric Investigation. 2011;**72**:152-156

[9] Valdés ER, Lattes KA, Muñoz HS, Cumsille M. Sex-hormone binding globulin (SHBG) levels dung pregnancy as predictors for pre-eclampsia and fetal growth restriction. Revista Médica de Chile. 2012;**140**:589-594

[10] Valdés E, Sepúlveda-Martínez A, Manukian B, Parra-Cordero M. Assessment of pregestational insulin resistance as a risk factor of preeclampsia. Gynecologic and Obstetric Investigation. 2014;**77**:111-116

[11] Miranda P, Javier P, Palacios T, Patricia L, Cueva C, Luis J, et al. Evelin Marcela Rol de la metformina en el tratamiento de la diabetes mellitus gestacional: situación actual. Archivos Venezolanos de Farmacología y Terapéutica. 2019;**38**(2)

[12] Valdés RE, Soto-Chacón E, Lahsen MR, Barrera HC, Candia PP. Effectiveness of oral hypoglycemic drugs in the metabolic control of patients with gestational diabetes. Revista Médica de Chile. 2008;**136**:915-920

[13] Zavaroni I, Bonini L, Gasparini P, et al. Hyperinsulinemia in a normal population as a predictor of non-insulin-dependent diabetes mellitus, hypertension, and coronary heart disease: The barilla factory revisited. Metabolism. 1999;**48**:989-994

[14] International Association of Diabetes and Pregnancy Study Groups Consensus Panel, Metzger BE, Gabbe SG, et al. Inter- national Association of Diabetes and Pregnancy Study Groups recommendations on the diagnosis and classification of hyperglycemia in pregnancy. Diabetes Care. 2010;**33**:676-682

[15] Brown MA, Lindheimer MD, de Swiet M, Van Assche A. Hypertensive disorders of pregnancy: Statement from the International Society for the Study of hypertension in pregnancy (ISSHP). Hypertension in Pregnancy. 2001;**20**:IXIV

[16] Valdés E, Sepúlveda-Martínez A, Candia P, Abusada N, Orellana R, Manukian B, et al. Metformin as a prophylactic treatment of gestational diabetes in pregnant patients with pregestational insulin resistance: A randomized study. The Journal of Obstetrics and Gynaecology Research. 2018;**44**(1):81-86

[17] Dumesic DA, Oberfield SE, Stener-Victorin E, Marshall JC, Laven JS, Legro RS. Scientific statement on the diagnostic criteria, epidemiology, pathophysiology, and molecular genetics of polycystic ovary syndrome. Endocrine Reviews. 2015;**36**:487-525

[18] Azziz R, Carmina E, Chen Z, Dunaif A, Laven JSE, Legro RS, et al. Polycystic ovary syndrome. Nature Reviews Disease Primers. 2016;**2**:16057

[19] Paschou SA, Shalit A, Gerontiti E, Athanasiadou KI, Kalampokas T, Psaltopoulou T, et al. Efficacy and safety of metformin during pregnancy: An update. Endocrine. 2024;**83**:259-269

[20] Rowan JA, Hague WM, Gao W, Battin MR, Moore MP. Metformin versus insulin for the treatment of gestational diabetes. (MIG). The New England Journal of Medicine. 2008;**358**(19):2003-2015. DOI: 10.1056/NEJMoa0707193

[21] Bao LX, Shi WT, Han YX. Metformin versus insulin for gestational diabetes: A systematic review and meta-analysis. Journal of Maternal-Fetal and Neonatal Medicine. 2021;**16**:2741-53n 8, 834-44 (2020). DOI: 10.1016/S2213-8587(20)30310-70000004526

[22] Ainuddin N, Karim S, Zaheer S, Sanwer Ali A, Ara Hasan. Metformin Treatment in Type 2 Diabetes in Pregnancy: An Active Controlled, Parallel-Group, Randomized, Open Label Study in Patients with Type 2 Diabetes in Pregnancy. 2015. 10.1155/2015/325851

[23] Guo L, Ma J, Tang J, Hu D, Zhang W, Zhao X. Comparative efficacy and safety of metformin, glyburide, and insulin in treating gestational diabetes mellitus: A meta-analysis. Journal Diabetes Research. 2019;**2019**(9084708). DOI: 10.1155/2019/9804708

[24] Feig DS, Donovan LE, Zinman B, Sanchez JJ, Asztalos E, Ryan EA, et al. Metformin in women with type 2 diabetes in pregnancy (MiTy): A multicentre, international, randomised, placebo-controlled trial. BMC Pregnancy and Childbirth. Oct 2020

[25] Tosti G, Barberio A, Tartaglione L, Rizzi A, Di Leo M, Viti L, et al. Lights and shadows on the use of metformin in pregnancy: From the preconception phase to breastfeeding and beyond. Frontiers in Endocrinology. 2023;**14**. DOI: 10.3389/fendo.2023.1270472

[26] Chiswick C, Reynolds RM, Denison F, Drake AJ, Forbes S, Newby DE, et al. Effect of metformin on maternal and fetal outcomes in obese pregnant women (EMPOWaR): A randomised, double-blind, placebo-controlled trial. The Lancet Diabetes and Endocrinology. 2015;**10**:2015. DOI: 10.1016/S2213-8587(15)00219-3

[27] Kalafat E, Sukur Y, Thilaganathan B, Khalil. Metformin for prevention of hypertensive disorders of pregnancy in women with gestational diabetes or obesity: Systematic review and

meta-analysis of randomized trials. Ultrasound in Obstetrics and Gynecology. 2018;**52**:706-714

[28] Balsells M, García-Patterson A, Solà I, Roqué M, Gich I, Corcoy R. Glibenclamide, metformin, and insulin for the treatment of gestational diabetes: A systematic review and meta-analysis. BMJ. 2015;**350**. DOI: 10.1136/BMJ.H102

[29] Zeng X-L, Zhang Y-F, Tian Q, Xue Y, An R-F. Effects of metformin on pregnancy outcomes in women with polycystic ovary syndrome a meta-analysis. Medicine. 2016;**95**. DOI: 10.1097/MD.000000

[30] Tarry-Adkins L, Aiken CE, Ozanne SE. Neonatal, infant, and childhood growth following metformin versus insulin treatment for gestational diabetes: A systematic review and meta-analysis. PLoS Medicine. 2019;**16**. DOI: 10.1371/JOURNAL.PMED.1002848

[31] Gorgal R, Gonçalves E, Barros M, Namora G, Magalhães Â, Rodrigues T, et al. Gestational diabetes mellitus: A risk factor for non-elective cesarean section. The Journal of Obstetrics and Gynaecology Research. 2012;**38**:154-159. DOI: 10.1111/J.1447-0756.2011.01659.X

[32] Waiyanikorn R. Emergency cesarean section rate between women with gestational diabetes and normal pregnant women. Taiwanese Journal of Obstetrics and Gynecology. 2016;**55**:64-67. DOI: 10.1016/J.TJOG.2015.08.024

[33] Ehrenberg HM, Durnwald CP, Catalano P, Mercer BM. The influence of obesity and diabetes on the risk of cesarean delivery. American Journal of Obstetrics and Gynecology. 2004;**191**:969-974. DOI: 10.1016/J.AJOG.2004.06.057

[34] Rø TB, Ludvigsen HV, Carlsen SM, Vanky E. Growth, body composition and metabolic profile of 8-year-old children exposed to metformin in utero. Scandinavian Journal of Clinical and Laboratory Investigation.

[35] Brand KMG, Saarelainen L, Sonajalg J, Boutmy E, Foch C, Vääräsmäki M, et al. Metformin in pregnancy and risk of adverse long-term outcomes: A register-based cohort study. BMJ Open Diabetes Research and Care. 2022;**10**:2363. DOI: 10.1136/BMJDRC-2021-002363

[36] Gordon HG, Atkinson JA, Tong S, Mehdipour P, Cluver C, Walker SP, et al. Metformin in pregnancy and childhood neurodevelopmental outcomes: A systematic review and meta-analysis. American Journal of Obstetrics and Gynecology. 2024;**231**:308-314

[37] Tertti K, Ekblad U, Koshinen P, Vahlberg T, Ronnemaa T. Metformin vs. insulin in gestational diabetes. A randomized study characterizing metformin patients needing additional insulin. Diabetes, Obesity and Metabolism. 2013;**15**(3):246-251

[38] Wong VW, Jalaludin B. Gestational diabetes mellitus: Who requires insulin therapy? Australian and New Zealand Journal of Obstetrics and Gynaecology. 2011;**51**(5):432-436

[39] Gante I, Melo L, Dores J, Ruas L, Almeida MDC. Metformin in gestational diabetes mellitus: Predictors of poor response. European Journal of Endocrinology. 2018;**178**(1):129-135

[40] Spaulonci CP, Bernardes LS, Trindade TC, Zugain M, Francisco RP. Randomized trial of metformin vs insulin in the management of gestational diabetes. American

Journal of Obstetrics and Gynecology. 2013;**209**(1):34.e1-7

[41] Ashoush S, El-Said M, Fathi H, Abdelnaby M. Identification of metformin poor responders, requiring supplemental insulin, during randomization of metformin versus insulin for the control of gestational diabetes mellitus. The Journal of Obstetrics and Gynaecology Research. 2016;**42**(6):640-647

Section 3

Gynecological Cancer

Chapter 9

Management of Cervical Cancer and Human Papillomavirus in Pregnancy

María Fernanda Calderón León, María Eugenia Ugarte Vega, Germania Elizabeth Yugcha Andino, Paula Andrea Vásquez Jaramillo, Germán Arturo Vélez Sáenz, Joel Paul Vargas Caicedo, Moraima Elizabeth Pazmiño Iñiga, Alfredo Guillermo Chong Viteri, Angélica María Apolo Montero and Nataly del Carmen Quisiguiña Jarrín

Abstract

Cervical cancer during pregnancy is the most commonly detected malignant tumor. It has become a public health problem, 99% related to human papillomavirus (HPV) infection, making it the only gynecological malignant tumor of clear etiology in the world. It is diagnosed at any stage of pregnancy. Its initial presentation is observed as transvaginal bleeding in all three trimesters associated with HPV infection. If the metastasis is negative in the lymph nodes, it improves. At an early stage the prognosis is favorable, management consists of preserving pregnancy, neoadjuvant chemotherapy can be used to treat cervical cancer in pregnancy, in cases of viable pregnancies between 27- and 31-weeks' gestation chemotherapy may be performed depending on the staging, caesarean section at 35 weeks, radical surgery and systemic chemotherapy may achieve good results depending on the stage of the tumor.

Keywords: cervical cancer, squamous intraepithelial lesions of the cervix, cancer screening, human papillomavirus (HPV), treatment, pregnancy

1. Introduction

Cervical cancer is a highly preventable and curable pathology, if diagnosed and treated in a timely manner, ranking as the third most common cancer in women worldwide and the second most common cancer in developing countries, where more than 85% of deaths from this cause occur. Considering that it is necessary to employ prevention strategies, since it has become a public health problem, 99% related to infection by the human papillomavirus (HPV), making it the only gynecological malignant tumor of clear etiology in the world. In addition, recent studies have established an association between vaginal microbiota composition, HPV infection, and progression to cervical dysplasia and cancer [1–4].

Cervical cancer is a gynecological malignancy that is most frequently diagnosed during pregnancy, being a major challenge for women and medical specialists to make the right decisions about the therapy for the women to receive during the gestation period, which must be individualized [5]. The biomolecular test of the human papillomavirus can detect 30–100% more cancer precursors than conventional cytology and 20–50% more than cytology in liquid medium, taking into account that a woman with a positive HPV test must be studied carefully because she may have a high-grade cervical intraepithelial neoplasm or cancer, despite having a colposcopy with minimal alterations. It should be noted that a good sample for cervical cytology is also a good sample for DNA testing for human papillomavirus [6].

The polymerase chain reaction (PCR) test is used to detect HPV DNA in various forms, with a predictive value greater than 99%, being a prevalent virus in the young and sexually active population with an incidence of up to 20%, where screening should be suggested from the age of 25, the virus generates a transient infection with a duration of 8 months in low-risk HPV cases. From 10 to 40 years later, the HPV screening test continues to increase, being part of the usual control, in Europe and other countries it is used less frequently, the objective is to perform this test as routine and that it is part of the gynecological control, but there are socioeconomic factors that need to improve so that the entire population has access to these tests [7].

Genetic and molecular advances consist of new screening strategies, such as DNA methylation, to locate high-grade epithelial lesions in HPV-positive women. Detection of long non-coding RNA (lncRNA), which functions as a tumor biomarker for the diagnosis and prognosis of patients, plays an important role in the regulation of gene expression at various levels. Cuproptosis plays a role in tumorigenesis and cancer progression, in addition to the development of other biomarkers such as programmed cell death ligand 1 (PD-L1), which predict cervical cancer outcomes, risk of recurrence, and assessment of response to immunotherapy (**Table 1**) [13–15].

Cervical cancer accounts for 8.7% of all cancers diagnosed during pregnancy, treatment is complicated by pathophysiological changes in the relationship between the reproductive organs and the developing fetus, so relevant aspects such as termination of pregnancy are treated to administer treatment. The administration of chemotherapy treatment will depend on the stage of the cancer, fetal viability by weeks of gestation at the time of diagnosis [16].

The International Federation of Gynecology and Obstetrics (FIGO) staging of cervical cancer patients is based on clinical examination, imaging, and potential surgical findings [17]. Cervical cancer is directly related to carcinogenesis and its treatment in pregnancy is of great importance [18].

The stage of cervical cancer in pregnancy is essential to determine individual management (**Table 2**) [23].

- Stage I: the cancer is found only in the cervix. It is divided into two sub classifications.
    - IA1: the tumor has spread to a depth of 3 mm or less into the tissues of the cervix.
    - IA2: the tumor has spread to a depth of more than 3 mm, but not more than 5 mm into the tissues of the cervix.

Carcinogenesis	New findings
Long non-coding RNA (lncRNA)	The identification of lncRNA is involved with cuproptosis and the pathogenesis of chemotherapy resistance, both cuproptosis and chemotherapy resistance play a role in carcinogenesis and progression. Non-coding RNAs (ncRNAs) are closely related to cancer initiation and development due to their critical role in gene expression and epigenetic modulation.
Oncoproteins	The oncogenic potential of HPV depends on the oncoproteins E6 and E7 that are expressed in cells infected by the virus and alter the cell cycle. They are considered usable biomarkers in the treatment of women with positive results, and these proteins disrupt the cell cycle
DNA methylation	It is an epigenetic process that adds a methyl group to the DNA, regulates the expression of genes, in the face of a genetic modification during its division, methylation modifies the function of DNA and acts as a regulator of gene transcription, and it allows us to know which cells present molecular changes to develop cervical cancer
Checkpoint inhibitors	Third-line treatment in metastatic cervical cancer with programmed death protein 1 (PD-1) blockade.
Differentially expressed genes	A prognostic model of risk for cervical cancer based on differentially expressed genes that are driven by histocompatibility locus antigen complex, class I, G (human) (HLA-G), and this showed a great ability to predict the overall survival of patients with cervical cancer.
Elaboration: Dr. María Fernanda Calderón León.	

Table 1.
Genetic and molecular advances in cervical cancer identified in HPV-associated cervical cancer [8–12].

- IB stage:
    - IB1: the tumor is 2 cm or smaller and has spread more than 5 mm deep.
    - IB2: the tumor is larger than 2 cm, but not larger than 4 cm.
    - IB3: the tumor is larger than 4 cm.
- Stage II: the tumor has spread from the uterus to the stroma of the cervix, but not to other parts of the body.
- Stage III: cancer has spread beyond the cervix and upper vagina, but not to the pelvic wall or lower vagina.
- Stage IV: cancer has spread to the pelvic wall, lower vagina, bladder, or rectum, or affected distant organs such as the lungs or liver.

Cervical cancer has three stages, the early stage has a survival rate of 92.5–93.1%, so it is vitally important to screen, detect, and treat it early [24, 25], cervical cancer, in the locally advanced stage, accounts for about 37% of cervical cancers, the median survival for this type is 15.5 months [26, 27]. In advanced, recurrent, or metastatic cervical cancer, the overall survival at 3 years is only 33% [28].

In a review of 14 pregnancies, the use of paclitaxel combined with cisplatin resulted in the birth of 14 live births, without miscarriages, with a complete response

Author	Manipulation	Results	Staging malignant tumors	Gestational age and recommendations
Beharee et al. [20]	Conization of the cervix	Conization is an appropriate and relatively safe treatment for cervical cancer patients	Treatment of stage I A1 cervical cancer	22–25 weeks pregnant
	Let the pregnancy progress and postpone treatment, until fetal maturity is reached.	When the lymph nodes are not involved and the diameter of the tumor is less than 2 cm	I A2–I B1	Before 22–25 weeks gestation
	Termination of pregnancy is recommended	Patients with lymph node involvement and a tumor diameter of less than 2 cm	I A2–I B1	Before 22–25 weeks gestation
	If the lymph node is negative or the patient has a strong desire to continue pregnancy, neoadjuvant chemotherapy may be used, until the fetus matures and is born.	The diameter of the tumor is greater than 2 cm, if the lymph node is positive, termination of pregnancy is recommended	Stage I B1	Before 22–25 weeks gestation
	Adjuvant chemotherapy to stabilize the tumor, prevent tumor progression and spread.	Adjuvant chemotherapy may be used at this stage, until fetal maturity is reached	I B2	Older than 22–25 weeks gestation
Rouen [22]	Treatment may be postponed between 20 and 33 weeks of pregnancy, until a cesarean section is performed to promote lung maturation of the fetus. The initial treatment time of delayed treatment should not exceed 32–34 weeks of pregnancy, and the pregnancy may be terminated after fetal lung maturation	Neoadjuvant chemotherapy may be used, until fetal maturity is reached.	FIGO 2018 IB1 or IIA	For patients with 14 ~ 20 weeks of pregnancy
Hammer et al. [21]	If indicated, definitive surgery is performed during the same period, delivery is performed by cesarean section	The tumor may block the birth canal. The placenta is sent for histological examination to rule out metastasis.	Women who have not received treatment.	Vaginal delivery is not chosen, as there is an increased risk of damage to the tumor, a high risk of bleeding, and a risk of spreading malignant cells

Author	Manipulation	Results	Staging malignant tumors	Gestational age and recommendations
Teoh et al. [19]	In the absence of clinical or histological suspicion of invasive cancer, excision procedures during pregnancy are not recommended.	Colposcopy is recommended skipping endocervical sampling every trimester, and an excision procedure is performed after delivery.	Cervical adenocarcinoma *in situ* (AIS).	Conization, usually for the evaluation of biopsy-diagnosed AIS, is not recommended during pregnancy unless invasive cancer is suspected.

Elaboration: Dr. María Fernanda Calderón León.

Table 2.
Management of cervical cancer in pregnancy according to gestational age, clinical stage of cancer [19–22].

to treatment in 7.2% and a partial response in 92.9% of pregnant women with cervical cancer. Taxane treatment after the first trimester of pregnancy demonstrated obstetric and fetal outcomes that enable the treatment of cervical cancer during pregnancy [29, 30].

The goal of the chapter is to understand how to stage and treat cervical cancer during pregnancy.

2. Genetic and molecular advances in the field of cervical cancer identified in HPV-associated cervical cancer

The main advances are genetic and molecular in cervical cancer associated with the human papillomavirus [8–12].

Table 1 describes the genetic and molecular mechanisms associated with carcinogenesis caused by human papillomavirus in the cervix. Genetic and molecular advances consist of new screening strategies, such as DNA methylation, to locate high-grade epithelial lesions in high-risk HPV-positive women. Detection of long non-coding RNA (lncRNA), which functions as a tumor biomarker for patient diagnosis and prognosis, plays an important role in the regulation of gene expression at various levels. Cuproptosis plays a role in tumorigenesis and cancer progression, in addition to the development of other biomarkers such as programmed cell death ligand 1 (PD-L1), which predicts cervical cancer outcomes, risk of recurrence, and assessment of response to immunotherapy.

3. Management of tumor staging according to gestational age and current recommendations

Current strategies have made it possible to provide treatment during pregnancy in some common histological types of gynecological cancer, since within the search of the literature a published clinical case was found, it is a 29-year-old Chinese woman who went to the hospital after presenting intermittent vaginal bleeding since the 16th week of gestation. Reporting a history of papillary thyroid carcinoma with metastases

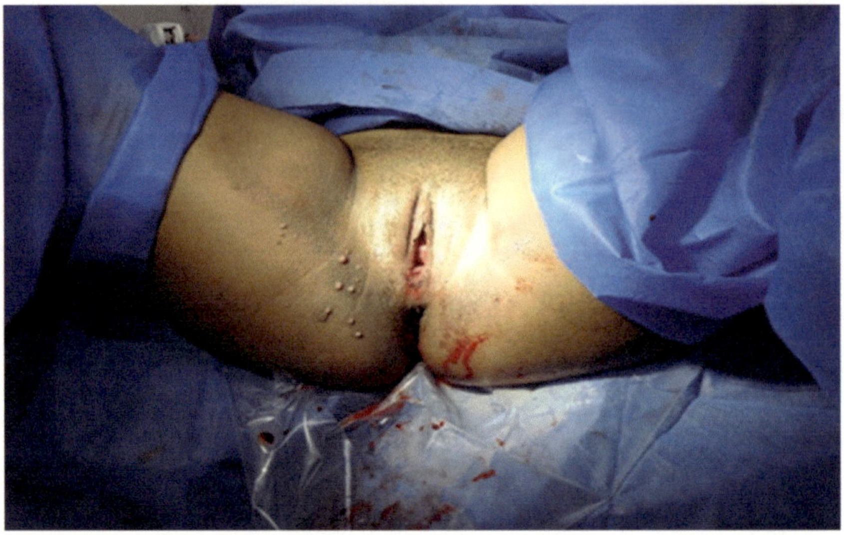

Figure 1.
Patient in lithotomic position after vaginal delivery. Multiple genital warts are present in the right perineal region. Source: Dr. María Fernanda Calderón León.

to the lymph nodes in the neck, she indicates that she underwent radical surgery 3 years earlier. Regular postoperative examinations showed no signs of recurrence until the current admission. Gynecological examination revealed an exophytic lesion of 3 × 1 × 2 cm on the posterior lip of the cervix without invasion of the parametrium or the fundus of the vaginal sac. The patient had persistent human papillomavirus type 18 (HPV-18) infection and a serum alpha-fetoprotein (AFP) level of 235.55 ng/ml. Pathological examination of the lesion revealed large cell neuroendocrine carcinoma (LCCD) with adenocarcinoma of the cervix, which showed positive immunoreactivity for CK, cytokeratin 7, synaptophysin (Syp), chromogranin A (CgA), P16 proteína supresora tumoral, molécula de adhesión de células neuronales CD-56, and proteína Ki67 (>90%). The tumor was classified as clinical stage IB2, according to the FIGO (2018) cervical cancer staging. The patient's wish was to continue the pregnancy, so neoadjuvant chemotherapy with cisplatin and etoposide was administered at 27 and 31 weeks, respectively. During observation of the pregnancy, there were no signs of toxicity or fetal malformation. At 35 weeks, a single live product was obtained by cesarean section with an Apgar score of 9 at 1 minute and 10 at 5 minutes, and then the patient underwent a radical hysterectomy combined with bilateral salpingectomy, with bilateral ovarian biopsy and sentinel node biopsy (**Figure 1**) [16].

Table 2 describes the current management of cervical cancer in pregnancy [19–22].

4. Conclusions

Cervical cancer is closely related to infection by the human papillomavirus, since it is of great importance to carry out adequate screening during prenatal and gynecological control, for which there are a series of biomolecular tests whose sample collection is easy, the same as taking a sample for conventional cytology with an endocervical brush. It helps us to determine if there is HPV infection, in addition to informing what subtype it is, if it is of high, medium, and low degree of malignancy, in order to, according to the results, promote vaccination against the virus and prevent its spread. If we detect a patient with signs and symptoms of cervical cancer during prenatal care, we must take a therapeutic approach according to the gestational stage in which the patient is, and also according to the stage of the tumor. It has now been shown that pregnant women can receive chemotherapy during pregnancy without the need to delay treatment, obtaining encouraging results.

Acknowledgements

To God and to my parents.

Conflict of interest

The authors declare that they have no conflict of interest.

Acronyms and abbreviations

HPV	human papillomavirus
FIGO	International Federation of Gynecology and Obstetrics

Author details

María Fernanda Calderón León[1*], María Eugenia Ugarte Vega[2], Germania Elizabeth Yugcha Andino[3], Paula Andrea Vásquez Jaramillo[4], Germán Arturo Vélez Sáenz[5], Joel Paul Vargas Caicedo[6], Moraima Elizabeth Pazmiño Iñiga[7], Alfredo Guillermo Chong Viteri[8], Angélica María Apolo Montero[9] and Nataly del Carmen Quisiguiña Jarrín[10]

1 Hospital Universitario de Guayaquil-Universidad Católica de Santiago de Guayaquil, Ecuador

2 Bilingual Educational Unit of the Immaculate Conception, Guayaquil, Ecuador

3 Faculty of Medical Sciences, Nursing Career, University of Guayaquil, Ecuador

4 Universidad Laica Eloy Alfaro de Manabí-Hospital de Especialidades de Portoviejo, Ecuador

5 Universidad Laica Eloy Alfaro de Manabí, Portoviejo, Ecuador

6 University of Guayaquil, Ecuador

7 Centro Médico de Especialidades Virgen del Cisne, Guayaquil, Ecuador

8 University Hospital of Guayaquil, Ecuador

9 Hospital del Norte IESS Ceibos, Guayaquil, Ecuador

10 Hospital Clínico Médico Metropolitano Specialized in Gynecology and Obstetrics, Riobamba, Ecuador

*Address all correspondence to: dracalderonleon@hotmail.es

References

[1] Ye J, Zheng L, He Y, Qi X. Human papillomavirus associated cervical lesion: Pathogenesis and therapeutic interventions. MedComm (2020). 14 Sep 2023;**4**(5):e368. DOI: 10.1002/mco2.368

[2] Suzuki Y, Sukegawa A, Ueda Y, Sekine M, Enomoto T, Melamed A, et al. The effect of a web-based cervical cancer survivor's story on parents' behavior and willingness to consider human papillomavirus vaccination for their daughters: A randomized controlled trial. JMIR Public Health Survey. 2022;**8**(5):E34715. DOI: 10.2196/34715

[3] Zhang J, Cheng K, Wang Z. Prevalence and distribution of human papillomavirus genotypes in cervical intraepithelial neoplasia in China: A meta-analysis. Archives of Gynecology and Obstetrics. 2020;**302**(6):1329-1337. DOI: 10.1007/S00404-020-05787-W. Epub 2020 Sep 10

[4] Norenhag J, Du J, Olovsson M, Verstraelen H, Engstrand L, Brusselaers N. Vaginal microbiota, human papillomavirus and cervical dysplasia: A systematic review and network meta-analysis. BJOG: An International Journal of Obstetrics and Gynaecology. 2020;**127**(2):171-180. DOI: 10.1111/1471-0528.15854. Epub 2019 Jul 17

[5] Brun-Micaleff E, Coffy A, Rey V, Didelot MN, Combecal J, Doutre S, et al. Cervical cancer screening by human papillomavirus cytology and testing during pregnancy in French women with poor adherence to regular cervical screening. Journal of Medical Virology. 2014;**86**(3):536-545. DOI: 10.1002/jmv.23764. Epub 2013 Sep 23

[6] Pujade-Lauraine E, Tan DSP, Leary A, Mirza MR, Enomoto T, Takyar J, et al. Comparison of global treatment guidelines for locally advanced cervical cancer to optimize best care practices: A systematic and exploratory review. Gynecologic Oncology. 2022;**167**(2):360-372. DOI: 10.1016/j.ygyno.2022.08.013

[7] Borghi C, Biagioli E, Mauro J, Roberto A, Borghese M, Buda A. Neoadjuvant chemotherapy prior to radical hysterectomy in locally advanced cervical cancer: A systematic review and meta-analysis. The International Journal of Gynecology Cancer. 2023;**34**:35-46. DOI: 10.1136/ijgc-2023-004863

[8] Downham L, Jaafar I, Rol ML, Nyawira Nyaga V, Valls J, Baena A, et al. Accuracy of HPV E6/E7 oncoprotein tests for detecting high-grade cervical lesions: A systematic review of the literature and meta-analysis. British Journal of Cancer. 2024;**130**:517-525. DOI: 10.1038/s41416-023-02490-w

[9] Kong X, Xiong Y, Xue M, He J, Lu Q, Chen M, et al. Identification of cuproptosis-related lncRNA to predict prognosis and immunotherapeutic response in cervical cancer. Scientific Reports. 2023;**13**(1):10697. DOI: 10.1038/s41598-023-37898-0

[10] Modabber N, Mahboub SS, Khoshravesh S, Karimpour F, Karimi A, Goodarzi V. Evaluation of long non-coding RNA (LncRNA) in the pathogenesis of chemotherapy resistance in cervical cancer: Diagnostic approach and prognosis. Molecular Biotechnology. 2023. DOI: 10.1007/S12033-023-00909-6

[11] Xia L, Wang J, Wang C, Zhang Q, Zhu J, Rao Q, et al. Efficacy and safety of zimberelimab monotherapy (GLS-010) in patients with recurrent or metastatic cervical cancer: A multicenter, single-arm, phase II study. The International

Journal of Gynecology Cancer. 2023;**33**(12):1861-1868. DOI: 10.1136/ijgc-2023-004705

[12] Chen J, Pang L, He L, Li T, Cheng X. Whether a specific genetic characteristic predicted the efficacy of immunotherapy: A case report. Medicine (Baltimore). 2024;**103**(2):E36922. DOI: 10.1097/MD.0000000000000036922

[13] Pisano G, Wendler T, Valdés Olmos RA, Garganese G, Rietbergen DDD, Giammarile F, et al. Molecular image-guided surgery in gynecologic cancer: Where are we? European Journal of Nuclear Medicine and Molecular Imaging. 2024. DOI: 10.1007/S00259-024-06604-1

[14] Salta S, Lobo J, Magalhães B, Henrique R, Jerónimo C. DNA methylation as a triage marker for colposcopic shunt in HPV-based cervical cancer screening: A systematic review and meta-analysis. Clinical Epigenetics. 2023;**15**(1):125. DOI: 10.1186/s13148-023-01537-2

[15] Fu H, Fu Z, Mao M, Si L, Bai J, Wang Q, et al. Prevalence and prognostic role of PD-L1 in patients with gynecologic cancers: A systematic review and meta-analysis. Critical Reviews in Oncology/Hematology. 2023;**189**:104084. DOI: 10.1016/j.critrevonc.2023.104084

[16] Geyang D, Gaowen C, Xiaoxuan LI, et al. Maternal-fetal and pregnancy-preservation management in a patient with rare large neuroendocrine cell carcinoma of the cervix. Nan Fang yi ke da xue xue bao = Journal of Southern Medical University. 2021;**41**(1):1-9. DOI: 10.12122/j.issn.1673-4254.2021.01.01

[17] Mileshkin LR, Moore KN, Barnes EH, Gebski V, Narayan K, King MT, et al. Adjuvant chemotherapy after chemoradiation therapy as a primary treatment for locally advanced cervical cancer versus chemoradiation therapy OUTBACK: An international, open-label, randomized, phase 3 trial. The Lancet Oncology. 2023;**24**(5):468-482. DOI: 10.1016/S1470-2045(23)00147-X

[18] Kalliala I, Athanasiou A, Veroniki AA, Salanti G, Efthimiou O, Raftis N, et al. Incidence and mortality from cervical cancer and other malignancies after treatment of cervical intraepithelial neoplasia: A systematic review and meta-analysis of the literature. Annals of Oncology. 2020;**31**(2):213-227. DOI: 10.1016/j.annonc.2019.11.004

[19] Teoh D, Musa F, Salani R, Huh W, Jiménez E. Diagnosis and management of adenocarcinoma in situ: A review and evidence-based recommendations from the Society of Gynecologic Oncology. Obstetrics and Gynecology. 2020;**135**(4):869-878. DOI: 10.1097/AOG.0000000000000003761

[20] Beharee N, Shi Z, Wu D, Wang J. Diagnosis and treatment of cervical cancer in pregnant women. Cancer Medicine. 2019;**8**(12):5425-5430. DOI: 10.1002/cam4.2435

[21] Hammer A, Haubjerg L, Gibrael HS, Winther A, Pedersen LH, Fuglsang K, et al. Detection, diagnosis, and treatment of cervical cancer in pregnancy. Ugeskrift for Laeger. 2022;**184**(35):V03220187

[22] Ruan X. Chinese expert consensus on ovarian function and fertility preservation of cervical cancer in pregnancy. Frontiers in Endocrinology (Lausanne). 2023;**14**:1280631. DOI: 10.3389/fendo.2023.1280631

[23] Howe T, Lankester K, Kelly T, Watkins R, Kaushik S. Cervical cancer

in pregnancy: Diagnosis, staging, and treatment. The Obstetrician and Gynecologist. 2022;**24**:31-39. DOI: 10.1111/tog.12783

[24] Mauro J, Viveros-Carreño D, Vizzielli G, De Ponti E, Fanfani F, Ramírez PT, et al. Survival after sentinel lymph node biopsy alone in early-stage cervical cancer: A systematic review. International Journal of Gynecology & Obstetrics. 2023;**33**(9):1370-1375. DOI: 10.1136/ijgc-2023-004692

[25] Smits A, Ten Eikelder M, Dhanis J, Moore W, Blake D, Zusterzeel P, et al. Finding the sentinel lymph node in early cervical cancer: When is it unusual not uncommon? Gynecologic Oncology. 2023;**170**:84-92. DOI: 10.1016/j.ygyno.2022.12.013

[26] Xing Y, Yasinjan F, Du Y, Geng H, Zhang Y, He M, et al. Immunotherapy in cervical cancer: From the point of view of scientometric analysis and clinical trials. Frontiers in Immunology. 2023;**2**:1094437. DOI: 10.3389/fimmu.2023.1094437

[27] Li K, Chen J, Hu Y, Wang YZ, Shen Y, Chen G, et al. Neoadjuvant chemotherapy plus camrelizumab for locally advanced cervical cancer (NACI study): Single-arm, multicenter phase 2 trial. The Lancet Oncology. 2024;**25**(1):76-85. DOI: 10.1016/S1470-2045(23)00531-4

[28] Sousa LG, Rajapakshe K, Rodriguez Canales J, Chin RL, Feng L, Wang Q, et al. ISA101 and nivolumab for HPV-16+ cancer: Updated clinical efficacy and immunological response correlates. Journal for Immunotherapy of Cancer. 2022;**10**(2):E004232. DOI: 10.1136/JITC-2021-004232

[29] Zagouri F, Korakiti AM, Zakopoulou R, Kyriazoglou A, Zografos E, Haidopoulos D, et al. Taxanes during pregnancy in cervical cancer: A systematic review and pooled analysis. Cancer Treatment Reviews. 2019;**79**:101885. DOI: 10.1016/j.ctrv.2019.08.001

[30] Aranda-Gutierrez A, Ferrigno Guajardo AS, Vaca-Cartagena BF, Gonzalez-SanchezDG,Ramirez-CisnerosA, Becerril-Gaitan A, et al. Obstetric and neonatal outcomes after taxane use during pregnancy: A systematic review. BMC Cancer. 2024;**24**(1):9. DOI: 10.1186/s12885-023-11704-6

Chapter 10

The Need for Audiological Care for Cervical Cancer Patients in South Africa

Jessica Paken

Abstract

Cisplatin chemotherapy, a standard treatment for cervical cancer, may result in ototoxicity. Given the paucity of information on ototoxicity amongst cervical cancer patients, this chapter describes the findings of a study that investigated the extent of cisplatin-associated ototoxicity and the feasibility of an ototoxicity monitoring programme (OMP) amongst this cohort. This study, conducted at a hospital in South Africa, revealed that, while the audiologist was considered a part of the oncology team, provision for ototoxicity monitoring in the chemotherapy protocols was not evident, nor was any OMP in place. Prospective recruitment of cervical cancer cases and regular audiological assessments revealed a 98% incidence of ototoxicity (cumulative cisplatin dose 150 mg/m^2). HIV seropositivity (53.7%) was significantly associated with the NCI-CTCAE Grading Scale at 3- ($p = 0.022$) and 6-month ($p = 0.023$) post-treatment. Feasibility assessment revealed that key stakeholders found the OMP beneficial. Costs to the service provider (equipment, personnel) and patient (transport, daily loss of income) were paramount to successfully implementing and continuing the programme. This study highlights cisplatin's ototoxic effect and provides clear evidence for the need for an OMP. Through meaningful engagements with, and considerations from, patients and service providers regarding planning, delineation of responsibilities, and cost implications, such a programme is feasible.

Keywords: cisplatin, ototoxicity, cervical cancer, HIV, South Africa, ototoxicity monitoring programme

1. Introduction

Cervical cancer is the second most prevalent cancer in African [1] and South African women [2]. The high incidence of this cancer in South Africa and other developing countries can be attributed to socio-economic factors (poverty, poor hygiene) and cultural norms (early or polygamous marriages, monogamous marriages with husbands engaging in extramarital affairs) [3]. Early sexual debut and multiple sexual partnerships are leading causes of Human Papillomavirus (HPV) infection, causally associated with cervical cancer [4] and partially responsible for some of the stigma associated with this cancer [5, 6]. This stigma can result in late screening and/

or diagnosis of this disease [7], which may warrant brachytherapy and chemotherapy containing cisplatin [8]. This poses a challenge for South Africa, as the country has the largest population of people living with HIV, the greatest percentage being Black African women [9]. With HIV infection known to increase the rate of HPV infection and its persistence, it is not surprising that cervical cancer considered an AIDS-defining illness, is so prevalent in the Black South African population [10].

This previously marginalised ethnic group, therefore, is at an increased risk for ototoxicity due to the double-barrelled effect of combined cisplatin [11–14] and antiretroviral therapy (ART) exposures [15, 16], which are both known to result in a high-frequency sensorineural hearing loss [17, 18]. Given the permanency yet invisible nature of high-frequency sensorineural hearing loss, its effect on the affected individual's quality of life cannot be underestimated, especially since international literature reports the incidence rate to vary from 50% to 100% [19]. A diagnosis of cervical cancer brings with it many challenges, as "the toll of cervical cancer in the African region is particularly high as the disease tends to affect women at a time of their lives when being in good health is so critical to the social and economic stability of families" ([20], p. 11). Furthermore, a woman's role goes beyond childbearing, as it is still the mother who shoulders most of the responsibilities, and her health largely determines the health and well-being of her children and sometimes grandchildren (in the case of HIV/AIDS orphans). The role of the female now extends beyond that of nurturer, caregiver, and manager of food security. They are also now wage earners [21]. Therefore, the added burden of acquiring hearing loss during this period may have devastating effects on the lives of the affected individual and family members. While some may argue that hearing loss may be a small price to pay for achieving a cure for cancer, it may still have a significant adverse effect on the survivor's quality of life [22]. Upon completion of treatment, this female will not only live with the fear of cancer returning [23] but will also have to deal with the repercussions of hearing loss, for example, the loss of employment and difficulty in communicating with partners, which in the South African context may mean increasing the risk of domestic violence. Therefore, the early identification and management of ototoxic hearing loss should be an essential component of the holistic treatment of a patient with cervical cancer.

Furthermore, hearing loss, especially if undiagnosed or not appropriately managed, can result in psychosocial and physical health problems, depression, and social isolation [24]. The many roles taken on by women are then affected, resulting in hearing loss becoming a disability and eventually a handicap. Therefore, healthcare personnel working within a biopsychosocial model should endeavour to reduce the challenges affecting the cancer patient's quality of life because women with disabilities are also at a greater risk for all forms of violence, including Gender-Based Violence [25]. Therefore, the implementation of an ototoxicity monitoring programme is essential not only for these individuals' hearing health but also for their safety and functioning within the community and society and, essentially, their quality of life.

However, ototoxicity monitoring is not commonplace in South Africa, with the recent guidelines by the Health Professions Council of South Africa (HPCSA) [26] being based on programmes and policies developed for first-world countries [27, 28], and not necessarily considering contextual relevance [29]. There has also been an absence of context-specific research to expedite the implementation of an accountable and effective ototoxicity monitoring programme (OMP) in this country, particularly for this patient population. Identifying the need for such a programme through prospective data on the extent and severity of cisplatin-associated ototoxicity in

South Africa would serve as motivation to amalgamate audiological clinical practice within the oncology context, employing a team approach.

Therefore, a recent real-world study, guided by the "Conceptual Framework for Implementation Outcomes" [30], investigated the extent of cisplatin-associated ototoxicity in cervical cancer patients receiving chemotherapy and the feasibility of an audiological monitoring programme in a public health care facility in KwaZulu-Natal that epitomises the South African context. In attempting to inform a contextually relevant ototoxicity monitoring programme, this concurrent embedded study adopted a structured approach to achieve its aim, with each objective feeding into the other. The first two objectives: (1) to describe the perspectives and practices of healthcare professionals in relation to cisplatin-associated ototoxicity at an institution treating patients with cancer, and (2) to evaluate the extent and severity of ototoxicity amongst patients with cervical cancer receiving cisplatin-based chemotherapy, served as the foundation to achieve objective 3, that is, to evaluate the ototoxicity monitoring programme with the feasibility of integration into the clinical environment. In so doing, the study offered key considerations for a locally responsive ototoxicity monitoring programme.

2. Objective 1: Perspectives and practices of healthcare professionals in relation to cisplatin-associated ototoxicity at an institution treating patients with cancer

While policies and guidelines, such as those of the HPCSA, matter and make a difference, they are inadequate on their own as they must be implemented with change occurring through stakeholders and processes. Therefore, using literature [31] as a framework for the key responsibilities of the healthcare personnel (see **Figure 1**), a concurrent triangulation mixed-methods approach was used in this phase to gain insights into the current perspectives of cisplatin ototoxicity and the practices in identifying and managing ototoxic hearing loss in the study setting [32].

This was achieved through the use of questionnaires completed by nine oncology nurses, seven clinicians, and 13 pharmacists, as well as interviews with four audiologists. There is no doubt that there are numerous studies related to this area that have been conducted in South Africa, but they mainly focus on oncologists, audiologists, and general practitioners in isolation [29, 33–35]. None have reported on the variation in practices and awareness of other healthcare professionals in the team about cisplatin ototoxicity, especially with a single-facility managing patients with cancer. While single-facility studies are often frowned upon and considered limited, such research must be conducted, as such a study site provides an ideal environment for implementing an ototoxicity monitoring programme to maximise patient outcomes while being cognisant of facility-specific constraints, infrastructure, and resources [32].

Quantitative data from the questionnaires were descriptively analysed, while **Table 1** reflects the themes and subthemes emerging from the interviews.

While all participant oncologists and pharmacists reported awareness of certain chemotherapy drugs causing hearing loss, this awareness was reported by 33% of the nursing personnel. Effects of comorbid conditions and their subsequent treatment, that is, ARTs were unfortunately not identified as detrimental to a patient's hearing health by all audiologists. Participant audiologists, even more surprisingly, did not identify themselves as having a role in pre-treatment counselling despite knowing the ototoxic effect of the treatment. Referrals for hearing assessments were made only

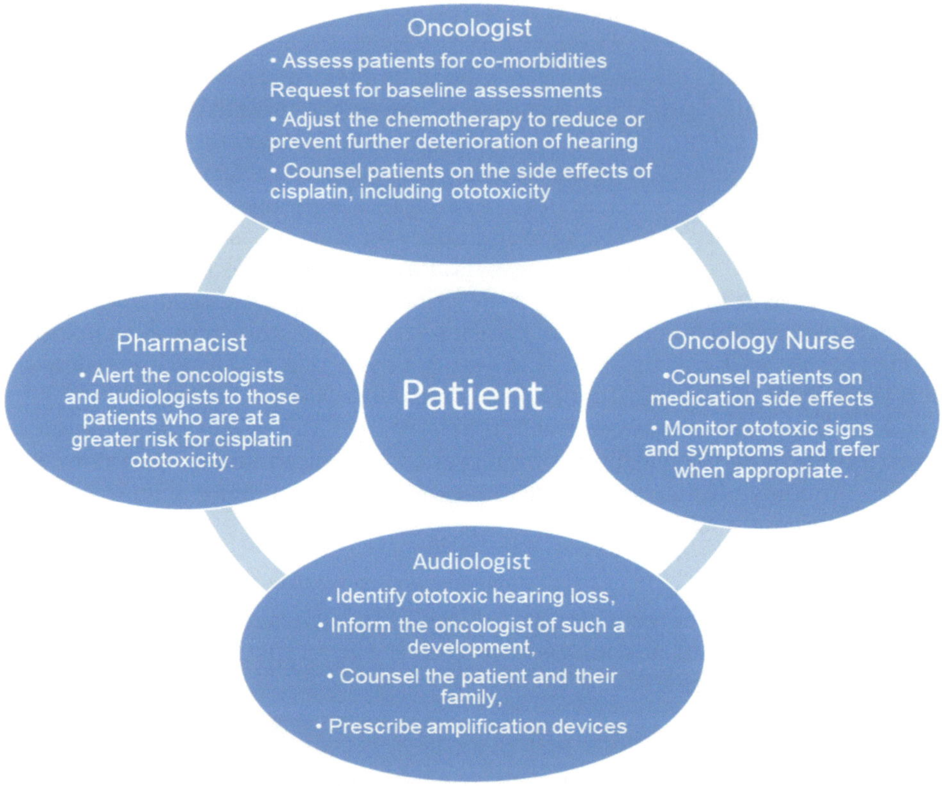

Figure 1.
Key responsibilities of health care team managing ototoxicity in cancer patients. Adapted from Paken et al. [32].

after patient complaints of difficulty hearing, and most participants correctly identified the clinician as being responsible for this task. Responses from participant audiologists also highlighted the need for greater awareness by audiologists around the elements of ototoxicity monitoring. An essential component to a successful ototoxicity monitoring programme was identified as including an awareness of healthcare personnel's roles and responsibilities within the multidisciplinary team, with each member aware of their tasks with regards to referring, counselling, identifying, and appropriately managing the patient receiving ototoxic treatment for cancer, as only 82% of healthcare personnel considered the audiologist a part of the oncology team. Furthermore, provision for ototoxicity monitoring in the chemotherapy protocols was not evident, nor was any OMP in place. This phase emphasised the audiologist's key role in training healthcare personnel within this multidisciplinary team and also allowed for the identification of topics that should be addressed in *in-service* training before implementing an ototoxicity monitoring programme, namely:

- Signs and symptoms of cisplatin-associated ototoxicity,
- Risk factors for cisplatin-associated ototoxicity,
- Ototoxicity monitoring programme, and
- Responsibilities of healthcare personnel in the team managing ototoxicity.

Themes	Sub-themes
Awareness of chemotherapy-associated ototoxicity	• Identification of common ototoxic medication
Patient-reported symptoms	• Reduced hearing sensitivity • Tinnitus
Responsibilities of healthcare personnel	• Team approach in ototoxicity monitoring • Pre-treatment counselling • Referrals
Ototoxicity monitoring programme	• Awareness of ototoxicity monitoring at the hospital • Elements of an ototoxicity monitoring programme
Current practices of healthcare personnel in ototoxicity monitoring	• Identification of at-risk patients • Referrals • Audiologist's role

Table 1.
Themes and subthemes. Adapted from Paken et al. [32].

Signs and symptoms of cisplatin-associated ototoxicity include hearing loss and tinnitus. Hearing loss is more likely to be experienced in both ears; however, it may not necessarily be symmetrical. The rare diagnosis of unilateral hearing loss is generally due to the location of the tumour and surgical or radiation therapy on the affected side. Irrespective of whether the hearing loss is unilateral or bilateral, it is usually permanent and progressive. However, the tinnitus, often described as buzzing or ringing in the ears and/or head, may resolve a few weeks after treatment [31].

The likelihood and extent of cisplatin-associated ototoxicity is often related to the dose with higher cumulative doses likely to result in a greater ototoxic effect [36]. Other factors influencing the degree of hearing loss include the duration, number of cycles administered [37], and method of administration [38]. While cranial radiation therapy is also known to influence cisplatin-associated ototoxicity [39], females with cervical cancer are most likely to be spared from this increased risk, as the site exposed to radiation is further away from the head and neck area. However, exposure to concomitant noise [40] and other ototoxic medications, as well as presenting with renal insufficiency [41], may also increase one's risk for cisplatin-associated ototoxicity. Age and pre-exposure hearing ability are also known risk factors, with younger children [41] and older adults (older than 46 years) [42] presenting with a greater severity of ototoxic damage.

With numerous risk factors, monitoring for cisplatin-associated ototoxicity should be an inherent part of the cervical cancer patient's holistic management. Audiological evaluations conducted at specific time points are unfailing in detecting ototoxicity before patients experience the symptoms [31]. These time points may differ based on the ototoxicity monitoring guidelines used, but all guidelines are common in that a comprehensive audiological assessment should be conducted before commencing with and upon completion of chemotherapy. As per HPCSA guidelines [26], this entails a detailed case history, otoscopic examination, immittance audiometry, speech audiometry, Distortion Product Otoacoustic Emission (DPOAEs), and conventional and extended high-frequency audiometry, with auditory brainstem response testing conducted for those patients who are too ill or too young to respond. Modifications of the comprehensive audiological monitoring may occur during chemotherapy and post-completion of chemotherapy.

3. Objective 2: Evaluating the extent and severity of ototoxicity amongst patients with cervical cancer receiving cisplatin-based chemotherapy

This objective involved the comprehensive audiological assessment of 82 participants with cervical cancer at five-time points, namely baseline, after three cycles of cisplatin chemotherapy, and at 1-, 3- and 6-month post-treatment. The patients with cervical cancer underwent the following audiological tests comprising case history, otoscopic examination, immittance audiometry (tympanometry and acoustic reflex threshold testing), pure tone audiometry (conventional and high-frequency audiometry), speech audiometry (speech reception threshold testing and word recognition score testing), and DPOAE testing. Study findings [43] revealing cisplatin's detrimental effect on hearing as a significant ototoxic change, using the American Speech-Language-Hearing Association (ASHA) criteria, was evident in 98% of participants at the mid-cycle audiological assessment. A significant association between HIV status and the National Cancer Institute-Common Terminology Criteria for Adverse Events (NCI-CTCAE) Grading Scale was evident at 3- ($p = 0.022$) and 6-month ($p = 0.023$) post-cisplatin treatment, thus, indicating that HIV-positive patients with cervical cancer present with a greater severity of ototoxic change. Significant differences in the CTCAE grading scale were evident between the low dosage (150–200 mg/m^2) and high dosage (250–300 mg/m^2) groups at 1- ($p = 0.017$), 3- ($p = 0.01$), and 6-months ($p = 0.015$) post-treatment; thus, revealing that increased cumulative cisplatin dosage results in increased severity of ototoxicity, as reflected in **Figure 2**.

Multiple Tobit regression revealed a dose effect bilaterally, especially evident from 9000 Hz and above in the right ear, while a plateau effect was visible at 250 mg/m^2 in the left ear after adjustment for the effect of age and HIV status. Increasing cumulative cisplatin dosage significantly increased hearing thresholds in the high and extended high-frequency ranges. While adjusting for age, multiple Tobit

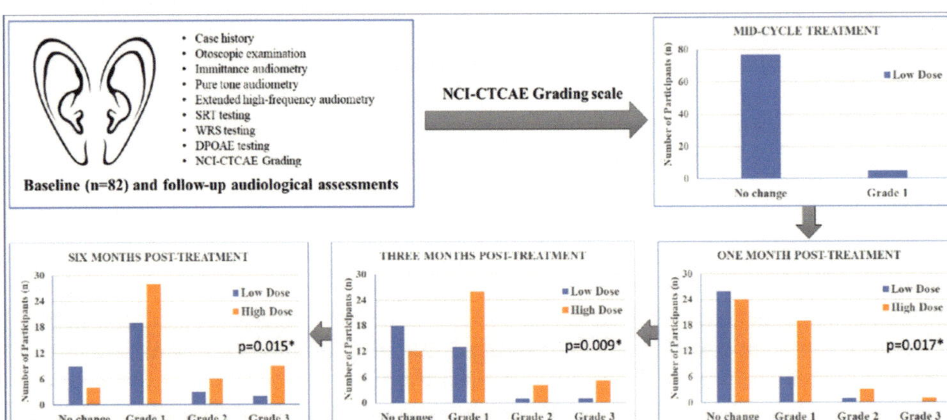

* denotes statistical significance in the relationship between Cisplatin dose and Grade (Fisher's exact test)
At mid-cycle, all patients received 3 cycles of cisplatin (150 mg/m^2) – stratified as Low Dose only.

Figure 2.
Temporal variation in severity of ototoxicity according to NCI-CTCAE classification. Source: Paken et al. [43].

regression was also used to compare the effect of cisplatin dosage in HIV-positive and HIV-negative patients. HIV-positive patients were affected with hearing change to a greater degree at similar cisplatin doses compared to the HIV-negative stratum (see **Table 2**) [43].

Presenting with diabetes and/or hypertension, despite being identified as risk factors [44], did not significantly increase a participant's risk for ototoxic hearing loss during and after the course of cisplatin treatment; however, this was most likely due to the small number of participants in each of these subgroups. Despite the 100% incidence of ototoxicity by the end of the follow-up period, most participants did not report difficulties in hearing, possibly due to them presenting with mild to moderate degrees of hearing loss and the deterioration in hearing thresholds being more evident in the extended high-frequency range.

This study, being the first to use a prospective cohort design on the African continent, emphasised the need for early and effective identification of ototoxicity in these previously marginalised women through a structured, acceptable, and appropriate ototoxicity monitoring programme. There is a higher incidence of significant ototoxic change in the current study than in other international studies despite the use of a lower cumulative dosage of the treatment. The potential contributor to this high incidence is the HIV burden in the country and the subsequent treatment with ART. Noting that women in Africa endure a large portion of the global burden of disease [20], the added imposition of hearing loss is likely to increase their challenges. Therefore, the implementation of an ototoxicity monitoring programme becomes invaluable for this patient population, especially since the affected individuals do not experience difficulties hearing until the communication problems become evident. This calls for audiological monitoring to be incorporated as part of the standard care for patients with cancer receiving cisplatin, especially if there is a high incidence of people living with HIV.

Follow-up	HTV status	NCI-CTCAE Grading Scale, n (%)				p-Value
		No change	Grade 1	Grade 2	Grade 3	
Mid-cycle	Negative	35 (92.1)	3 (7.9)	0	0	0.659
	Positive	42 (95.5)	2 (4.5)	0	0	
One-month post-treatment	Negative	26 (70.3)	10 (27.0)	0	1 (2.7)	0.124
	Positive	24 (55.8)	15 (34.9)	4 (9.3)	0	
Three-month post-treatment	Negative	20 (54.1)	13 (35.1)	1 (2.7)	3 (8.1)	0.022*
	Positive	10 (23.3)	26 (60.5)	4 (9.3)	3 (6.9)	
Six-month post-treatment	Negative	10 (27.0)	22 (59.4)	1 (2.7)	4 (10.8)	0.023*
	Positive	3 (7.0)	25 (58.1)	8 (18.6)	7 (16.3)	

**Fisher's Exact Test revealed a significant association between HIV status and the NCI-CTCAE Grading Scale at 3- and 6-month post-cisplatin treatment.*
Source: Paken et al. [43].

Table 2.
Severity of ototoxicity by HIV status at each audiological assessment (NCI-CTCAE Grading Scale).

4. Objective 3: Evaluation of the ototoxicity monitoring programme

Through real-world experience, this concurrent triangulation mixed-methods study aimed to inform the implementation of an ototoxicity monitoring programme with the feasibility of integration into the clinical environment by focusing on the audiological monitoring conducted within the prospective cohort study. The study findings [45] revealed the ototoxicity monitoring programme as being feasible within this setting and possible extension to other low/middle income countries (LMICs). The success of the ototoxicity monitoring programme is evident in stakeholder responses, with 91% of healthcare personnel and 89% of patients reporting it to be beneficial. With eight patients being assessed weekly, the audiologist can allocate one 8-hour workday to assess patients with cervical cancer. The approximate cost of setting up such a programme includes the purchase of equipment and the appointment of an audiologist. The approximate costs to patients included transport costs and the loss of income for the day, calculated at the minimum wage per hour if employed. Creative scheduling and detailed, easy-to-understand counselling improved patient compliance with the programme.

Key findings in this study, as reflected in **Figure 3**, were seen as the essential factors critical to an ototoxicity monitoring programme for women with cervical cancer. A multidisciplinary team approach, employing a collaborative partnership, evidence-based practice, *in-service* training for all healthcare personnel provided by the audiologist, the consideration of patient context (costs, time) and costs to the service provider, selection of the audiological tests most sensitive to ototoxicity monitoring are some of the factors identified as vital for a contextually relevant patient-centred ototoxicity monitoring programme for these previously marginalised and often stigmatised women (see **Figure 3**).

While the ototoxicity monitoring programme is feasible for women with cervical cancer, it is not without threats to its success. Gender bias in care-seeking and

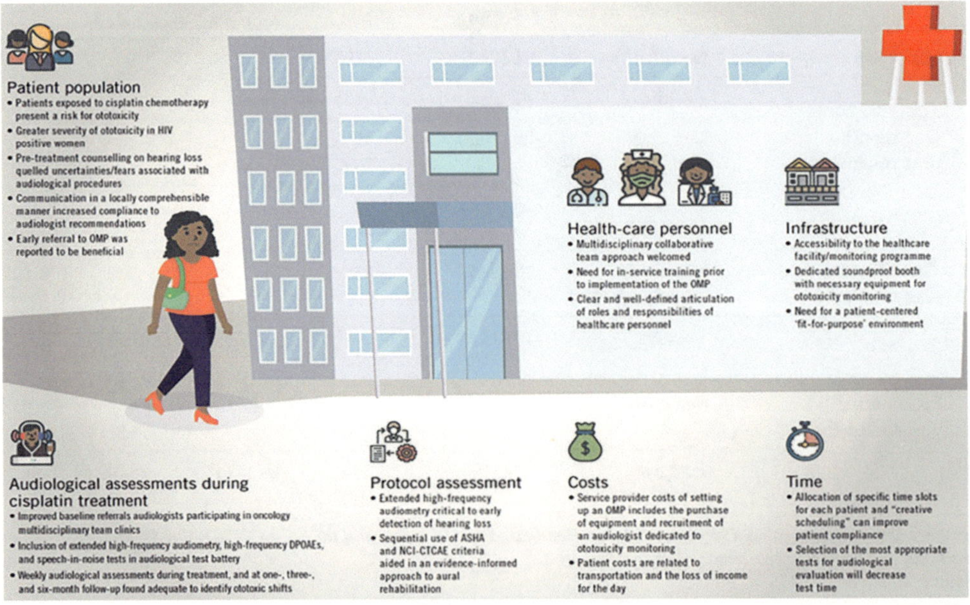

Figure 3.
Key findings informing the implementation of the ototoxicity monitoring programme.

treatment completion for long-term illness, together with stigma and information gaps [21], inhibit the successful implementation of such programmes. Complicating the situation further is that oncology services are generally provided at a tertiary or district-level hospital, which may be a great distance away from their residences. Therefore, women who usually play many roles in the household, community, and society may not always have the time or finances to attend consultations and treatment sessions [21], such as that required for both cervical cancer and the ototoxicity monitoring programme.

Furthermore, South Africa's dual health system lends itself to variations in respect of accessibility [10]. This previously marginalised group is most likely to access services at a public hospital, as 84% of the South African population access the public sector [46]. However, public hospitals in South Africa experience varying shortages of medical equipment, with it being higher in rural hospitals than in urban hospitals [47]. With audiological diagnosis being essentially an equipment-based practice, poor maintenance, poor repair, and limited financial resources hinder effective clinical practice, such as in an ototoxicity monitoring programme. While the study site was a well-resourced hospital, which ensured that equipment was timeously calibrated and repaired to ensure the best possible service delivery, this may not be the case in all facilities offering the service, as a national healthcare facilities baseline audit conducted in 2012 revealed public hospitals in South Africa generally scored below 50% for medical equipment [47].

The shortage of healthcare personnel in Sub-Saharan Africa is another well-known challenge that could potentially hinder an ototoxicity monitoring programme. Sub-Saharan Africa's health personnel/population ratios are the lowest globally [48]. While the ratios of medical doctors and nurses to the population in South Africa are better than the Sub-Saharan African continent's average, they are still lower than those in comparable developing countries such as India and Korea. Additionally, South Africa's health worker density per 100,000 population is lower than in its benchmarked countries, namely Brazil, Russia, India, and China [48]. This shortage of healthcare personnel in the country is potentially worsened by unequal access between urban and rural public sector users, with a recent national study revealing an inverse relationship between the location of audiologists and speech-language therapists and the number of persons with disabilities the Western Cape and Gauteng have the highest number of audiologists and speech-langauge therapists but the lowest population of persons with disabilities [46]. The shortage of human resources is a huge stumbling block to an ototoxicity monitoring programme, which requires a collaborative multidisciplinary team approach to managing women with cervical cancer receiving cisplatin chemotherapy. If oncology clinics are understaffed, oncologists in public hospitals may be too busy to manage the patient holistically and may be narrowly focused only on their oncological needs, with nurses also not necessarily informing and querying about medication side effects. Referrals to the ototoxicity monitoring programme may be subsequently delayed, and ototoxicity goes unnoticed until a communication problem becomes evident.

Lack of audiologists may result in ototoxic hearing loss, if even identified, not being appropriately managed. This raises a valid question about the value and ethical positioning of the identification of ototoxicity, especially where rehabilitative resources are limited [49]. In addition, a lack of patient counselling may reduce patient adherence to treatment. Furthermore, if information on hearing conservation strategies to reduce the synergistic effects of toxins to the ear (excessive noise) is not imparted to patients, there may be a greater progressive deterioration in hearing, subsequently raising rehabilitation costs significantly.

Another financial implication that may be detrimental to a resource-constrained country such as South Africa is the admission of all patients receiving cisplatin into the ototoxicity monitoring programme. While HPCSA [26] proposes that all patients receiving cisplatin need to be enrolled in an ototoxicity monitoring programme, such a suggestion may only be workable if the programme caters to one type of cancer. However, cisplatin is used to treat a variety of cancers and would, therefore, possibly necessitate the use of a screening tool for use by nurses and oncologists to identify patients presenting with risk factors for ototoxic hearing loss. Such a tool could potentially be a short questionnaire administered by healthcare personnel other than the audiologist, who can then refer the patient to the ototoxicity monitoring programme.

Additionally, the patient could also screen their own hearing through a screening application on their mobile devices [50]. This method of service provision, referred to as tele-audiology, has the potential to revolutionise how audiology services are provided [51] and bridges the gap between limited resources, restricted access, and lack of trained professionals [52], especially important in resource-constrained countries with more prevalent ototoxic effects [53]. With the advantage of remote synchronous and asynchronous assessments, Tele-audiology has played a crucial role in audiological service provision amid the global crisis of COVID-19 [54]. The pandemic has fast-tracked eHealth trends that were already starting to shape the future of healthcare and audiology [55], as is evident in a study by Saunders and Roughley [56], which reflected this increasing trend. Before the COVID-19 pandemic, only 30% of audiologists utilised tele-audiology; this increased to 98% during the pandemic, of whom 86% indicated that they would continue this method of service provision even after the pandemic. While studies conducted in South Africa have displayed the use of tele-audiology in ototoxicity monitoring [57, 58], the exorbitant data costs [59], and connectivity issues, especially in rural areas, have not been expanded on.

Despite these limitations, early identification of an ototoxic hearing loss provides oncologists with an opportunity to adjust the chemotherapy regimen in order to reduce or prevent further deterioration of hearing [27], especially since, none of the oto-protective agents researched have been found to unequivocally prevent cisplatin ototoxicity and no agent is currently recommended for routine use [60]. However, further research is needed to explore the intra-tympanic administration of oto-protective agents into the inner ear without potentially reducing the efficacy of the cisplatin treatment [31].

5. Conclusion

Cervical cancer, which is largely preventable by Human Papillomavirus vaccination [1], maintains its stronghold on the South African female population. This cancer often results in psychological and physical morbidities, with a consequent negative impact on the affected woman's quality of life. Marital discordance and waning partner support during treatment and survival are contributing factors to this psychological morbidity [61]. Therefore, these women are grateful for the treatment with cisplatin, which is considered the most potent anti-cancer therapy [62], despite its expansive toxicity profile, which includes ototoxicity. An acquired hearing loss earlier in one's life course, especially if undiagnosed, can result in this sensory impairment becoming a disability, which would only further add to the innumerable challenges faced by these women in South Africa. This study shows the extent and severity of cisplatin-associated ototoxicity in this cohort, with an incidence of 98% at a cumulative dose of

150 mg/m^2, after completion of three cycles. However, it leads one to question whether this high incidence will receive as much attention as other debilitating illnesses, largely because of the competing priorities in treatment outcomes. With numerous barriers to equality faced by women, a diagnosis of cervical cancer and hearing loss should not further disadvantage them [63]. Therefore, audiologists need to ensure that ototoxicity monitoring is implemented to minimise the effects of ototoxic hearing loss on the affected individual's quality of life. Adopting and implementing ototoxicity monitoring protocols by professionals and governments is not optional, considering that these are vital for improving the patient's quality of life; "they should form the minimum standards of care in ototoxicity management" ([63], p. 81).

This study shows that the ototoxicity monitoring programme for South African cancer patients treated with cisplatin chemotherapy is feasible. Despite this evidence and the known benefits of the early identification of ototoxic hearing loss, the implementation of ototoxicity monitoring programmes will continue to remain a challenge in South Africa if audiologists are complacent with the current status quo. Implementing and maintaining such a programme requires institutional support, political advocacy, and funding, which can be challenging, especially in a country like South Africa, where much of its limited resources are directed towards competing healthcare priorities, including infectious and other chronic diseases. Therefore, audiologists should advocate for audiological monitoring to be incorporated into the holistic management of women with cervical cancer through a political advocacy strategy that involves healthcare activism, gender-based care, poverty, and rehabilitation. This advocacy is especially essential in light of the World Health Organisation [63] recently indicating that the field of audiology requires not only professionals who are able to provide quality services at the individual level but can also address the subject at public policy levels.

With the recent COVID-19 pandemic stealing the limelight away from other diseases, it is improbable that ototoxicity monitoring for these women with cervical cancer will receive the necessary attention and support it calls for. This lack of attention can, however, be avoided through more contextual research that reveals the extent and severity of cisplatin ototoxicity in other populations within the scope of audiological services in South Africa. Such information may garner governmental support towards incorporating and implementing contextually relevant audiological monitoring programme into the holistic management of cancer patients and survivors. The ultimate goal is to have a contextually relevant, cost-effective, nationally accepted ototoxicity monitoring programme that can reduce the impact of cisplatin-associated hearing loss, as women experience numerous challenges in their lives, and hearing loss should not further weigh them down.

6. Recommendations

Recommendations relating to the academic, clinical, and research community are reflected below:

- Undergraduate audiology programmes in South Africa need to focus on audiology practice within the burden of disease framework and include more practical components in ototoxicity monitoring to build the student audiologist's knowledge and confidence in being the principal member of the multidisciplinary team.

- Practising audiologists need to market their profession to the various disciplines within the medical fraternity and highlight the importance of hearing to an individual's quality of life which in turn may encourage a collaborative multidisciplinary team approach to managing patients receiving cisplatin chemotherapy. This may consequently encourage the referral to an ototoxicity monitoring programme as part of standard oncological care.

- The audiology profession should develop standard pamphlets or information documents in English and the country's native languages to be shared with the necessary stakeholders. Pamphlets on ototoxicity and the effects of undiagnosed hearing loss distributed to patients will encourage informed decision-making.

- All audiologists should be motivated to purchase high-frequency audiometers and high-frequency DPOAEs, considering the high burden of disease and related ototoxicity in the country.

- Audiologists should also incorporate speech-in-noise tests in the audiological test battery for patients receiving ototoxic medication but score well in "speech in quiet tests."

- Tertiary, academic, and district hospitals in South Africa are the sites for oncological care and also tend to have audiology departments and, therefore, serve as ideal contexts to provide comprehensive audiological coverage to patients with cancer, especially those from disadvantaged communities. Therefore, audiologists working at these facilities should initiate and drive the process of implementing an ototoxicity monitoring programme.

- Referring all patients receiving cisplatin chemotherapy may not be feasible, especially for newly/recently implemented ototoxicity monitoring programmes. Therefore, oncologists and oncology nurses should use a simple screening tool such as a questionnaire to identify patients at increased risk for ototoxicity.

- With advancements in technology, more public hospitals should strive to utilise electronic/digital patient records that may allow the pharmacist to easily identify patients who are receiving ototoxic medication.

- The current study focused on the effect of cisplatin treatment on hearing and the implementation of an ototoxicity monitoring programme. However, there has been no focus on how these affect the South African patient's quality of life. A longitudinal study that focuses on the patient's quality of life from the time of a cancer diagnosis can inform clinicians and policymakers of the challenges experienced by the patient and consequently provide them with an opportunity to include other healthcare personnel in the multidisciplinary team. This will facilitate more holistic management of the oncology patient, reducing the sometimes devastating effects on the patient's quality of life.

- Cisplatin retention in the cochlea has been reported to be indefinite [14]. Therefore, a longitudinal study tracking the auditory status of patients for a longer period post-cisplatin may inform clinicians of the possible need for a longer formalised duration for ototoxicity monitoring.

- All study participants in the current study were responsive. Therefore, an investigation into the feasibility of implementing an ototoxicity monitoring programme for patients who have limited responsiveness or are non-responsive using an appropriate test audiological test battery, including the auditory brainstem response test, is warranted.

- Screening for ototoxicity by healthcare personnel other than the audiologists may require a quick, inexpensive tool such as a questionnaire. The development and validation of such a tool would be beneficial to identify those patients at an increased risk for ototoxicity to reduce the burden of oversubscription to a newly implemented ototoxicity monitoring programme.

- The use of tele-audiology has increased significantly during the COVID-19 pandemic. Therefore, investigating the feasibility of using this alternate method of service provision in an ototoxicity monitoring programme would be beneficial, as it would allow the ototoxicity monitoring programme to proceed uninterrupted.

- Perspectives of both patients and healthcare personnel regarding their acceptance of an existing ototoxicity monitoring programme should be obtained through one-on-one interviews and possible focus group studies to obtain more detailed information to inform policymakers.

- More studies exploring key attributes to enhance the success of such programmes, while highlighting the barriers, gaps, and local needs not identified/investigated in this study, are required to build on the evidence base. This can be achieved through further qualitative research methodologies, such as one-on-one and focus group interviews, which would allow for data enrichment and data saturation.

Acknowledgements

This study was supported by the South African Medical Research Council of South Africa in terms of the National Health Scholarship Programme provided for this purpose by the National Department of Health, the Oticon Foundation as well as the University of KwaZulu-Natal.

Vikash Sewram, Cyril D. Govender, and Mershen Pillay are thanked for their supervision, mentorship and critical appraisal of the project.

Author details

Jessica Paken
University of KwaZulu-Natal, Durban, South Africa

*Address all correspondence to: pakenj@ukzn.ac.za

References

[1] Denny L, Kuhn L. Cervical cancer prevention and early detection from a South African perspective. In: Padarath A, Barron P, editors. South African Health Review 2017. South Africa: Health Systems Trust; 2017. pp. 189-196. Available from: http://www.hst.org.za/publications/south-african-health-review-2017

[2] Ferlay JEM, Lam F, Laversanne M, et al. Global Cancer Observatory: Cancer Today. Lyon, France: International Agency for Research on Cancer; 2024. Available from: https://gco.iarc.who.int/today

[3] Maree JE, Moitse KA. Exploration of knowledge of cervical cancer and cervical cancer screening amongst HIV-positive women. Curationis. 2014;**37**(1):e1-e10. DOI: 10.4102/curationis.v37i1.1209

[4] Bosch FX, Lorincz A, Muñoz N, Meijer CJLM, Shah KV. The causal relation between human papillomavirus and cervical cancer. Journal of Clinical Pathology. 2002;**55**(4):244-265. DOI: 10.1136/jcp.55.4.244

[5] Nyblade L, Stockton M, Travasso S, Krishnan S. A qualitative exploration of cervical and breast cancer stigma in Karnataka, India. BMC Women's Health. 2017;**17**(1):58. DOI: 10.1186/s12905-017-0407-x

[6] Shepherd MA, Gerend MA. The blame game: Cervical cancer, knowledge of its link to human papillomavirus and stigma. Psychology & Health. 2013;**29**(1):94-109. DOI: 10.1080/08870446.2013.834057

[7] Marlow LAV, Waller J, Wardle J. Barriers to cervical cancer screening among ethnic minority women: A qualitative study. The Journal of Family Planning and Reproductive Health Care. 2015;**41**(4):248. DOI: 10.1136/jfprhc-2014-101082

[8] Marnitz S, Schermeyer L, Sea D. Age-corrected hearing loss after chemoradiation in cervical cancer patients. Strahlentherapie und Onkologie. 2018;**194**:1039-1048. DOI: 10.1007/s00066-018-1347-6

[9] Mabaso M, Makola L, Naidoo I, Mlangeni LL, Jooste S, Simbayi L. HIV prevalence in South Africa through gender and racial lenses: Results from the 2012 population-based national household survey. International Journal for Equity in Health. 2019;**18**(1):167. DOI: 10.1186/s12939-019-1055-6

[10] Olorunfemi G, Ndlovu N, Masukume G, Chikandiwa A, Pisa PT, Singh E. Temporal trends in the epidemiology of cervical cancer in South Africa (1994-2012). International Journal of Cancer. 2018;**143**(9):2238-2249. DOI: 10.1002/ijc.31610

[11] Arora R, Thakur JS, Azad RK, Mohindroo NK, Sharma DR, Seam RK. Cisplatin-based chemotherapy: Add high-frequency audiometry in the regimen. Indian Journal of Cancer. 2009;**46**(4):7. DOI: 10.4103/0019-509X.55551

[12] Nader M-E, Gidley PW. Challenges of hearing rehabilitation after radiation and chemotherapy. Journal of Neurological Surgery Part B. 2019;**80**(02):214-224. DOI: 10.1055/s-0039-1677865

[13] Choe WT, Chinosornvatana N, Chang KW. Prevention of cisplatin ototoxicity using transtympanic

N-acetylcysteine and lactate. Otology & Neurotology. 2004;**25**(6):910-915. DOI:10.1097/00129492-200411000-00009

[14] Breglio AM, Rusheen AE, Shide ED, et al. Cisplatin is retained in the cochlea indefinitely following chemotherapy. Nature Communications. 2017;**8**(1):1654. DOI: 10.1038/s41467-017-01837-1

[15] Bisht M, Bist SS. Ototoxicity: The hidden menace. Indian Journal of Otolaryngology and Head & Neck Surgery. 2011;**63**(3):255-259. DOI: 10.1007/s12070-011-0151-8

[16] van der Westhuizen Y, Swanepoel DW, Heinze B, Hofmeyr LM. Auditory and otological manifestations in adults with HIV/AIDS. International Journal of Audiology. 2013;**52**(1):37-43. DOI: 10.3109/14992027.2012.721935

[17] Rybak L, Ramkumar V. Ototoxicity. Kidney International. 2007;**72**(8):931-935. DOI: 10.1038/sj.ki.5002434

[18] Schacht J, Talaska AE, Rybak LP. Cisplatin and aminoglycoside antibiotics: Hearing loss and its prevention. The Anatomical Record. 2012;**295**(11):1837-1850. DOI: 10.1002/ar.22578

[19] Paken J, Govender CD, Sewram V. Research protocol: Cisplatin-associated ototoxicity amongst patients receiving cancer chemotherapy and the feasibility of an audiological monitoring program. BMC Women's Health. 2017;**17**(1):129. DOI: 10.1186/s12905-017-0486-8

[20] World Health Organization. Addressing the Challenge of Womens Health in Africa. Regional Office for Africa: World Health Organization; 2012. Available from: https://www.afro.who.int/sites/default/files/2017-06/report-of-the-commission-on-womens-health-in-the-african-region-who_acsummary-comp.pdf

[21] Tsu VD, Levin CE. Making the case for cervical cancer prevention: What about equity? Reproductive Health Matters. 2008;**16**(32):104-112. DOI: 10.1016/S0968-8080(08)32411-2

[22] Haugnes HS, Stenklev NC, Brydøy M, Dahl O, Wilsgaard T, Laukli E, et al. Hearing loss before and after cisplatin-based chemotherapy in testicular cancer survivors: A longitudinal study. Acta Oncologica. 2018;**57**(8):1075-1083. DOI: 10.1080/0284186X.2018.1433323

[23] Islam J, Harris GD. Cancer survivor health needs for women. Primary Care. 2018;**45**(4):659-676. DOI: 10.1016/j.pop.2018.07.005

[24] Fausti AS, Wilmington DJ, Helt PV, Helt WJ, Konrad-Martin D. Hearing health and care: The need for improved hearing loss prevention and hearing conservation practices. Journal of Rehabilitation Research and Development. 2005;**42**(s2):45-62. DOI: 10.1682/JRRD.2005.02.0039

[25] Van der Heijden I, Harries J, Abrahams N. Barriers to gender-based violence services and support for women with disabilities in Cape Town, South Africa. Disability & Society. 2019;**35**(442):1-21. DOI: 10.1080/09687599.2019.1690429

[26] Health Professions Council of South Africa. Audiological Management of Patients on Treatment That Includes Ototoxic Medications: Guidelines. 2018. Available from: https://www.hpcsa.co.za/Uploads/SLH/Guidelines%20for%20Audiological%20Management%20of%20Patients%20on%20Treatment%20that%20includes%20Ototoxic%20Medications.pdf

[27] American Academy of Audiology. American Academy of Audiology Position Statement and

Guidelines: Ototoxicity Monitoring. 2009. Available from: https://audiology-web.s3.amazonaws.com/migrated/OtoMonGuidelines.pdf_539974c40999c1.58842217.pdf

[28] American Speech-Language-Hearing Association. Audiologic Management of Individuals Receiving Cochleotoxic Drug Therapy. 1994. Available from: https://www.asha.org/policy/gl1994-00003/

[29] Khoza-Shangase K, Masondo N. What are the current audiological practices for ototoxicity assessment and management in the South African Healthcare Context? International Journal of Environmental Research and Public Health. 2020;**17**(7):1-14. DOI: 10.3390/ijerph17072613

[30] Proctor EK, Landsverk J, Aarons G, Chambers D, Glisson C, Mittman B. Implementation research in mental health services: An emerging science with conceptual, methodological, and training challenges. Administration and Policy in Mental Health. 2009;**36**(1):24-34. DOI: 10.1007/s10488-008-0197-4

[31] Paken J, Govender CD, Pillay M, Sewram V. Cisplatin-associated ototoxicity: A review for the health professional. Journal of Toxicology. 2016;**2016**:13. DOI: 10.1155/2016/1809394

[32] Paken J, Govender CD, Pillay M, Sewram V. Perspectives and practices of ototoxicity monitoring. The South African Journal of Communication Disorders. 2020;**67**(1):e1-e10. DOI: 10.4102/sajcd.v67i1.685

[33] de Andrade V, Khoza-Shangase K, Hajat F. Perceptions of oncologists at two state hospitals in Gauteng regarding the ototoxic effects of cancer chemotherapy: A pilot study. African Journal of Pharmacy and Pharmacology. 2009;**3**(6):307-318. DOI: 10.5897/AJPP.9000214

[34] Khoza-Shangase K, Jina K. Ototoxicity monitoring in general medical practice: Exploring perceptions and practices of general practitioners about drug-induced auditory symptoms. Innovations in Pharmaceuticals and Pharmacotherapy. 2013;**1**(3):250-259. Available from: http://www.innpharmacotherapy.com/VolumeArticles/FullTextPDF/50_17IPPSAOct2013.pdf

[35] Wium A, Gerber B. Ototoxicity management: An investigation into doctors' knowledge and practices, and the roles of audiologists in a tertiary hospital. The South African Journal of Communication Disorders. 2016;**63**(1):1-15. DOI: 10.4102/sajcd.v63i1.174

[36] Dutta A, Venkatesh M, Kashyap R. Study of the effects of chemotherapy on auditory function. Indian Journal of Otolaryngology and Head & Neck Surgery. 2005;**57**(3):226-228. Available from: https://pmc.ncbi.nlm.nih.gov/articles/PMC3451338/pdf/12070_2008_Article_BF03008019.pdf

[37] Allen GC, Tiu C, Koike K, Ritchey AK, Kurs-Lasky M, Wax MK. Transient-evoked otoacoustic emissions in children after cisplatin chemotherapy. Otolaryngology-Head and Neck Surgery. 1998;**118**(5):584-588. Available from: https://aaoh-nsfjournals.onlinelibrary.wiley.com/doi/epdf/10.1177/019459989811800504

[38] Kopelman J, Budnick AS, Sessions RB, Kramer MB, Wong GY. Ototoxicity of high-dose cisplatin by bolus administration in patients with advanced cancers and normal hearing. The Laryngoscope. 1988;**98**(8):858-864. Available from: https://onlinelibrary.wiley.com/doi/epdf/10.1288/00005537-198808000-00014

[39] Theunissen EAR, Zuur CL, Jóźwiak K, Lopez-Yurda M, Hauptmann M, Rasch CRN, et al. Prediction of hearing loss due to cisplatin chemoradiotherapy. JAMA Otolaryngology. Head & Neck Surgery. 2015;**141**(9):810-815. Available from: https://www.researchgate.net/publication/281140309_Prediction_of_Hearing_Loss_Due_to_Cisplatin_Chemoradiotherapy#fullTextFileContent

[40] Gratton MA, Salvi RJ, Kamen BA, Saunders SS. Interaction of cisplatin and noise on the peripheral auditory system. Hearing Research. 1990;**50**(1):211-223. DOI: 10.1016/0378-5955(90)90046-R

[41] Coradini PP, Cigana L, Selistre SG, Rosito LS, Brunetto AL. Ototoxicity from cisplatin therapy in childhood cancer. Journal of Pediatric Hematology/Oncology. 2007;**29**(6):355-360. Available from: https://journals.lww.com/jpho-online/fulltext/2007/06000/ototoxicity_from_cisplatin_therapy_in_childhood.2.aspx

[42] Helson L, Okonkwo E, Anton L, Cvitkovic E. Cis-platinum ototoxicity. Clinical Toxicology. 1978;**13**(4):469-478

[43] Paken J, Govender CD, Pillay M, Feyasa M, Sewram V. Cisplatin-associated ototoxicity amongst cervical cancer patients: A prospective cohort study in South Africa. PLoS ONE. 2023;**18**(4):e0283639. DOI: 10.1371/journal.pone.0283639

[44] Paken J, Govender CD, Pillay M, Ayele BT, Sewram V. Baseline audiological profiling of South African females with cervical cancer: An important attribute for assessing cisplatin-associated ototoxicity. BMC Women's Health. 2021;**21**(1):164. Available from: https://bmcwomenshealth.biomedcentral.com/articles/10.1186/s12905-021-01313-5

[45] Paken J, Govender CD, Pillay M, Sewram V. Cisplatin-associated ototoxicity: Perspectives from a single institution cervical cancer cohort and implications for developing a locally responsive monitoring programme in a public healthcare setting. BMC Health Services Research. 2022;**22**(1):791. DOI: 10.1186/s12913-022-08099-8

[46] Pillay M, Tiwari R, Kathard H, Chikte U. Sustainable workforce: South African audiologists and speech therapists. Human Resources for Health. 2020;**18**(1):47. DOI: 10.1186/s12960-020-00488-6

[47] Moyimane MB, Matlala SF, Kekana MP. Experiences of nurses on the critical shortage of medical equipment at a rural district hospital in South Africa: A qualitative study. The Pan African Medical Journal. 2017;**28**(100):1-8. DOI: 10.11604/pamj.2017.28.100.11641

[48] Essack SY. Models for increasing the health workforce. South African Medical Journal. 2012;**102**(11):830-832. DOI: 10.7196/SAMJ.5779

[49] Khoza-Shangase K, Stirk M. Audiological testing for ototoxicity monitoring in adults with tuberculosis in state hospitals in Gauteng, South Africa. Southern African Journal of Infectious Diseases. 2016;**31**(2):44-49. DOI: 10.1080/23120053.2016.1128143

[50] Swanepoel DW, Sousa KC, Smits C, Moore DR. Mobile applications to detect hearing impairment: Opportunities and challenges. Bulletin of the World Health Organization. 2019;**97**(10):717-718. DOI: 10.2471/BLT.18.227728

[51] Swanepoel DW. eHealth technologies enable more accessible hearing care. Seminars in Hearing. 2020;**41**(2):133-140. DOI: 10.1055/s-0040-1708510

[52] Swanepoel DW, Clark JL, Koekemoer D, Hall JW, Krumm M, Ferrari DV, et al. Telehealth in audiology: The need and potential to reach underserved communities. International Journal of Audiology. 2010;**49**(3):195-202. DOI: 10.3109/14992020903470783

[53] Vijayasingam A, Frost E, Wilkins J, Gillen L, Premachandra P, McLaren K, et al. Tablet and web-based audiometry to screen for hearing loss in adults with cystic fibrosis. Thorax. 2020;**75**(8):632. DOI: 10.1136/thoraxjnl-2019-214177

[54] Coco L. Teleaudiology: Strategies, considerations during a crisis and beyond. The Hearing Journal. 2020;**73**(5):26-28. Available from: https://journals.lww.com/thehearingjournal/toc/2020/05000

[55] Ratanjee-Vanmali H, Swanepoel DW, Laplante-Lévesque A. Strengthening the role of the audiologist in the digital age. The Hearing Journal. 2020;**73**(6):38-39. DOI: 10.1097/01.HJ.0000669892.80715.e1

[56] Saunders GH, Roughley A. Audiology in the time of COVID-19: Practices and opinions of audiologists in the UK. International Journal of Audiology. 2020;**60**(4):1-8. DOI: 10.1080/14992027.2020.1814432

[57] Bornman M, Swanepoel W, De Jager LB, Eikelboom RH. Extended high-frequency smartphone audiometry: Validity and reliability. Journal of the American Academy of Audiology. 2019;**30**(3):217-226. DOI: 10.3766/jaaa.17111

[58] Brittz M, Heinze B, Mahomed-Asmail F, Swanepoel W, Stoltz A. Monitoring hearing in an infectious disease clinic with mHealth technologies. Journal of the American Academy of Audiology. 2019;**30**(6):482-492. DOI: 10.3766/jaaa.17120

[59] Bottomley E. SA has some of Africa's most expensive data, a new report says—But it is better for the richer. Business Insider South Africa. 2020. Available from: https://www.businessinsider.co.za/how-sas-data-prices-compare-with-the-rest-of-the-world-2020-5

[60] Rybak LP, Mukherjea D, Ramkumar V. Mechanisms of cisplatin-induced ototoxicity and prevention. Seminars in Hearing. 2019;**40**(2):197-204. Available from: https://pmc.ncbi.nlm.nih.gov/articles/PMC6486366/pdf/10-1055-s-0039-1684048.pdf

[61] Finocchario-Kessler S, Wexler C, Maloba M, Mabachi N, Ndikum-Moffor F, Bukusi E. Cervical cancer prevention and treatment research in Africa: A systematic review from a public health perspective. BMC Women's Health. 2016;**16**(1):29. DOI: 10.1186/s12905-016-0306-6

[62] Gómez-Ruiz S, Maksimović-Ivanić D, Mijatović S, Kaluđerović GN. On the discovery, biological effects, and use of Cisplatin and metallocenes in anticancer chemotherapy. Bioinorganic Chemistry and Applications. 2012;**140284**:9. DOI: 10.1155/2012/140284

[63] World Health Organization. World Report on Hearing. 2021. Available from: https://cdn.who.int/media/docs/default-source/documents/health-topics/deafness-and-hearing-loss/world-report-on-hearing/wrh-executive-summary.en.pdf?sfvrsn=feb8d533_30&download=true

Chapter 11

Understanding Cervical Cancer in Mozambique: Insights from Patients, Partners, and Families

Iva Duval, Salma Chidassicua, Arminda Eugenio and Jose Chidassicua

Abstract

Cervical cancer (CC) is a significant public health issue in Mozambique, being the most common malignancy among women. This study explores the perceptions of patients, partners, and family members regarding the diagnosis and treatment of CC at the Central Hospital of Maputo. Methods: A qualitative research study was conducted at the Central Hospital of Maputo, involving 18 participants (6 women with CC, 6 partners, and 6 family members). Data were collected through semi-structured interviews and analyzed using thematic analysis. Women exhibited limited awareness of CC and HPV, while partners acknowledged the diagnosis but had a poor understanding of the disease. Family support was generally positive; however, emotional distress and changes in marital relationships were noted. It is essential to implement public health policies focused on educational initiatives regarding CC, involving patients, partners, and family members, as well as to promote preventive campaigns about HPV and the use of condoms.

Keywords: cervical cancer, patient perceptions, HPV awareness, qualitative research, family support

1. Introduction

Cervical cancer (CC) is recognized as a significant global public health problem, being particularly prevalent in developing countries. According to Globocan [1], CC ranks fourth among the most frequent types of cancer among women, with approximately 530 thousand new cases and 265 thousand deaths per year. The reality is alarming, especially in Africa, where the mortality rate is 23 per 100,000 women [2]. Mozambique stands out in this scenario, with CC accounting for about a third of cancer cases among women, partly due to the high prevalence of Human Papillomavirus (HPV) infection [3, 4]. HPV, which can not only cause cervical cancer but also affect male sexual health, has a high spread among the young population, with significant infection rates reported among young women aged 20 to 30 years [5].

Early detection of CC is a crucial aspect to minimize the mortality associated with the disease. Although there are effective screening methods, such as cervical cytology (Pap smear), late diagnosis is still a worrying reality, with about 80% of cases being inoperable at the time of diagnosis [6]. A study by Lorenzoni et al. [7] points out that cervical cancer represents the most common malignant neoplasm among women in central hospitals in Mozambique. The situation is aggravated by the lack of knowledge about the routes of HPV transmission by men, who play a key role not only in the spread of the virus but also in women's reproductive health [8].

In addition to the clinical aspects, the emotional impact of a cancer diagnosis is profound and multiform, affecting not only patients but also their partners and families. Trombini et al. [9] describe the diagnosis period as a time of intense emotional charge, where feelings of fear, dread, and depression are frequently reported. Family and partner support, in turn, is essential in the treatment and recovery phases. Salci and Marcon [10] emphasize that emotional, social, and financial support is vital to overcome the difficulties imposed by the disease.

This study aims to investigate the perception of cancer patients and their partners and family members in relation to the diagnosis and treatment of CC at the Maputo Central Hospital, one of the main health referral centers in Mozambique. Through this research, it is expected to better understand attitudes and knowledge about the disease, as well as the psychological and social impact that CC generates in families. The identification of these aspects can contribute to the development of more effective support and intervention strategies, providing an approach that not only treats the disease but also considers the integral well-being of women and their support network.

2. Methodology

This is a descriptive exploratory study, with a qualitative approach, through which we sought to know in depth the universe of meanings and attitudes of women with cancer and their partners and family members in relation to the diagnosis and treatment of CC at the Maputo Central Hospital. Data collection was carried out during the months of September to November 2022 in the oncology ward of Maputo Central Hospital, which usually admits patients with CC. It is a quaternary level hospital, of national reference, located in the center of Maputo city with the following geographical limitations (north – AV. Agostinho Neto; south – AV. Eduardo Mondlane; to this – AV. Tomás Nduda; and to the west – AV. Salvador Allende).

Data collection began after the women, their partners, and family members were informed of the importance and purpose of the research by signing the Informed Consent Form (ICF). Semi-structured interviews were used as a technique to capture data, and the interviews were recorded and transcribed in full after the participants' consent using the MP4 player as an instrument. An interview script was prepared with the following guiding questions: What are the perceptions of cancer patients, their partners, and family members in relation to the diagnosis and treatment of cervical cancer in the oncology service of the Maputo Central Hospital. This instrument included sociodemographic data for women, their partners, and family members, in which the participants had the opportunity to discuss the theme, addressing aspects such as knowledge about the mode of transmission and attitudes of women, their partners, and family members toward the diagnosis and treatment of CC (See Appendix).

DOI: http://dx.doi.org/10.5772/intechopen.1008177

Through convenience sampling, defined by the criterion of data saturation and recurrence of information, but taking into account those that were not repetitive, the total size of research subjects to be interviewed was composed of 18 participants, 6 women with CC, 6 partners of women diagnosed with CC, and 6 family members.

For data analysis, the theme of content analysis proposed by Bardin was used. For the purpose of understanding and preserving the confidentiality of the women's identity, their partners and family members were identified by the letters "EN" added to the sequential number of the interviews.

The research project was approved by the Institutional Committee of Bioethics for Health of the Higher Institute of Health Sciences - ISCISA (CIBS - ISCISA) under number TFCSPID20/19 and respected the principles of the Declaration of Helsinki that establish the criteria for research involving human beings. All the information obtained during this study was handled confidentially by the researcher responsible for the study.

3. Results and discussion

3.1 Sociodemographic characteristics of the participants

The study involved interviews with six women diagnosed with cervical cancer (CC), six partners, and an equal number of family members, all of whom were admitted to the Oncology service at Maputo Central Hospital. Among the women, half were over 40 years old; all were employed in the informal sector, and five identified as evangelical Christians. Two women had completed primary education, two had completed secondary education, and two had attained higher education (**Table 1**).

These findings are consistent with research conducted by Dejeane Barro and Regina Lopes [11], which noted that the incidence of cervical cancer is rare in women under 30 years of age, peaking between the ages of 45 and 50. Additionally, a study by Allanda Santos et al. [12] highlighted that HPV infections tend to regress spontaneously in women under 30, whereas persistent infections are more commonly observed

Variables	Features	Women	Partners	Family
Acts	30–39 years	3	0	6
	40–49	3	6	0
Education level	Primary	2	0	0
	Secondary	2	1	1
	Academic	2	5	5
Profession	Formal	0	1	3
	Informal	6	5	3
Religion	Catholic	1	1	1
	Evangelical	5	3	5
	No	0	2	0
Total		**6**	**6**	**6**

Table 1.
Characteristics of participants.

in older women. Moreover, Allanda Santos et al. [12] indicated that limited access to health information may be correlated with low educational attainment, potentially resulting in delayed health-seeking behavior and subsequently late CC screening.

The partners of the women interviewed ranged in age from 40 to 50 years. Five partners had completed high school and were employed in the informal sector, and three identified as evangelical Christians. Family members were all under 40 years old; five had completed high school and identified as evangelical Christians (**Table 1**).

3.2 Women's knowledge about cervical Cancer

All interviewed women reported having heard about cervical cancer at some point in their lives, although most lacked detailed knowledge about the disease. These findings align with the research conducted by Santos et al. [13], which indicated that 45% of women surveyed had heard of cervical cancer but could not articulate its specifics.

> *"I just know it's an infection..." (EN02)*
> *"I heard... but heee I've already made it happen..." (EN03)*

Knowledge of cervical cancer is essential for women to prevent this pathology through early screening. When asked about their understanding of cervical cancer, the majority of women (five out of six) demonstrated some awareness of the disease. Allan Santos et al. [13] noted similar findings, suggesting that knowledge about cervical cancer is generally low among women due to inadequate information and deficiencies in educational programs that promote effective health actions. These conclusions are consistent with those of Allan Santos et al. [13], who found that many women approached health facilities primarily for symptomatic concerns rather than for preventive measures.

Responses from participants included:

> *"I can't say what it is; I just know that it's a disease that affects the uterus." (EN01)*
> *"It is a disease that enters through the uterus and sometimes causes problems, making the belly swell due to accumulating blood." (EN05)*
> *"This disease attacks the uterus and causes bleeding." (EN03)*

Concerning the transmission mode, all interviewed women expressed a lack of understanding regarding how cervical cancer is transmitted. Al-Naggar et al. [14] reported that over 50% of participants in their study were unaware of HPV transmission methods.

> *"To tell the truth, I can't say." (EN01)*
> *"Honestly, I don't know how to get this disease." (EN04)*
> *"Hiiii, I don't know; maybe if I had known, I would have avoided it." (EN02)*

All participants reported that they neither smoked nor consumed alcoholic beverages. However, they exhibited uncertainty and fear regarding how they contracted cervical cancer.

Luciana Buosis [15] noted that tobacco can exacerbate HPV-infected tissues' susceptibility to mutations while reducing Langerhans cells, which play a critical role in the immune response. Research by Sang-Soo Seo et al. [16] demonstrated that women who consume alcohol while being exposed to tobacco have a higher risk of persistent HPV infection, while those not exposed to these substances have a lower risk. Therefore, the participants' denial of smoking and alcohol use may indicate an attempt to dissociate from socially stigmatized risk factors.

3.3 Sexual and reproductive health

The average age for the onset of sexual activity among participants was 18 years. Allan Dantas dos Santos et al. [13] similarly found that the average age of sexual debut among their interviewees was approximately 17.8 years, corroborating our findings. Early initiation of sexual activity (prior to age 18) is associated with an increased risk of cervical cancer due to greater exposure to carcinogenic agents [17].

Most participants reported having between two and five children, a reflection of societal values where larger families are often perceived as a sign of prosperity. These findings align with a systematic review by Tekalegn Yohannes et al. [18], which indicated an elevated risk of cervical cancer among women with multiple pregnancies.

Participants were also questioned about their number of sexual partners in lifetime: two indicated they had only one sexual partner, one reported seven, and three reported three sexual partners. Studies suggest that women with more than two sexual partners face a five-fold increase in the incidence of cervical HPV lesions [19].

Sakshi Basoya and Ashish Anjankar [20] posited that the use of condoms during sexual intercourse is a primary preventative measure against cervical cancer by mitigating HPV infection risks. While all women reported using condoms at the onset of sexual activity, they eventually discontinued their use due to trust in their partners.

> *"At first, we used it, but after the first child, we didn't."* (EN01)
> *"He's my husband; we don't use it."* (EN02)
> *"We used it at first, yes."* (EN03)

Sexually transmitted infections (STIs) are recognized as contributing factors to cervical cancer development [21]. All interviewed women acknowledged having had STIs in the past, which were treated at local health facilities. One participant reported never using a contraceptive method, while the others cited using Depo-Provera or oral contraceptive pills. Oral contraceptive use may influence HPV genome transcription, as noted by Adriane Cristina Bovo et al. [22].

3.4 Women's attitudes toward the diagnosis and treatment of cervical cancer

Most participants expressed feelings of anguish, despair, fear, and melancholy. Similar results have been reported in studies conducted by Dinah Kassaman et al. [23] and Patience Asante et al. [24], which find that many women not only experienced fear and despair but also harbored doubts about the effectiveness of available treatments.

Upon receiving a diagnosis of CC, patients described the experience as arduous, marked by feelings of sadness and dread, as well as fear of death and an existential questioning of their circumstances. As one participant articulated,

> *"I was desperate, I put everything in God's hands."* (EN02)

Another shared,

> *"I was very sad, I cried a lot."* (EN03)

A third participant noted,

> *"(...) I was very distressed and desperate, I don't even know how I got home." (EN04)*

Regarding challenges encountered during treatment, all women reported that they were managing well overall. However, two participants mentioned experiencing symptoms such as diarrhea, mucositis, myalgias, and anemia. It was also observed that some women experienced a decline in self-esteem attributed to physical weakness as well as other factors. Research has indicated that chemotherapy can lead to various physiological changes, with common side effects including hair loss, anxiety, nausea, vomiting, anemia, fatigue, and digestive disturbances [25, 26].

All participants unanimously expressed appreciation for the support they received from their families, including their partners, and they conveyed satisfaction with this support. According to Emma Ream et al. [27], family support during such challenging times is paramount, as it assists individuals in making decisions to persevere with treatment despite its side effects and the associated challenges.

3.5 Partners' knowledge about cervical cancer

Understanding the experiences of the partners of women with CC is critical, as they play a fundamental role in providing care and support during challenging health crises [28]. Partners were queried about their knowledge of their partner's cancer diagnosis. Most men recognized that their partners had cancer but could not specify the type, with only one correctly identifying it as cervical cancer. This aligns with findings by Charity Binka [28], which highlighted men's limited awareness of their partners' cervical cancer diagnoses.

Responses included:

> *"I know it's just cancer". (EN01)*
> *"My wife has cancer" (EN02).*
> *"She suffers from uterine cancer." (EN03)*

Partners' awareness of cervical cancer transmission paths was also assessed. Unprotected sexual activity is recognized as a primary transmission pathway for cervical cancer [29]; however, all partners interviewed could not specify these routes, despite numerous public health campaigns by the Mozambique Ministry of Health.

Similar findings were observed by Hae Kim et al. [30], who noted that none of the 12 men interviewed could identify cervical cancer transmission routes. Likewise, Pedro Pedreira et al. [8] reported that men held misconceptions surrounding cervical cancer and were largely uninformed regarding transmission pathways.

Responses from men included:

> *"No, I don't know how it is transmitted." (ENO4)*
> *"I've never heard of how this disease originates." (EN05)*
> *"I can't say how a woman gets this disease." (EN06)*

3.6 Support from partners at diagnosis of cervical cancer

It is crucial for men to accompany their partners to health units, as a cervical cancer diagnosis presents significant challenges in the couple's marital life. When asked, all partners stated that they were not present when their partners received their cervical cancer diagnosis. Many were busy with work or family responsibilities. This finding supports previous research demonstrating that many men fail to accompany their partners to health appointments due to various obstacles, including time constraints, hostility from healthcare professionals, transportation issues, and uncertainty regarding how to provide support following a diagnosis [31–33].

Statements from participants included:

"I was at work." (EN01)
"That day, I couldn't go with her." (EN02)
"I had too much work and couldn't be there." (EN03)

3.7 Partner support following cervical cancer diagnosis

Although all men stated they were not present at the time of diagnosis, they reported actively participating in their partners' treatment process. All indicated helping to acquire medications, providing transportation for hospital visits, and seeking blood donors. These findings echo those of Charity Binka et al. [28], in Ghana, where many men reported providing financial, material, social, and emotional support to their partners.

Responses included:

"I've been coming here day after day, haaaaa, now I'm coming here, let's go there" (EN01)
"Always, I come to the hospital, when they prescribe medication I do everything" (EN02)
"When I need blood donors, I go out to look for them" (EN03)"

3.8 Implications of cervical cancer on marital life

All partners reported that cervical cancer led to a cessation of sexual activity due to the pain experienced by women during intercourse. Changes in the couple's daily routine were noted, particularly concerning the time that women spent receiving treatment. Statements from participants included:

"We had to stop, she suffers to have sex, xii... pains" (EN04)
"What has changed is not being at ease, all the time in the hospital, there are a lot of things that are damaged at home" (EN05)
"It changed our routine at home" (EN06)

These findings align with results from Suelem Magalhães [34], in Brazil, where 90% of women with cervical cancer reported negative effects on their marital life. Furthermore, many men indicated that their sexual lives had changed due to their partner's health condition [28, 35]. Leucorrhea with an unpleasant odor, a common symptom of cervical cancer, has also contributed to the reduction of sexual contact between couples [28].

3.9 Extramarital relationships

In the Mozambican context, where polygamy [36, 37], is culturally "accepted," maintaining regular sexual activity is vital for marital stability. Due to their partner's health condition, most men reported having other sexual partners, and all but one acknowledged not using condoms in these extramarital relationships. Such behaviors increase the risk of HPV transmission and subsequent cases of cervical cancer.

Statements from participants included:

> *"I have a girlfriend." (EN02)*
> *"I have someone; I don't use condoms." (EN03)*
> *"I have someone on the side; no condom." (EN06)*

Parallel findings were reported by Charity Binka et al. [28], where men acknowledged engaging in extramarital relationships due to their partner's illness. Men's sexual behaviors, characterized by multiple partners and a lack of condom use, pose additional health risks to women, as they may facilitate HPV transmission [38]. Unprotected sex and having multiple sexual partners are recognized risk factors for cervical cancer [19].

3.10 Family perspectives

According to Dwi Kurniasih et al. [39], knowledge about cervical cancer and its progression can significantly enhance the support provided by families to patients. Family members were queried about their familiarity with cervical cancer. Most participants reported having heard of the disease but demonstrated limited understanding of its specifics. For some, cervical cancer was perceived as a "wound in the uterus," while others regarded it as a form of bleeding.

These findings are consistent with research conducted by Zintle Gwavu et al. [40] and Allan Santos et al. [13], where many interviewees could not articulate the nature of cervical cancer but had heard of it.

Responses included:

> *"Cervical cancer, as I understand, is an incurable infection, but treatment can lead to recovery if diagnosed early." (EN01)*
> *"I cannot explain it well; I only know that cervical cancer exists." (EN02)*
> *"I have heard of it because my mother has the same condition; I think it's a sore in the uterus." (EN03)*
> *"I know it's a disease that causes significant bleeding in women and is often fatal." (F04)*

3.11 Knowledge of family members regarding the causes of cervical cancer

Half of the family members interviewed were unable to identify causes of cervical cancer, while the other half attributed it to sexual contact and/or sexually transmitted infections. Human Papillomavirus (HPV) is the primary risk factor for precursors of cervical cancer [41, 42]. None of the family members interviewed could accurately specify its causes.

Responses included:

> *"I don't know, but my mother when this disease started they said they were fibroids, until now they say she has cancer, but I don't know what causes it" (EN01)*
> *"I always ask myself this question, is it through the discharge? DTS? From sex, the positions we do? I don't know" (EN03)*
> *"Maybe the person gets beaten through sex" (EN04)*

3.12 Knowledge of family members regarding transmission routes of cervical cancer

Family members offered divergent opinions regarding transmission pathways. Some linked transmission with poor genital care or hygiene, while others mentioned sexual intercourse or expressed uncertainty.

Responses included:

> *"Maybe it can be through sex" (EN04)*
> *"Is it from sex? I don't know" (EN05)*
> *"When the woman does not have good hygiene perhaps" (EN06)*

The divergent opinions among family members regarding the transmission pathways of cervical cancer reveal gaps in knowledge, particularly around the understanding of HPV.

The reference to hygiene as a potential risk factor could reflect broader socio-cultural misconceptions about women's health, where cleanliness is wrongly associated with cancer prevention. The health education interventions that clarify the nature of HPV transmission can help to demystify these beliefs and shift the focus toward evidence-based preventive measures such as vaccination and regular Pap tests [43].

3.13 Attitudes of family members toward the diagnosis

According to Livia Urtiga et al. [44], family support is crucial for ensuring that patients with cervical cancer can navigate their diagnosis in a secure and calm environment. Family members expressed feelings of pain, fear, and despair upon hearing about their loved one's diagnosis while simultaneously conveying hope and faith in their recovery. Their religious beliefs provided significant emotional support during this challenging time [44].

Responses included:

> *"We were shocked and fearful; I wondered if I would face this too." (EN02)*
> *"It was very shocking and a lot to handle; I pray daily for skilled doctors to assist." (EN03)*
> *"We were distressed and confused, as I thought cervical cancer was incurable." (EN04)*

3.14 Attitudes of family members toward treatment

Family support is crucial for cervical cancer patients to maintain hope and commitment to treatment [39, 45, 46]. Family members affirmed that they provided social, economic, spiritual, and emotional support. These findings corroborate studies highlighting the significance of family encouragement in enabling patients to face treatment challenges.

Responses included:

> *"I talk to her and encourage her not to give up." (EN01)*
> *"I ensure she makes it to chemotherapy sessions." (EN02)*
> *"When blood donations are needed, we actively seek donors." (EN03)*

Despite encountering various side effects from chemotherapy, such as mood swings, nausea, and lack of appetite, family members reported offering necessary assistance, including medications for nausea and emotional support.

Responses included:

> *"She gets irritable and sensitive; we help by providing water and medication." (EN02)*
> *"She has been complying with treatment but suffers from nausea and loss of appetite; we buy suitable foods for her." (EN03)*
> *"Her physical appearance has changed drastically; she doesn't eat well and has been vomiting." (EN04)*

4. Conclusion

Cervical cancer poses a significant public health challenge in developing countries such as Mozambique, predominantly affecting women from lower socioeconomic backgrounds. The limited awareness of cervical cancer among women, along with their family members, underscores the urgent need for enhanced educational initiatives regarding the importance of early screening.

This study indicates that women with cervical cancer, along with their partners and families, displayed limited knowledge regarding the disease. This necessitates governmental and partner engagement in comprehensive educational programs focused on primary prevention and awareness, especially in schools and community settings.

Upon receiving a cervical cancer diagnosis, women and their families often experience feelings of anguish, fear, and self-doubt. Psychosocial support is essential for navigating these difficult experiences. Despite potentially adverse reactions to chemotherapy, the women reported receiving emotional, spiritual, financial, and social support from their partners and families. Family and community support systems play pivotal roles in helping cervical cancer patients approach their diagnosis with hope and resilience.

The repercussions of cervical cancer extend to marital relationships, often resulting in reduced sexual activity and increases in extramarital relations among partners, contributing to heightened risks associated with HPV transmission. Without adequate protective measures, these patterns pose additional public health risks and underscore the need for comprehensive approaches to cervical cancer prevention and treatment.

Appendix

A. Interview guide

B. Appendix 1: Interview guide for women

B.1 Participants' background information

Demographic information:

B.2 Age

- Gender:
- Educational Level:

- Occupation:
- Marital Status:
- Number of Children (if applicable):

CC Knowledge

1. Have you ever heard of CC? If so, in your opinion what is CC?
2. Could you tell me how you knew you have CC? In your opinion, how does CC appear?

Risk factors

1. Do you consume any alcohol or tobacco?
2. How old were you when did you have your first sexual intercourse?
3. How many children do you have and how old did you have your first child?
4. I am now going to ask a sensitive question, but I would like you to answer me honestly. Could you tell me how many men you had sexual involvement with before the disease you have been diagnosed?
5. Did you always use condoms in your sexual relations? If not why?
6. Have you ever contracted a sexually transmitted disease? If so, how many times? Did you go to the health unit for treatment? Have you ever used oral contraceptive? For how long?

Diagnosis of CC.

1. On the day you went to the health facility for cervical screening or consultation, did you go alone, or did someone accompany you?
2. At the time you received the diagnosis that you have CC, what was your reaction?
3. When you learned of the diagnosis, who was the first person who revealed your health condition? Why?
4. Have you revealed to your husband that you have CC? If not why? If so, what was your partner's reaction?
5. In addition to your partner, have you revealed to other family members that you have CC? If so, what was the family's reaction?

Treatment of CC.

1. Could you tell me how the treatment is going? Is there any difficulty you face in relation to treatment? If so, which ones?

2. Regarding treatment, have you received any support/encouragement from your partner and your family? If so, which ones?

Women's attitudes toward diagnosis and treatment

1. Are you satisfied with the support of your family and your partner? If yes or no, why?

2. Do you want to ask me any questions? Thank you very much for your time.

Future perspectives and suggestions

1. What recommendations would you make for improving awareness and education about cervical cancer in your community?

2. What additional support do you believe is necessary for women diagnosed with cervical cancer and their families?

Closing:

- Thank you for your time and insights today. Is there anything else you would like to add regarding your experiences with cervical cancer, or any questions you have for us?

C. Appendix 2: interview guide for (men) partners

C.1 Relationship context

- How are you related to the woman diagnosed with cervical cancer? (e.g., partner, family member)

- How long have you known the wife diagnosed with cervical cancer?

Knowledge of CC.

1. What do you understand about cervical cancer and its causes?

2. What are your thoughts on how cervical cancer is transmitted?

3. Have you had any conversations with the woman about her diagnosis? What was discussed?

Diagnosis of CC.

1. Were you with your wife at the time the diagnosis was made? If not, why?

2. What was your reaction at that moment?

3. Could you tell me what implications this disease has brought to your married life?

4. What changes did this disease bring to the family?

Treatment and support experience

1. Have you accompanied your wife at the time of treatment? If not why?

2. How did you feel when your partner was diagnosed with cervical cancer?

3. What kind of support do you believe you provided to her?

Risk factor

1. I am now going to ask a sensitive question, but I would like you to answer it truthfully. Do you have other sexual partners? If so, do you use condoms in these relationships?

Future perspectives and suggestions

1. What recommendations would you make for improving awareness and education about cervical cancer in your community?

2. What additional support do you believe is necessary for women diagnosed with cervical cancer and their families?

Closing:

- Thank you for your time and insights today. Is there anything else you would like to add regarding your experiences with cervical cancer, or any questions you have for us?

Thank you very much for your time

D. Appendix 3: interview guide for family members

D.1 Relationship context

- How are you related to the woman diagnosed with cervical cancer? (e.g., partner, family member)

- How long have you known the woman diagnosed with cervical cancer?

Knowledge of CC.

1. To begin with, I would like to know in your perception, what is cervical cancer?

2. In your opinion, what is the cause of CC?

3. What are the routes of transmission of CC?

Diagnosis of CC.

1. When she revealed that she has CC in her family, how did you feel? What came to your mind? What was the reaction that the family had when they learned that she had this disease?

2. What changes did this disease bring to the family?

Treatment experiences

1. Have you/family joined her for any treatments? What has that experience been like?

2. How have you or family supported her during this process?

3. What are the difficulties she has faced to continue with the treatment? Can you explain whether these difficulties are related to the effects of the medication, or the type of work it does or some other reason? How has it overcome these difficulties?

Changes in relationships and daily life

1. How has your family dynamic changed since the diagnosis?

2. Are there any noticeable changes in the way you interact with the diagnosed woman?

Future perspectives and suggestions

1. What recommendations would you make for improving awareness and education about cervical cancer in your community?

2. What additional support do you believe is necessary for women diagnosed with cervical cancer and their families?

Closing:

Thank you for your time and insights today. Is there anything else you would like to add regarding your experiences with cervical cancer, or any questions you have for us?

Author details

Iva Duval[1], Salma Chidassicua[2], Arminda Eugenio[3] and Jose Chidassicua[4*]

1 Central Hospital Maputo - HCM, Mozambique

2 Federal University of Alfenas – UNIFAL, MG, Brazil

3 Pact Saude, Mozambique

4 National Institute of Health, Eduardo Mondlane University, Mozambique

*Address all correspondence to: jchidassicua@gmail.com

References

[1] GLOBOCAN. Cervix uteri source: Globocan 2020. International Agency for Research Cervic Uteri. 2020;**419**:1-10

[2] Bray F, Ferlay J, Soerjomataram I, Siegel RL, Torre LA, Jemal A. Global cancer statistics 2018: GLOBOCAN estimates of incidence and mortality worldwide for 36 cancers in 185 countries. CA: a Cancer Journal for Clinicians. 2018;**68**(6):394-424

[3] ICO, IARC. Human Papillomavirus and Related Diseases Report: Mozambique [Internet]. Lyon, France: ICO, IARC; 2023

[4] Menendez YA, Cambaco O, Mindú C, Nhantumbo H, Uamusse T, Matsinhe G, et al. Lay knowledge of cervical cancer in Manhiça district, Mozambique: A qualitative study. Reproductive Health. 2020;**17**(1):1-12

[5] Gravdal BH, Lönnberg S, Skare GB, Sulo G, Bjørge T. Cervical cancer in women under 30 years of age in Norway: A population-based cohort study. BMC Womens Health [Internet]. 2021;**21**(1):1-8. DOI: 10.1186/s12905-021-01242-3

[6] Dasgupta S. The efficiency of cervical pap and comparison of conventional pap smear and liquid-based cytology: A review. Cureus. 2023;**15**(11):1-16

[7] Lorenzoni CF, Ferro J, Carrilho C, Colombet M, Parkin DM. Cancer in Mozambique: Results from two population-based cancer registries. International Journal of Cancer. 2020;**147**(6):1629-1637

[8] Pedreira PWF, JMC DS, Monteiro BKSM, Dias JMG. Man's perception of the human papillomavirus infection - HPV. Revista Médica Minas Gerais. 2015;**25**(3):322-329

[9] Trombini C, Mattos D, Velloso S, Oliveira S, Tavares M. Percepção da mulher frente ao diagnóstico e tratamento do câncer do colo do útero - Subsídios para o cuidado de enfermagem. Revista Pró-UniverSUS. 2012;**5**:27-35

[10] Salci MA, Marcon SS. Enfrentamento do câncer em família. Texto Context - Enferm. 2011;**20**(spe):178-186

[11] de Barros DO, RLM L. Mulheres com câncer invasivo do colo uterino: suporte familiar como auxílio. Revista Brasileira de Enfermagem. 2007;**60**(3):295-298

[12] Rodrigues Santos AM, de Lima B, Holanda J, De e Marques Oliveira Silva J, dos Pereira Santos AA, Melo Silva E. Câncer de colo uterino: conhecimento e comportamento de mulheres para prevenção. Rev Bras em promoção da Saúde. 2015;**28**(2):153-159

[13] Santos A, de Maria Andrade Santos P, Bezerra Santos M, dos María Dantas Santos A. Conhecimento De Mulheres Sobre O Câncer De Colo Uterino Em Um Município Do Nordeste Do Brasil. Revista Iberoamericana de Educación e Investigación Enfermería. 2015;**5**(3):64-76

[14] Al-Naggar RA, Low WY, Isa ZM. Knowledge and barriers towards cervical cancer screening among young women in Malaysia. Asian Pacific Journal of Cancer Prevention. 2010;**11**(4):867-873

[15] Buosi L. A abordagem do parceiro de mulheres diagnosticadas com HPV. Brasilia, DF: Escola Superior de Ciências da Saúde; 2007

[16] Seo SS, Oh HY, Kim MK, Lee DO, Chung YK, Kim JY, et al. Combined effect of secondhand smoking and alcohol drinking on risk of persistent human papillomavirus infection. BioMed Research International. 2019;**2019**:1-9

[17] Mekonnen AG, Mittiku YM. Early-onset of sexual activity as a potential risk of cervical cancer in Africa: A review of literature. PLOS Global Public Health [Internet]. 2023;**3**(3):1-13. DOI: 10.1371/journal.pgph.0000941

[18] Tekalegn Y, Sahiledengle B, Woldeyohannes D, Atlaw D, Degno S, Desta F, et al. High parity is associated with increased risk of cervical cancer: Systematic review and meta-analysis of case–control studies. Women's Health. 2022;**18**:1-11

[19] Huang Y, Wu X, Lin Y, Li W, Liu J, Song B. Multiple sexual partners and vaginal microecological disorder are associated with HPV infection and cervical carcinoma development. Oncology Letters. 2020;**20**(2):1915-1921

[20] Basoya S, Anjankar A. Cervical cancer: Early detection and prevention in reproductive age group. Cureus. 2022;**14**(11):1-7

[21] Cunha MMCM. Normas nacionais para prevenção do cancro do colo uterino. MISAU - Programa Nacional de prevenção e Control do cancro do colo uterino e da mama; 2007

[22] Bovo AC, Pedrão PG, Guimarães YM, Godoy LR, Resende JCP, Longatto-Filho A, et al. Combined oral contraceptive use and the risk of cervical cancer: Literature review. Revista Brasileira de Ginecologia e Obstetrícia. 2023;**45**(12):E818-E824

[23] Kassaman D, Mushani T, Kiraithe P, Brownie S, Barton-Burke M. Fear, faith and finances: Health literacy experiences of English and Swahili speaking women newly diagnosed with breast and cervical cancer. Ecancermedicalscience. 2022;**16**:1-21

[24] Okyere Asante PG, Owusu AY, Oppong JR, Amegah KE, Nketiah-Amponsah E. The psychosocial burden of women seeking treatment for breast and cervical cancers in Ghana's major cancer hospitals. PLoS One [Internet]. 2023;**18**(8 August):1-14. DOI: 10.1371/journal.pone.0289055

[25] Society AC. Treating Cervical Cancer. American Cancer Society. [Internet]. 2021. Available from: https://www.cancer.org/cancer/types/cervical-cancer/treating.html [Accessed: September 15, 2024]

[26] Anand U, Dey A, Chandel AKS, Sanyal R, Mishra A, Pandey DK, et al. Cancer chemotherapy and beyond: Current status, drug candidates, associated risks and progress in targeted therapeutics. Genes & Diseases. 2023;**10**(4):1367-1401

[27] Ream E, Richardson A, Lucas G, Marcu A, Foster R, Fuller G, et al. Understanding the support needs of family members of people undergoing chemotherapy: A longitudinal qualitative study. European Journal of Oncology Nursing [Internet]. 2021;**50**(November 2019):1-10. DOI: 10.1016/j.ejon.2020.101861

[28] Binka C, Doku DT, Nyarko SH, Awusabo-Asare K. Male support for cervical cancer screening and treatment in rural Ghana. PLoS One. 2019;**14**(11):1-10

[29] Petca A, Borislavschi A, Zvanca M, Petca RC, Sandru F, Dumitrascu M. Non-sexual HPV transmission and role of

vaccination for a better future (review). Experimental and Therapeutic Medicine. 2020;**20**(6):1-1

[30] Kim HW, Kim DH, Kim Y. Men's awareness of cervical cancer: A qualitative study. BMC Women's Health. 2018;**18**(1):1-10

[31] Adeniran AS, Aboyeji AP, Fawole AA. Male partner's role during pregnancy, labour and delivery: Expectations of pregnant women in Nigeria. International Journal of Health Sciences (Qassim). 2015;**9**(3):301-309

[32] Muloongo H, Sitali D, Zulu JM, Hazemba AN, Mweemba O. Men's perspectives on male participation in antenatal care with their pregnant wives: A case of a military hospital in Lusaka, Zambia. BMC Health Services Research. 2019;**19**(1):1-9

[33] Nesane K, Maputle SM, Shilubane H. Male partners' views of involvement in maternal healthcare services at Makhado municipality clinics, Limpopo Province, South Africa. African Journal of Primary Health & Family Medicine. 2016;**8**(2):1-5

[34] Magalhães SVD, dos Moreira CS, TGGG C. Estudo da relação conjugal no contexto da doença crônica de um dos cônjuges. Revisão Integrativa. 2019;**8**:1-7

[35] Rosser JI, Zakaras JM, Hamisi S, Huchko MJ. Men's knowledge and attitudes about cervical cancer screening in Kenya. BMC Women's Health. 2014;**14**(1):1-7

[36] Carlos A, Frederico M, Dade A. Tendências e Factores Associados à Maternidade Precoce em Moçambique. Maputo, Mozambique: Center for African Studies; 2015. 31 p

[37] Tiago JA. Conflitos de género em niketche de paulina chiziane. Maputo, Mozambique: UEM; 2014

[38] Ampofo AG, Boyes AW, Asibey SO, Oldmeadow C, Mackenzie LJ. Prevalence and correlates of modifiable risk factors for cervical cancer and HPV infection among senior high school students in Ghana: A latent class analysis. BMC Public Health [Internet]. 2023;**23**(1):1-12. DOI: 10.1186/s12889-022-14908-w

[39] Kurniasih D, Titihalawa EM, Tiningsih SVR. Family support in cervical cancer patients treated: A qualitative case study. Malahayati International Journal of Nursing And Health Science. 2023;**6**(5):399-404

[40] Gwavu Z, Murray D, Okafor UB. Perception of women's knowledge of and attitudes towards cervical cancer and papanicolaou smear screenings: A qualitative study in South Africa. Healthcare. 2023;**11**(14):1-4

[41] Fantin C, Freitas JB, Teles HFM, Oliveira BAS, Brito DV. High prevalence of HPV 18 and multiple infections with oncogenic HPV genotypes in women at risk of cervical cancer examined in Manaus, Brazil. Brazilian Journal of Medical and Biological Research. 2023;**56**:1-7

[42] Mariño JM, Rocha DAP, dos Reis RS, de Souza MG, SCC S, JCA P, et al. HPV-positive women living in isolated areas in Amazonas, Brazil: Clinical–epidemiological profile and cytological findings. Cad Saúde Coletiva. 2024;**32**(1):1-9

[43] Krokidi E, Rao AP, Ambrosino E, Thomas PPM. The impact of health education interventions on HPV vaccination uptake, awareness, and acceptance among people under 30 years old in India: A literature review

with systematic search. Frontiers in Reproductive Health. 2023;**5**(May):1-13

[44] Vardar O, Ozkan S. Spirituality and religion in coping in cancer patients and caregivers. JERN. 2021;**18**:462-4666

[45] Yunitasari E. Optimizing of family support in improving resilience of cervical cancer client post radikal hysterectomy and bilateral salpingo oophorectomy which is getting. Chemotherapy. 2017;**3**(Inc):219-222

[46] Yumni FL. The relationship between family support and quality of life of cervical cancer patients in Rumah Singgah Sasana Marsudi Husada Indonesia. Critical Medical and Surgical Nursing Journal. 2023;**12**(1):14-18

Section 4

Gynecology Endocrinology

Chapter 12

Empowering Women in Priority Attention Zones of Tijuana: A Transdisciplinary Participatory Intervention to Address Socioeconomic and Cultural Vulnerabilities and Promote Gender Equity

Jimmy Emmanuel Ramos Valencia and Martha Cecilia Jaramillo Cardona

Abstract

This chapter focuses on the unique vulnerabilities and inequalities faced by women in the Priority Attention Zones (ZAP) of Tijuana, areas marked by significant socioeconomic and cultural challenges. The research aims to address gender inequity through a transdisciplinary participatory social intervention, enhancing women's capacities, skills, and knowledge to improve their health and well-being with a gender equity approach. The methodology includes situational analysis, identification of ZAP, pre-intervention diagnostics, and the implementation and evaluation of an intervention-action plan. The chapter underscores the importance of public policies that facilitate access to education, employment, health, and security, promoting women's well-being and rights. Additionally, it reviews relevant literature supporting the effectiveness of participatory interventions in women's health and well-being, emphasizing the need for holistic strategies that recognize the complexity and diversity of women's needs. This research aims to demonstrate significant improvements in quality of life and gender equity through the practical application of these models and theories in Tijuana.

Keywords: gender equity, participatory social intervention, Priority Attention Zones, women empowerment, well-being

1. Introduction

In the ongoing global pursuit of gender equity, substantial barriers remain that restrict the empowerment and holistic development of women. This research is positioned within a critical context where gender equality transcends being an aspirational goal and emerges as an urgent requirement for sustainable development and the protection of fundamental human rights. The study zeros in on the Priority Attention Zones (ZAP) of Tijuana, regions defined by distinct socioeconomic and cultural challenges, where women are particularly vulnerable and face unique inequalities.

This research specifically targets the gender inequities that manifest as social and labor disparities within Tijuana's Priority Attention Zones (ZAP). By employing a transdisciplinary and participatory socio-educational intervention, the study aims to strengthen the social fabric, with a focused effort on enhancing the capacities, competencies, and knowledge of women. The initiative seeks to improve women's health and well-being within a framework of gender equality, directly addressing the specific needs and expectations of women residing in these zones.

The importance of this project is underscored by its potential to narrow gender gaps at the local level, with broader implications for advancing global gender equity. The study operates on the hypothesis that a participatory social intervention, centered on women and informed by the identification of their specific needs, can serve as an effective mechanism to improve their quality of life and foster their development. To achieve this, the research aims to conduct a comprehensive diagnosis of the needs and expectations of women in the ZAP, with the ultimate goal of designing and implementing a participatory social intervention that empowers women across various dimensions of social and economic life.

The methodology proposed for this study is both comprehensive and innovative, integrating situational analysis with the identification and delimitation of the ZAP, followed by the execution of pre-intervention diagnostics. This is further supported by the implementation and impact assessment of an intervention-action plan. This methodological framework emphasizes the necessity for public policies that prioritize improving the quality of life for women, facilitating access to education, employment, health, and security in an environment that supports their well-being and upholds their rights.

Grounded in the belief that full access to human rights is essential for achieving equality and living a dignified life, this project advocates for a holistic approach that positions public policies and these rights at its core. The project's structure meticulously outlines each phase, from situational analysis to the evaluation of the intervention's impact, with the dual aim of enhancing the lives of women in Tijuana's ZAP and contributing to global knowledge and practices in the fields of social intervention and gender equity. Consequently, this study represents a significant contribution to social and political research, with the potential to influence public policies and practices both locally and nationally.

2. Addressing gender inequality through participatory social interventions in Tijuana's Priority Attention Zones

Since 2015, the team from the Faculty of Economics and International Relations at the Autonomous University of Baja California has played a crucial role in supporting

DOI: http://dx.doi.org/10.5772/intechopen.1007166

social-based microenterprises in the state of Baja California. This effort has led to the formalization of 12,000 businesses, of which 70% are led by women. The experience accumulated over these years has enabled the team to develop a robust methodology for assistance and training, which has not only been successfully implemented in these microenterprises but has also been shared in various academic forums and scientific publications [1].

The present project, titled "Social Intervention for the Pursuit of Well-being with Equity in Women Living in Priority Attention Zones," arises from the need to address the deep gender inequalities that persist in the Priority Attention Zones (ZAP) of Tijuana. These areas, characterized by high levels of poverty and social exclusion, present unique challenges that disproportionately affect women, limiting their access to opportunities for economic, educational, and social development.

The research methodology adopted in this project is transdisciplinary and participatory, focused on identifying the specific needs and expectations of women in these zones. The objective is to design and implement public policies that not only mitigate existing inequalities but also strengthen the capacities and competencies of these women, thereby promoting their overall well-being. This approach is based on the premise that a social intervention actively involving the beneficiaries in diagnosing and solving their problems has a greater potential to generate sustainable and significant changes.

The project is structured into several stages, each with clear objectives and expected outcomes. In the first stage, the ZAPs are selected according to the criteria established by CONEVAL[1], and a detailed diagnosis is conducted on the needs and expectations of the women in these areas. This information will be used to design a social intervention that addresses economic, political, educational, cultural, social security, infrastructure, and environmental dimensions. In subsequent stages, the designed interventions will be implemented, their impact evaluated, and necessary adjustments made to improve outcomes.

Additionally, the project includes a component for the social appropriation of knowledge, aimed at ensuring that the findings and lessons learned are shared with the community, social organizations, and relevant public institutions. This will be achieved through workshops, discussion forums, and the dissemination of digital content that will enable women in the ZAPs and other social actors to understand and act on issues related to gender inequality.

In summary, this project not only seeks to improve the quality of life of women in the ZAPs of Tijuana but also to contribute to the development of more effective and equitable public policies. The successful implementation of this project has the potential to serve as a model for similar interventions in other regions, helping to close gender gaps and promoting a more just and sustainable social development.

---

[1] CONEVAL (National Council for the Evaluation of Social Development Policy) is an autonomous government agency in Mexico responsible for measuring poverty and evaluating social development programs and policies. Its primary function is to generate reliable, objective data and evaluations to assess the effectiveness of government interventions aimed at reducing poverty and inequality in Mexico. CONEVAL produces poverty measurements at the national and state levels and evaluates the impact of social programs to inform policy decisions. CONEVAL's official website: Available from: https://www.coneval.org.mx.

3. Empowerment through participatory health models: A transdisciplinary perspective for women's well-being

The literature on participatory interventions in women's health and well-being has utilized a variety of theoretical frameworks and conceptual models to explore and understand the effectiveness and impacts of these interventions [2–4]. A critical analysis of the current literature reveals a wide range of approaches and outcomes in the field of participatory interventions in women's health and well-being [5–7].

The diversity of approaches within the literature on participatory interventions in women's health and well-being reflects the broad perspective and interest in the efficacy of these strategies. A notable example is the Theory of Participation and Autonomy in Health, presented by Chor et al. [8], which highlights the critical importance of women's active participation in health programs. This theory emphasizes not only the improvement in autonomy and access to key services achieved through women's participation but also the importance of adequate training for health personnel. Particularly in the context of post-abortion care, this approach has proven fundamental in increasing women's satisfaction and safety in essential aspects of their reproductive health and contraceptive care, underscoring the need for policies and programs that recognize and strengthen effective and informed participation of women in their own healthcare.

Similarly, the Food Security and Nutritional Education Model presented by Ebadi-Vanestanagh et al. [9] addresses another crucial aspect of women's health: nutrition. This model proposes that nutritional education programs, especially when tailored to the cultural realities of women, can have a significant impact on their health and food security. Both approaches underscore the critical need for public policies and programs that not only address the physical aspects of women's health but also consider cultural and educational contexts for effective and empowering implementation.

The Food Security and Nutritional Education Model, proposed by Ebadi-Vanestanagh et al. [9], also focuses on nutrition, complements and enriches the landscape of interventions in women's health and well-being. This model emphasizes that nutritional education programs, when adapted to the specific cultural realities of women, can play a transformative role in improving their health and food security. Like the Theory of Participation and Autonomy in Health, these strategies highlight the urgency of policies and programs that encompass not only physical aspects of health but also educational and cultural contexts for the effective empowerment of women. Similarly, Maury et al.'s [10] focus on empowerment through education emphasizes the importance of education as a means to empower women, particularly those in vulnerable situations. This model demonstrates how well-designed and focused educational interventions can induce substantial changes in dietary habits and knowledge in critical areas such as diabetes management, reaffirming the positive influence of education in strengthening women's autonomy and well-being.

Additionally, the Social Support and Mental Health Model [11], which studies how the lack of social support can exacerbate mental health problems in older women, highlights the need to incorporate community support into the design of women-centered interventions. Like the previously mentioned models, this approach underscores the importance of considering mental and emotional well-being in the design of women-centered interventions. This approach complements previous perspectives by highlighting the need for a comprehensive approach that includes not only physical well-being but also the mental and emotional health of women. Integrating this model with nutritional education and empowerment through education approaches

DOI: http://dx.doi.org/10.5772/intechopen.1007166

offers a holistic framework for the design of policies and programs. This demonstrates that to achieve true advancement in women's well-being, it is essential to consider all facets of their lives, from nutrition and education to social support and mental health, thus recognizing the diversity and complexity of their needs.

The perspective of Ebadi-Vanestanagh et al. [9] on food security and nutritional education integrates seamlessly with Maury et al.'s [10] approach to female empowerment through education. Both models recognize the need for interventions that go beyond addressing physical health issues and also tackling educational and cultural aspects to achieve a lasting and significant impact on women's lives. While Ebadi-Vanestanagh et al. [9] focus on how nutritional education can transform women's health and food security, Maury et al. [10] highlight the influence of education in empowering women in vulnerable situations, such as those facing chronic illnesses. These approaches emphasize the importance of a holistic strategy in women's health, where education acts as a fundamental pillar for empowerment and the improvement of quality of life.

The combination of these models provides a comprehensive framework for the development of women's health and well-being policies and programs that integrate nutritional, educational, and social support aspects, highlighting the importance of addressing women's needs in a way that recognizes and respects their complexity and diversity.

Chor et al.'s [8] proposal for training female health workers in community contexts emphasizes the importance of training health workers in communities, where they can act as agents of change, suggesting that women's empowerment through education and training can have a multiplier effect on improving community health. This approach suggests that by training women as health workers in their communities, not only is access to health services improved, but their role as agents of change is also promoted. This training model has the potential to create a multiplier effect, where empowered women can lead and promote improvements in the health and well-being of their communities. The combination of these models and approaches provides a robust and multifaceted landscape for developing interventions and policies that comprehensively address women's well-being, thus promoting significant change at both the individual and community levels.

This approach stands out as a progressive strategy that empowers women within their own communities. It underscores the importance of health training, not only to improve access to health services but also to promote female leadership in the health sector. By training women as health workers, they are given a vital role as agents of change, enhancing their capacity to influence and improve the health and well-being of their communities. This approach highlights the potential for significant and sustainable change in community health, driven by empowered and educated women. Integrating this model with nutritional education and social support approaches offers a comprehensive framework for addressing women's health and well-being challenges in a community context.

In the context of Tijuana's Priority Attention Zones (ZAP), the implementation of these models and theoretical approaches takes on special relevance. Adapting participatory interventions, nutritional education, and social support in these areas can effectively address the needs and expectations of women. By applying these theoretical frameworks, it is possible to develop and implement social interventions that not only build and strengthen women's capacities and competencies in aspects of social and economic life but also promote their health and well-being. The practical application of these models in Tijuana has the potential to significantly improve the quality of life for women in these areas, thereby contributing to the reduction of gender inequalities in a context historically marked by vulnerability.

The synergy of these models and approaches in Tijuana's ZAPs may be key to achieving sustainable social and health transformation. By focusing on training female health workers in the community and combining it with nutritional education and social support, a conducive environment is created for the empowerment and well-being of women. These interventions, rooted in a deep understanding of local realities and women's needs, can establish a new standard in the development of health policies and programs. With such a comprehensive approach, it is possible not only to address immediate needs but also to build the foundations for lasting and equitable change, thus fostering a more just and healthy future for the women of Tijuana.

The application of these models and theories to Tijuana's Priority Attention Zones is particularly relevant. By considering participatory interventions, nutritional education, and social support in these areas, the needs and expectations of women in these environments can be effectively addressed. These theoretical frameworks provide a solid foundation for developing and implementing social interventions that build and strengthen capacities and competencies in various aspects of the social and economic lives of women in Tijuana. The application of these models in policy research and development can lead to a significant improvement in these women's quality of life and promote gender equity in a context historically marked by inequalities and vulnerabilities.

After examining the theoretical models and approaches in the literature on participatory interventions in women's health and well-being, the importance of applying this knowledge in a practical and targeted manner becomes evident. The transition toward the proposed methodology is based on the pressing need to implement effective strategies that respond to the specific conditions and needs of women in Tijuana's ZAPs. A deep understanding of these theories has not only illuminated the path toward more sensitive and adaptive interventions but also underscored the importance of an evidence-based approach to designing interventions that sustainably promote well-being and gender equity.

With this theoretical foundation, the next section addresses the practical application of these principles through a diagnostic tool designed to capture the complexities of the lived realities of women in the ZAPs. This methodological approach reflects a commitment to precision and relevance in research while emphasizing the active participation of affected communities in the process of identifying problems and solutions. The integration of research and practice, in this sense, becomes a critical step toward realizing interventions that are not only effective in the short term but also have the potential to generate positive and lasting change in the health and well-being of the women participating in the study.

4. Methodological proposal

This research is part of Project CF-2023-G-1287, approved by CONAHCYT under the Frontier Science 2023 Call. The initiative, titled "Social Intervention for the Pursuit of Well-being with Equity in Women Living in Priority Attention Zones," focuses on neighborhoods identified as Priority Attention Zones (ZAP) in Tijuana, Baja California. The study was conducted using a holistic and empirical approach, aimed at designing interventions based on the specific needs and realities of women in the ZAPs, following methodological proposals that emphasize mixed methods to develop empirical research on women's relationships with resources in vulnerable contexts [12].

DOI: http://dx.doi.org/10.5772/intechopen.1007166

Over an intensive three-month period, field teams engaged with the communities in the Priority Attention Zones on weekends, conducting a total of 250 surveys. To facilitate the participation of women in our research, weekend workshops were organized, focusing on women's economic and social empowerment [13]. These workshops not only encouraged participation in the survey process but also served as a platform for skill development in critical areas for their empowerment and autonomy [12, 14]. Interactions during these survey sessions and workshops highlighted the need for interventions aimed at achieving tangible progress in local infrastructure and removing barriers to accessing essential services.

The methodological component of this work involved several phases. In September 2023, an intensive training workshop was held, focusing on social security, violence against women, infrastructure, and the environment. The workshop at the Faculty of Economics and International Relations of the Autonomous University of Baja California, aimed to raise awareness and prepare students for fieldwork, acknowledging the substantial barriers to accessing education and other basic services faced by many women in these communities [15]. In October 2023, field visits to the Nido de las Águilas Priority Attention Zone provided students with firsthand observation of the living conditions of women, characterized by inadequate infrastructure, such as unpaved streets and insufficient drainage systems. This reinforced the importance of prioritizing effective access to resources and comprehensive training for the target population in intervention proposals [16].

During the fieldwork sessions, students expanded their practical experience by gaining a deeper understanding of the terrain [17]. This stage focused on addressing sensitive topics, emphasizing the importance of empathetic and reflective communication for effective interaction with women in the ZAP. These interactions were crucial for the students' learning and practical skill acquisition, highlighting the need to continuously adapt the data collection methodology [18]. To support this process, a field diary technique was implemented. The field diaries maintained by the students became a tool for reflection and analysis on field dynamics, significantly contributing to the design of more informed interventions aligned with the lived experiences of the women surveyed [19].

The responses obtained from the surveys provided vital information on the most urgent needs and expectations in terms of social promotion and development for women in the Nido de las Águilas and División del Norte neighborhoods. The objective was to structure support and technical assistance programs that effectively respond to these needs, with the aim of improving quality of life and promoting social development with gender equity [13].

The results of this applied methodology constitute a solid foundation for the formulation of public policies and programs [12, 14]. The project reflects a commitment to inclusion and equity, fostering a participatory approach that integrates the voices of affected women, their families, governmental institutions, and civil organizations in the process of improving living conditions and well-being in the ZAPs of Tijuana [13].

The database corresponding to the results of the project's first stage represents a fundamental compendium for analyzing the socioeconomic and health conditions of women in the Priority Attention Zones. This database includes demographic information, indicators of access to health services, education, social security, and employment, as well as data on perceptions of well-being and specific obstacles faced by women in Tijuana [15].

The data collection was carried out using a mixed-methods approach involving both quantitative and qualitative techniques [18]. The central instrument was a structured survey administered to a representative sample of women in the ZAPs, selected through a stratified random sampling process. The questionnaire included closed-ended questions for quantitative data collection and open-ended sections to allow for detailed expression of personal experiences, thus providing valuable qualitative insights [17].

During the field phase, data from 250 complete surveys were collected, ensuring adequate representation of the various subpopulations within the ZAPs. Additionally, focus groups and semi-structured interviews were conducted with selected participants to delve deeper into issues that emerged as relevant in the surveys. This ethnographic approach allowed for a richer understanding of the social and cultural contexts affecting the daily lives of women [20].

The data analysis phase involved a process of cleaning and coding, followed by descriptive and inferential statistical techniques. Qualitative analysis tools such as Maxqda (Analytics Pro Student, version 24.2.0) were used to identify patterns and themes within the narrative responses [21]. This facilitated a contextualized interpretation of the quantitative data, providing a holistic view of the needs and challenges faced by women in the ZAPs.

The analysis of data collected during the project's first phase has provided a detailed understanding of the multiple dimensions of women's lives in the Priority Attention Zones. Through descriptive statistics, this study has explored crucial relationships between various variables that directly influence women's well-being and autonomy. These include the type of social security and its relationship to healthcare service accessibility, the frequency of service use in the face of insurance coverage gaps, and how these conditions impact critical health-related decisions, such as attending medical appointments and purchasing medications.

The findings were reviewed in collaborative work sessions with experts in public health, social work, economics, and urban development, enriching data interpretation and informing recommendations for the second intervention stage. Critical intervention areas were identified, and pilot programs were designed, focusing on health promotion, human rights education, and economic capacity building.

The methodology applied for cross-referencing these variables was designed to identify not only existing correlations but also to delve into the underlying causes of observed inequalities. This approach enables researchers and policymakers to better understand the specific barriers women face in these areas and to design more effective interventions. By addressing issues such as depression and anxiety in relation to received treatment, and expectations regarding health policies versus social security types, this analysis highlights specific needs and areas of dissatisfaction that must be prioritized.

In the next section of the article, a detailed analysis of these variable cross-references will be presented. This discussion will focus on interpreting how existing support structures, or their absence, influence the daily lives and health decisions of women in the ZAPs. The analysis will seek to provide concrete recommendations for public policies that can effectively address the identified challenges, aiming to improve both gender equity and the quality of life for women in Tijuana. This transition from data analysis to practical recommendations underscores the project's commitment to sustainable, evidence-based change.

Entering the discussion phase, the research findings highlight the urgency of addressing deficiencies in access to and the quality of mental health services, as well as the critical need to expand social insurance coverage. These problematic areas, identified through comprehensive analysis, underscore the interconnectedness of mental health, physical well-being, and social security in promoting a dignified and fulfilling life for women in the ZAPs. Discussing these results not only allows for a better understanding of the complexities of health inequalities in Tijuana but also serves as a call to action for policymakers, health professionals, and the community at large. Considering these findings, the importance of designing and implementing public policies and programs that effectively respond to the identified needs is emphasized, promoting a more inclusive and equitable approach to the health and well-being of women in Tijuana.

5. Health access disparities and utilization patterns: Analyzing the impact of social security coverage on women's healthcare engagement

Delving into a detailed analysis of the data collected through this study reveals realities that demand immediate attention and well-directed strategies to address inequalities in access to and the quality of health services in the considered Priority Attention Zones (ZAP). The evidence gathered highlights critical patterns and significant challenges in the realms of mental health, social security coverage, and healthcare accessibility, which become the central focus of this discussion. This section aims to deepen the understanding of these issues and explore the implications of these findings for the development of policies and intervention programs that are not only effective but also inclusive and equitable for the women in these communities.

The variation in perceptions of healthcare accessibility, depending on the type of social security coverage, underscores the complexity of the healthcare system and the need to adopt differentiated approaches that consider the specific needs of each group of women. Similarly, the impact of a lack of insurance coverage on health-related decisions highlights a critical gap in social protection and access to essential care.

The data indicate that a large proportion of individuals with anxiety or depression have not received treatment, suggesting significant barriers to accessing mental health services. Moreover, the expectations for health services in relation to accessibility suggest that the more accessible the services, the greater the expectations in areas such as preventive care and mental health. This pattern underscores the need for policies that improve access to and the quality of mental health services, particularly in vulnerable communities.

The analysis of the impact of the lack of social security coverage reveals that the absence of this benefit leads to adverse health-related decisions, such as missing medical appointments and not purchasing medications. This underscores the critical importance of social security in facilitating access to healthcare and highlights the need to expand coverage to include the most vulnerable populations.

The analysis of **Figure 1** "Comparison of Social Security Type and Perceived Accessibility of Health Services in the Study Population" offers a compelling examination of the disparities in healthcare access among women based on their type of social security coverage. This data underscores the critical role that social security plays in determining the quality and accessibility of health services, revealing both strengths and significant gaps that need to be addressed to promote healthcare equity.

Figure 1 reveals that women covered by the Mexican Social Security Institute (IMSS) generally report better access to health services, with a considerable proportion finding these services either "Accessible" or "Very Accessible." This pattern suggests that IMSS provides a relatively robust healthcare infrastructure and perhaps clearer communication regarding the services available to its affiliates. However, the

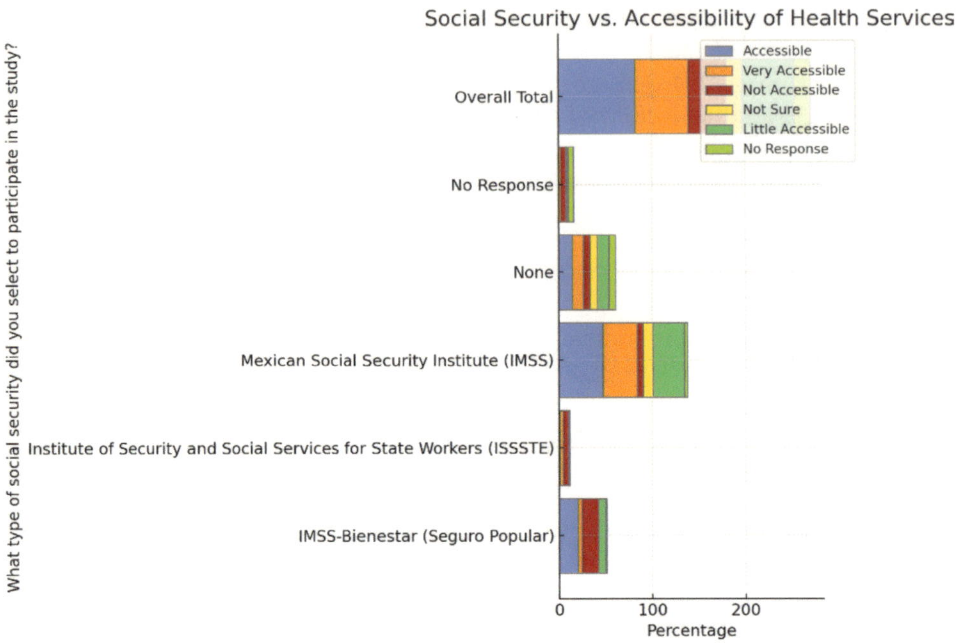

Figure 1.
Comparison of social security type and perceived accessibility of health services in the study population [22].

presence of a significant number of IMSS beneficiaries who find health services "Not Accessible" or "Little Accessible" highlights persistent systemic issues within the IMSS framework. These challenges might include bureaucratic inefficiencies, uneven service distribution, or regional disparities in healthcare infrastructure that continue to hinder equitable access to care for all IMSS beneficiaries.

In contrast, the perception of healthcare accessibility among women covered by IMSS-Bienestar (formerly Seguro Popular) is notably less favorable. A larger proportion of respondents in this group report difficulties in accessing health services, which points to potential deficiencies in the reach and quality of the services provided under this program. The lower accessibility could be attributed to a range of factors, including inadequate healthcare infrastructure, insufficient service coverage, and administrative barriers that disproportionately affect the most vulnerable populations who rely on public health programs. This finding is particularly concerning, as it underscores the need for targeted improvements within IMSS-Bienestar to ensure that its services meet the needs of all beneficiaries effectively.

The data also starkly contrasts the experiences of women with and without social security coverage. Those without any form of social security overwhelmingly report that health services are either "Not Accessible" or "Little Accessible." This disparity highlights a significant equity gap in healthcare access, where the absence of social security exacerbates existing barriers to essential health services. The findings reinforce the critical role that social security plays in mitigating these barriers and ensuring that healthcare is a universal right, rather than a privilege tied to employment or socioeconomic status.

Given these insights, policy interventions must be tailored to address the specific challenges faced by different groups. For IMSS, while the data suggests that it provides relatively better access to healthcare, there is still a need to streamline services and address the specific pain points that lead to reports of inaccessibility. This might involve improving communication strategies, simplifying bureaucratic processes, and expanding service availability in underserved regions to ensure that all beneficiaries can fully exercise their healthcare rights.

For IMSS-Bienestar, the data indicates a more urgent need for systemic reforms. With a significant proportion of its beneficiaries perceiving services as inaccessible, policy efforts should focus on strengthening the program's infrastructure, enhancing the quality and availability of services, and ensuring that beneficiaries are well-informed about how to access these services. Addressing these issues will be crucial for improving the effectiveness of IMSS-Bienestar and ensuring that it meets the healthcare needs of its diverse beneficiary base.

The analysis also underscores the necessity of expanding social security coverage to include the uninsured. The stark differences in accessibility perceptions between those with and without social security highlight the urgent need for innovative solutions that can bridge the access gap. Community-based health programs, mobile clinics, and partnerships with non-governmental organizations could play a vital role in providing essential services to uninsured populations. These efforts should be accompanied by advocacy for broader systemic reforms aimed at achieving universal health coverage, thereby ensuring that no one is left without access to the healthcare they need.

Figure 2 titled "Impact of Insurance Coverage on Frequency of Health Service Use Among Respondents" provides a compelling visual representation of the profound impact that social security coverage has on healthcare utilization among women. The data clearly illustrates that women who possess social security are more likely to access health services regularly, engage in preventive care, and maintain ongoing management of health conditions. This proactive approach to healthcare is essential for early detection and treatment, leading to better health outcomes and a reduction in the long-term costs associated with untreated conditions.

In contrast, **Figure 2** reveals a starkly different pattern among women without social security coverage. This group predominantly utilizes health services only when necessary, indicating a reactive rather than preventive approach to healthcare. Such

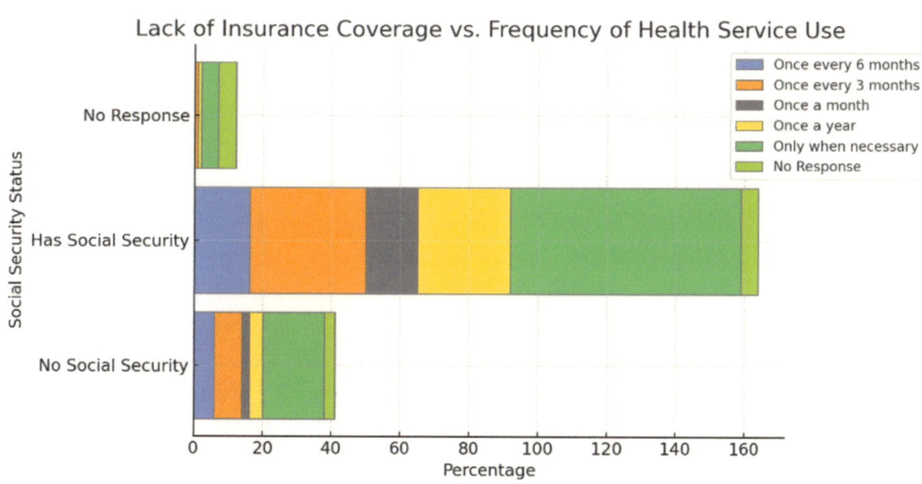

Figure 2.
Impact of insurance coverage on frequency of health service use among respondents [22].

behavior is often driven by financial constraints and the high out-of-pocket costs associated with uninsured healthcare visits. The reactive use of health services suggests that these women are more likely to delay care until their health issues become severe, increasing the risk of complications and more intensive, costly treatments. This pattern not only underscores the vulnerability of uninsured populations but also highlights the critical role that social security plays in enabling regular access to necessary healthcare services.

The disparities in healthcare access between insured and uninsured women are particularly concerning. The data clearly indicates that women with social security are better equipped to manage their health proactively, while those without coverage face significant barriers that limit their ability to access even basic healthcare. These disparities exacerbate existing health inequities and contribute to the overall burden on the healthcare system, particularly when preventable conditions go untreated due to lack of access.

Given these findings, there are significant policy implications. Expanding social security coverage to include all women, particularly those in marginalized communities, is essential for promoting equitable access to healthcare. Such expansion would likely result in more regular and preventive use of health services, improving health outcomes and reducing long-term healthcare costs. Moreover, public health initiatives should aim to educate uninsured populations about the importance of regular healthcare visits and the benefits of preventive care, even in the absence of insurance.

Furthermore, addressing the financial, geographic, and organizational barriers that prevent uninsured women from accessing healthcare is crucial. Innovative solutions such as mobile health clinics, community health workers, and subsidized healthcare services could help bridge these gaps, ensuring that all women could engage in proactive health management.

Figure 3 titled "Effect of Lack of Social Security Coverage on Health-Related Decisions" provides a stark illustration of the significant impact that the absence of social security coverage has on women's healthcare decisions. The data presented in the chart reveals troubling trends that highlight the barriers faced by uninsured women, which ultimately affect their ability to maintain their health and well-being.

A critical observation from **Figure 3** is that a substantial number of respondents did not attend medical appointments due to the lack of social security coverage.

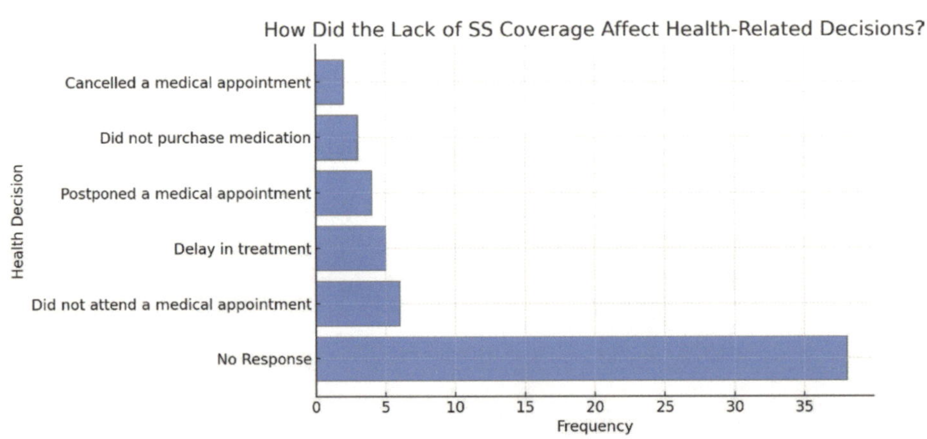

Figure 3.
Effect of lack of social security coverage on health-related decisions [22].

This decision, driven likely by financial constraints and the perceived or real cost of healthcare without insurance, is particularly concerning because it directly impedes early detection and timely treatment of health conditions. Skipping medical appointments can lead to the progression of untreated diseases, which not only compromises the health of these women but also increases the likelihood of more severe health complications in the future.

The chart further indicates that the absence of social security coverage has led many women to postpone medical appointments and delay necessary treatments. These delays can exacerbate treatable conditions, leading to poorer health outcomes and potentially requiring more intensive and expensive medical interventions later. Additionally, the decision to forgo purchasing necessary medications, as indicated by the chart, is another critical issue. Medication non-adherence can result in the deterioration of chronic conditions, reduce the effectiveness of treatment plans, and increase the risk of hospitalizations and emergency care visits.

The data presented underscores the multifaceted impact of lacking social security coverage on health-related decision-making. The choices to cancel or delay care, avoid purchasing medications, and skip medical appointments reflect broader systemic issues, including the inaccessibility of affordable healthcare services for uninsured populations. These trends are indicative of the broader public health implications, where the absence of social security coverage not only affects individual health outcomes but also places a greater strain on the healthcare system as untreated conditions escalate into emergencies.

Given these findings, the necessity for policy interventions becomes apparent. Expanding social security coverage to ensure that all women have access to affordable healthcare services is crucial. Such expansion would help mitigate the financial barriers that currently lead to the avoidance of necessary care. Moreover, public health campaigns should focus on educating women about the importance of regular medical care and adherence to prescribed treatments, even in the absence of social security. Providing information on available financial assistance programs and community health resources could help alleviate some of the burdens faced by uninsured women.

Figure 4 titled "Treatment Types Received by Individuals with Anxiety/Depression" provides a clear visual representation of a significant gap in the accessibility and utilization of mental health services. The data starkly illustrates that most individuals who report symptoms of anxiety or depression have not received any form of treatment. This is a deeply concerning finding, as untreated mental health conditions can lead to severe and long-lasting consequences, not only for the individuals affected but also for their families and communities.

The overwhelming proportion of respondents who indicate that they have not received treatment suggests several underlying issues. First, there may be substantial barriers to accessing mental health services, such as financial constraints, a lack of available services, or long waiting times. Additionally, this finding could reflect a lack of awareness or understanding of mental health issues and the importance of seeking treatment. Cultural factors and stigma associated with mental health may also play a significant role, deterring individuals from pursuing the help they need.

Figure 4 also shows that among those who have received treatment, therapy is slightly more common than medication. This could indicate a preference for therapeutic interventions or greater availability of counseling services compared to pharmacological options. It might also reflect a broader trend toward holistic approaches in managing mental health, where talking therapies are valued for their focus on addressing underlying psychological issues rather than just alleviating symptoms.

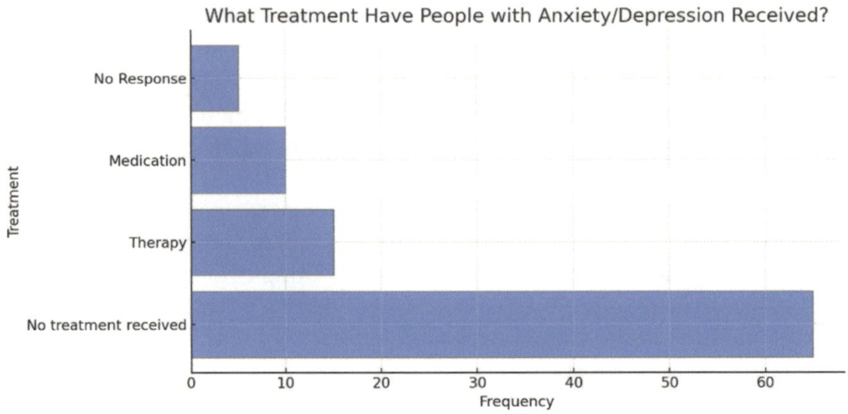

Figure 4.
Treatment types received by individuals with anxiety/depression [22].

However, the relatively low numbers of individuals receiving either therapy or medication highlight a critical underutilization of established treatment methods. This underutilization points to a disconnect between the availability of these services and their uptake, potentially due to issues such as inadequate mental health literacy, concerns about the side effects of medication, or the perceived ineffectiveness of therapy.

The presence of a significant "No Response" category further complicates the analysis, as it may suggest a lack of awareness about the available treatment options or reluctance to disclose personal information related to mental health. The stigma surrounding mental health conditions may lead to underreporting, which in turn makes it challenging to fully understand the extent of unmet treatment needs within the population.

This chart underscores the urgent need for comprehensive strategies to address the mental health treatment gap. Policymakers and healthcare providers must focus on improving access to mental health services by reducing financial barriers, expanding the availability of mental health professionals, and integrating mental health services into primary care settings. Additionally, public health campaigns should aim to raise awareness about the importance of mental health care and reduce the stigma associated with seeking treatment.

Figure 5 titled "Health Topics Expectations According to Social Security Type" provides a nuanced view of how women's health expectations vary depending on their type of social security coverage. This visualization reveals critical insights that can inform the design and implementation of targeted health interventions in the community.

The data indicates that regardless of the specific social security coverage, women universally express strong expectations for comprehensive reproductive health programs, preventive care, and access to medications and treatments. This broad demand suggests that existing health services might not be fully addressing the needs of women in these areas. For women with social security, such as those covered by IMSS and Seguro Popular, these expectations highlight the potential gaps in service delivery, particularly in reproductive health and preventive care. It is crucial for healthcare providers and policymakers to recognize these gaps and work toward enhancing the availability and quality of these services to meet the needs of their beneficiaries effectively.

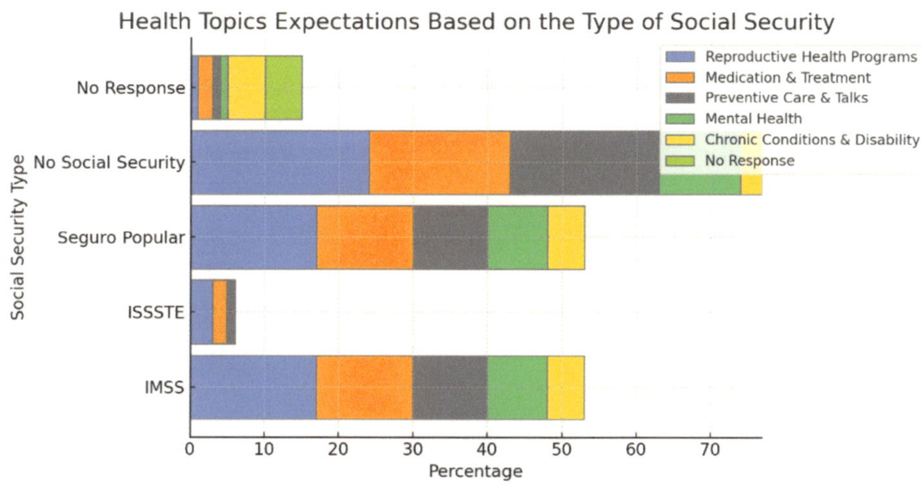

Figure 5.
Health topics expectations according to social security type [22].

A particularly noteworthy observation is that women without social security demonstrate a heightened concern for mental health services. This concern likely reflects significant barriers to accessing mental health care, including financial limitations, lack of service availability, and perhaps a greater burden of mental health issues within this group due to socioeconomic stressors. The strong emphasis on mental health among uninsured women underscores the urgent need for mental health services to be integrated into community health programs, especially in underserved areas. The inclusion of mental health care and counseling services in these programs could play a pivotal role in improving the overall well-being of women who lack social security.

Moreover, **Figure 5** shows that women across different types of social security coverage, including those under ISSSTE and IMSS, also express concerns about chronic conditions and disabilities. This indicates a broader need for health systems to prioritize long-term care management and support for chronic illnesses. The presence of these concerns across various social security types suggests that current healthcare provisions may not be sufficiently addressing the complexities of managing chronic conditions, which require continuous and specialized care.

The "No Response" category also merits attention, as it may reflect a lack of awareness or reluctance to engage with certain aspects of healthcare. This could indicate the need for improved health literacy and more effective communication strategies to ensure that women fully understand the health services available to them and feel empowered to utilize these services.

Overall, the chart highlights the critical importance of designing a multifaceted intervention strategy that addresses the specific needs and expectations of women based on their social security status. For women without social security, expanding access to mental health services and ensuring coverage for chronic conditions should be a priority. For those with social security, efforts should focus on closing the gaps in reproductive health and preventive care, as well as enhancing the quality of services related to chronic disease management.

Figure 6 titled "Health Care Expectations in Relation to Frequency of Health Service Use" provides an intricate view of how different health care expectations align

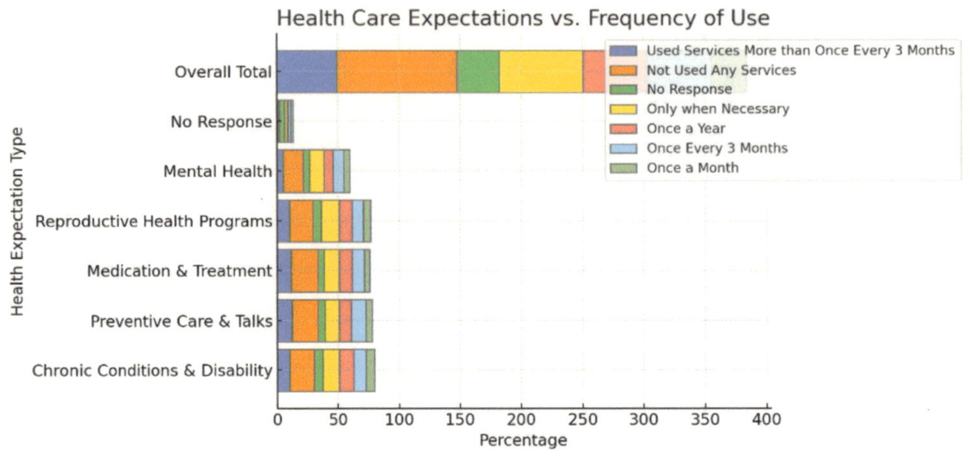

Figure 6.
Health care expectations in relation to frequency of health service use [22].

with the frequency of service utilization among women. This visualization is crucial in understanding not only the demands placed on the healthcare system but also the behaviors and challenges women face in accessing necessary services.

A notable observation from **Figure 6** is that across various healthcare expectation types—whether it be mental health, reproductive health programs, medication and treatment, preventive care, or care for chronic conditions—there is a consistent pattern of service underutilization. Many women appear to access services infrequently, with significant portions of respondents using services only when necessary or not at all. This pattern suggests that barriers such as financial constraints, lack of availability, or possibly even a lack of perceived need could be influencing the irregular use of health services.

Moreover, the "No Response" category present across all health expectation types indicates a potential gap in awareness or a reluctance to disclose information about health service use. This could stem from stigma, especially in areas such as mental health, or from a lack of engagement with the healthcare system altogether. The presence of this category across various expectations suggests that public health initiatives might need to focus more on outreach and education to ensure that women are both aware of and able to access the services they need.

Figure 6 also highlights the concerning trend of minimal service use for critical areas such as mental health and chronic conditions. These areas, which typically require ongoing and consistent care, are underrepresented in terms of frequent service utilization. This underuse is troubling, as it may lead to worsening conditions and higher long-term healthcare costs due to the need for more intensive interventions later.

Interestingly, the overall distribution of service use shows that while there is a segment of women who use services more than once every three months, this group is relatively small compared to those who use services infrequently or not at all. This disparity reinforces the idea that there are significant barriers to consistent healthcare access and that these barriers must be addressed to improve health outcomes.

The alignment between healthcare expectations and actual service use reveals a critical disconnect. Women have clear expectations for comprehensive care across various domains, yet the frequency with which they utilize these services does not meet these expectations. This disconnect points to the need for targeted interventions that not only expand access to healthcare but also encourage regular and proactive engagement with health services.

The data collected within this project reveals significant patterns in healthcare access and utilization among women, particularly concerning the disparities associated with social security coverage. The findings indicate that women with social security are more likely to engage in regular and preventive healthcare practices, whereas those without coverage tend to seek medical attention only when necessary. This difference suggests that social security plays a crucial role in enabling consistent access to healthcare services, which is essential for early detection and management of health conditions. The data highlights the importance of understanding how social security influences health behaviors and access to services, which is critical for informing public health policies.

Additionally, the data uncovers the varied health expectations among women based on their social security status. Regardless of the type of coverage, there is a notable demand for comprehensive reproductive health programs, preventive care, and access to medications and treatments. However, women without social security coverage express a heightened concern for mental health services, indicating a potential gap in the availability or accessibility of these services for uninsured populations. This finding points to the need for targeted interventions that address both the coverage and quality of health services, particularly in underserved communities where mental health care appears to be a significant unmet need.

The project also reveals a broader trend of underutilization of health services, even among women with social security coverage, which may reflect barriers beyond financial constraints, such as geographical access, awareness, and cultural factors. The presence of a substantial "No Response" category in the data suggests gaps in health literacy or a reluctance to engage with the healthcare system, which could be driven by stigma or mistrust. These results underscore the complexity of healthcare access and the need for multifaceted public policy approaches that not only expand coverage but also address the underlying factors that influence healthcare utilization.

6. Conclusions

The study's conclusions underscore the significant implications that the critical findings of this research have for the design of future policies and practices. A notable proportion of individuals with anxiety or depression have not received treatment, indicating substantial barriers to accessing mental health care. This highlights an urgent need to develop policies that not only improve the availability but also the quality of mental health services, particularly for vulnerable populations.

The relationship between social security coverage and health-related decisions emphasizes the pivotal role of social security as a key facilitator of access to medical care. The absence of coverage is associated with the avoidance of medical appointments and the purchase of medications, underscoring the need for an expansion of coverage that is inclusive of the most vulnerable segments of the population.

Social security coverage emerges as a fundamental factor affecting both the frequency of healthcare utilization and health-related decisions. Insufficient coverage leads to adverse consequences such as missed medical appointments and the inability to purchase necessary medications. The importance of expanding insurance coverage to include the most vulnerable is evident, and future policies should advocate for universal health coverage that enables access to essential services without the barrier of cost.

The perception of healthcare accessibility varies significantly between women affiliated with IMSS and those covered by Seguro Popular (now IMSS-Bienestar), with the latter group reporting more difficulties. This underscores the need for differentiated policies that consider the type of social security coverage and seek to strengthen women's capacity to navigate the social security system, as well as improve the infrastructure and processes of healthcare services.

The implications for future research include the need for more in-depth studies on the barriers to accessing and utilizing mental health services, as well as the effects of different types of insurance coverage on healthcare accessibility. Future practices should focus on developing interventions that enhance the accessibility, quality, and communication of healthcare services, and on promoting mental health education and preventive care.

In terms of limitations, the study faced challenges in collecting detailed responses regarding the use of mental health services due to the stigma associated with these issues, suggesting the need for awareness-raising and destigmatization strategies in future research and practice. Additionally, the self-selection of respondents and differences in the interpretation of accessibility may have influenced the results, indicating the need for more robust methodological approaches to fully understand the complexity of these issues.

Finally, the research underscores the importance of community intervention and the active participation of women in the design of health policies and programs that respond to their needs and expectations. The implementation of well-informed interventions and policies based on these findings can lead to significant improvements in the quality of life for women and advance toward greater health equity.

Author details

Jimmy Emmanuel Ramos Valencia[1*] and Martha Cecilia Jaramillo Cardona[2]

1 The Northern Border College (COLEF), Tijuana, Mexico

2 Autonomous University of Baja California, Tijuana, Mexico

*Address all correspondence to: jimmy.ramos@uabc.edu.mx

References

[1] Osorio-Novela G, Mungaray Lagarda A, Ramírez-Angulo N. Collaboration between university students and social business. Iberoamerican Journal of Higher Education. Higher Education. 2022;**13**(36):26-43. Epub 21 March 2022. DOI: 10.22201/iisue.20072872e.2022.36.1182

[2] Harris-Fry HA, Azad K, Younes L, Kuddus A, Shaha S, Nahar T, et al. Formative evaluation of a participatory women's group intervention to improve reproductive and women's health outcomes in rural Bangladesh: A controlled before and after study. Journal of Epidemiology and Community Health. 2016;**70**(7):663-670. DOI: 10.1136/jech-2015-205855

[3] Randolph SD, Golin C, Welgus H, Lightfoot AF, Harding CJ, Riggins LF. How perceived structural racism and discrimination and medical mistrust in the health system influences participation in HIV health services for black women living in the United States south: A qualitative, descriptive study. Journal of the Association of Nurses in AIDS Care. 2020;**31**(5):598-605

[4] Sabri B, Hartley M, Saha J, Murray S, Glass N, Campbell JC. Effect of COVID-19 pandemic on women's health and safety: A study of immigrant survivors of intimate partner violence. Health Care for Women International. 2020;**41**(11-12):1294-1312

[5] Ahuru RR. The influence of women empowerment on maternal and childcare use in Nigeria. International Journal of Healthcare Management. 2021;**14**(3):690-699

[6] Chinn JJ, Martin IK, Redmond N. Health equity among black women in the United States. Journal of Women's Health. 2021;**30**(2):212-219

[7] Kettel B. Women, Health and the Environment. En S. Sherwin y B. Paris, Women, Medicine, Ethics and the Law. Routledge, Taylor and Francis; 2020. pp. 23-35

[8] Chor J, Young D, Quinn M, Gilliam M. A novel lay health worker training to help women engage in Postabortion contraception and well-woman care. Health Promotion Practice. 2020;**21**(2):172-174

[9] Ebadi-Vanestanagh M, Molani-Gol R, Alizadeh M. Effects of the nutrition education intervention on food security, anthropometry, and body composition in women: A randomized controlled trial. Nutrition and Health. 2023. DOI: 10.1177/02601060231155538

[10] Maury A, Maury-Mena SC, Marín-Escobar JC, Marín-Benítez AC. Intervención educativa sobre la diabetes tipos 2 en una población sin hogar de Miami-Dade. Horizonte Sanitario. 2022;**21**(2):214-221. Epub 19 de abril de 2022. DOI: 10.19136/hs.a21n2.4746

[11] Vilar-Compte M, Giraldo-Rodríguez L, Ochoa-Laginas A, Gaitan-Rossi P. Association between depression and elder abuse and the mediation of social support: A cross-sectional study of elder females in Mexico City. Journal of Aging and Health. 2018;**30**(4):559-583. DOI: 10.1177/0898264316686432

[12] Dubois V. Critical policy ethnography. In: Fischer F, Torgerson D, Durnová A, Orsini M, editors. Handbook of Critical Policy Studies. Cheltenham, UK: Edward

Elgar Publishing; 2015. pp. 462-480. DOI: 10.4337/9781783472352.00005

[13] Charmaz K, Thornberg R, Keane E. Evolving grounded theory and social justice inquiry. In: Denzin NK, Lincoln YS, editors. The SAGE Handbook of Qualitative Research. sage; 2011

[14] Atkinson P, Hammersley M. What is ethnography? In: Hammersley M, Atkinson P, editors. Ethnography. Principles in Practice. 4rd ed. Routledge; 2019. DOI: 10.4324/9781315146027

[15] Mitchell JP. Ethnography. In: Turner SP, Outhwaite W, editors. The SAGE Handbook of Social Science Methodology. London: Sage; 2007. 640 p. ISBN: 9781446206454. Available from: http://digital.casalini.it/9781446206454. Casalini id: 4912554

[16] Murphy E, Dingwall R. The ethics of ethnography. In: Atkinson P, Coffey A, Delamont S, Lofland J, Lofland L, editors. Handbook of Ethnography. SAGE Publications Ltd; 2001. DOI: 10.4135/9781848608337

[17] Stanley L. Mass-Observation's fieldwork methods. In: Atkinson P, Coffey A, Delamont S, Lofland J, Lofland L, editors. Handbook of Ethnography. SAGE Publications Ltd; 2001. DOI: 10.4135/9781848608337

[18] Scott H. Data analysis: Getting conceptual. The Grounded Theory Review. 2009;**8**(2):89-110

[19] Mungaray Lagarda A, Ramírez Angulo N, Burgos Flores B, Ramírez Cervantes A, Ramírez Jiménez L. Los microempresarios sociales como modelo de referencia para emprendedores universitarios. Revista De La Educación Superior. 2024;**53**(209):125-143. DOI: 10.36857/resu.2024.209.2753

[20] Deterding NM, Waters MC. Flexible coding of in-depth interviews: A twenty-first-century approach. Sociological Methods and Research. 2021;**50**(2):1-32. DOI: 10.1177/0049124118799377

[21] Brinkmann S. The interview. In: Denzin NK, Lincoln YS, editors. The SAGE Handbook of Qualitative Research. 5th ed. SAGE Publications Ltd.; 2017. pp. 997-1038

[22] Jaramillo M et al. Analysis of the results of the survey applied in the project: Social intervention for the search of well-being with equity in women living in Priority Attention Zones. Project CF-2023-G-1287, funded by CONAHCYT. 2023

Chapter 13

Perspective Chapter: Oral Condition and Lifetime Hormonal Fluctuations

Mehrad Rafiei

Abstract

When you work in a dental health care service team, you must have seen women who say that the reason for their oral and dental problems is pregnancy, breastfeeding, or menopause. In this chapter, we will examine the role of hormonal changes during women's life on their oral health conditions. Hormonal fluctuations throughout a woman's life significantly impact her oral health. Key stages include puberty, menstruation, pregnancy, lactation, and menopause, where changes in estrogen and progesterone levels heighten susceptibility to oral issues, also we pay special attention to the periods of pregnancy and after, the periods which women have the most hormonal changes. Understanding these hormonal shifts is essential for addressing their implications, as they can lead to specific oral health issues such as gingivitis, dry mouth, and increased susceptibility to dental diseases. We also describe the effects of these hormonal changes on different oral conditions and represent the ways to deal with it.

Keywords: sex hormone, women, oral health, pregnancy, lactation

1. Introduction

Oral health is a key indicator of overall well-being, yet it is often studied in isolation from other physiological processes. In particular, the influence of hormonal fluctuations on oral health in women remains an underexplored area despite growing evidence suggesting that hormone levels significantly affect dental conditions. Throughout a woman's life, key hormonal milestones—puberty, menstruation, pregnancy, lactation, and menopause—bring marked changes in estrogen and progesterone levels. These shifts can increase the likelihood of developing certain oral health conditions, emphasizing the need for awareness among both healthcare providers and patients.

One of the earliest stages where hormonal influence on oral health becomes apparent is puberty. The increased levels of estrogen and progesterone at this stage can lead to gingival inflammation, heightened sensitivity, and increased plaque accumulation, even with consistent oral hygiene practices. Similarly, menstruation can trigger cyclic gingival changes due to hormonal surges, resulting in a condition known as menstrual gingivitis. Women may experience symptoms such as swollen, red gums, bleeding, and discomfort, highlighting the direct relationship between hormonal cycles and oral health.

During pregnancy, the body undergoes profound hormonal changes, particularly a surge in estrogen and progesterone, that significantly affect oral tissues. Pregnant women are at a higher risk of developing pregnancy gingivitis, characterized by inflammation, bleeding, and swelling of the gums. This condition can progress into more severe periodontal issues if not managed properly. Moreover, pregnancy can increase the risk of tooth erosion and dental caries due to increased acidity in the mouth from morning sickness and dietary changes. As a result, dentists recommend closer monitoring and preventive care for women during pregnancy to manage these risks.

Lactation is another period that impacts oral health. Hormonal adjustments after childbirth, especially during breastfeeding, can lead to decreased estrogen levels, which may influence bone density and gum health. Additionally, lactation-related dietary demands and potential changes in oral care routines can also affect oral health. Addressing these challenges with specific preventive measures can help protect women from developing long-term dental issues.

Finally, menopause represents a significant stage in a woman's life where hormonal declines bring new oral health challenges. Lower estrogen levels during menopause contribute to decreased saliva production, resulting in dry mouth, a condition that can increase susceptibility to cavities, gum disease, and other oral infections. Furthermore, postmenopausal women are more likely to experience osteoporosis, which can weaken jawbone density and exacerbate periodontal problems. Understanding and addressing these risks is crucial for maintaining oral health during this life stage.

This chapter aims to explore the cumulative effects of hormonal fluctuations on oral health, providing insights into how each stage of a woman's life can influence her susceptibility to various dental conditions. By reviewing these associations, we highlight the importance of preventive care and specialized management strategies tailored to each hormonal phase. This perspective chapter seeks to bridge the gap between dental and reproductive health, advocating for an integrated approach to oral care that accounts for hormonal influences.

2. Women's lifetime hormonal fluctuations

Women's lifetime hormonal fluctuations are influenced by various life stages, including puberty, menstrual cycles, pregnancy, and menopause. Hormonal fluctuations throughout a woman's life significantly influence her overall health, particularly oral health. These changes occur during various life stages, including puberty, menstruation, pregnancy, lactation, and menopause driven primarily by hormones such as estrogen, progesterone, luteinizing hormone (LH), and follicle-stimulating hormone (FSH), which regulate key physiological processes [1].

2.1 Puberty

Puberty typically begins between 9 and 14 years, and increased production of estrogen and progesterone leads to the development of secondary sexual characteristics, such as breast development and the onset of menstruation; also, puberty influences body composition. Hormonal changes can lead to mood swings and emotional challenges, affecting mental well-being [2].

2.2 Menstrual cycle

The menstrual cycle that occurs usually in 28 days, but can range from 21 to 35 days, comprises four main phases including menstrual, follicular, ovulatory, and luteal, each characterized by distinct hormonal profiles [3].

2.2.1 Menstrual phase

During the menstrual phase, which lasts from days 1 to 5 of the cycle, estrogen and progesterone levels are at their lowest. This drop may affect mood and energy levels. Nutrient-rich foods, particularly those high in iron and omega-3 fatty acids, can help alleviate menstrual symptoms and support overall health.

2.2.2 Follicular phase

The follicular phase occurs approximately from days 6 to 14, during which estrogen levels begin to rise, promoting the thickening of the uterine lining and often leading to improved mood and energy. Engaging in moderate exercise during this time can further enhance well-being. In some literatures, first two phases are considered as one.

2.2.3 Ovulatory phase

In the ovulatory phase, around day 14, estrogen peaks, triggering ovulation. This surge may contribute to increased libido and energy but can also lead to sensitivity in some women due to hormonal fluctuations.

2.2.4 Luteal phase

Following ovulation, the luteal phase (days 18 to 28) is marked by a rise in progesterone. This hormone prepares the body for a potential pregnancy but can also result in symptoms such as breast tenderness, mood swings, and fatigue. Nutritional choices during this phase should focus on complex carbohydrates to stabilize blood sugar levels, and calming exercises may be beneficial for managing stress and supporting hormonal balance.

Hormonal variations during the menstrual cycle can cause symptoms such as bloating, cramps, and fatigue. Fluctuations in estrogen and progesterone can influence muscle metabolism and strength, impacting physical performance.

2.3 Pregnancy

Pregnancy triggers significant hormonal shifts that affect various physiological systems, including the endocrine and oral health systems. The two primary hormones involved are estrogen and progesterone, which undergo dramatic increases during gestation. Estrogen, in particular, is produced in quantities exceeding those seen throughout a woman's non-pregnant life, playing a crucial role in uterine and placental development, as well as fetal maturation. The rise in estrogen levels peaks in the third trimester and is linked to symptoms such as nausea during the first trimester and breast development during the second trimester [4].

Hormonal shifts support fetal development but can also lead to discomfort, weight gain, and changes in body image. Pregnancy hormones can affect mood, leading to anxiety or depression in some women, especially during stressful periods like the COVID-19 pandemic. Recent studies reveal that hormonal changes during pregnancy produce profound effects on both the body and mind, due to high levels of hormones such as estrogen, progesterone, and oxytocin. These hormones orchestrate physiological changes that support fetal development and prepare the body for childbirth, while also influencing the brain to adjust for motherhood [5].

2.3.1 Physical effects

In terms of physical effects, hormonal surges trigger changes such as increased blood volume, altered immune responses, and redistribution of body fat. Estrogen and progesterone are especially active, promoting uterine growth, enhancing blood flow, and adjusting immune function to protect the fetus. In the brain, these hormones contribute to neuroplasticity, meaning the brain adapts and reorganizes itself in preparation for caregiving tasks. These findings highlight pregnancy as a period of intense physiological and psychological adaptation, with implications for understanding maternal health and potential support strategies for maternal mental well-being during and after pregnancy.

During pregnancy, hormonal changes lead to a series of major physical adaptations that help prepare the body to support the fetus and undergo childbirth. Here are some key areas affected:

2.3.2 Cardiovascular changes

Increased blood volume: By the second trimester, blood volume increases by about 40–50% to meet the oxygen and nutrient needs of the developing fetus. This requires the heart to work harder, often increasing heart rate by around 10–20 beats per minute.

Lowered blood pressure: Progesterone causes blood vessels to relax, which can initially lower blood pressure. However, blood pressure may return to normal or increase slightly as the pregnancy progresses [6].

2.3.3 Respiratory changes

Increased oxygen demand: Estrogen helps expand the rib cage and increases lung capacity, enabling the mother to take in more oxygen. Additionally, progesterone enhances breathing efficiency, allowing the mother's body to take in more air with each breath.

Shortness of breath: Toward the later stages of pregnancy, the uterus presses against the diaphragm, contributing to sensations of breathlessness, especially with exertion [6].

2.3.4 Immune system modulation

Adjustments to prevent fetal rejection: Since the fetus contains genetic material from both parents, the maternal immune system adapts to avoid attacking it.

Progesterone plays a major role in creating an immune environment that both protects the fetus and prevents maternal illness. This can, however, make pregnant women more susceptible to certain infections [6].

2.3.5 Metabolic changes

Increased caloric demand: Pregnancy significantly boosts metabolism, requiring additional caloric intake, particularly in the second and third trimesters. Hormones like human placental lactogen alter the way the mother's body processes carbohydrates, fats, and proteins to ensure an adequate energy supply for fetal development [6].

2.3.6 Musculoskeletal adaptations

Joint and ligament relaxation: The hormone relaxin is released to relax ligaments, particularly around the pelvis, to prepare the body for labor. This also affects other joints, making pregnant women more prone to injuries or discomforts such as lower back pain.

Postural changes: The growing uterus shifts the mother's center of gravity, leading to postural adjustments that can contribute to strain in the lower back and pelvis. These physiological shifts showcase how hormonal changes allow the body to support fetal development while preparing for the demands of labor and delivery [6].

2.3.7 Mental and emotional effects

Mental changes during pregnancy include structural shifts in the brain that may impact emotional processing, memory, and social behaviors. For example, recent imaging studies show that pregnancy causes a reduction in gray matter volume in certain brain regions associated with social cognition and empathy, which may facilitate a stronger mother-infant bond. This neuroplasticity during pregnancy appears linked to hormonal fluctuations and is thought to enhance caregiving instincts, though it can also make some mothers more vulnerable to mood disorders such as postpartum depression if hormonal and physical demands overwhelm these adaptive changes [7].

2.4 Postpartum period and lactation

Hormonal changes in the postpartum period: The postpartum period, which follows childbirth, is marked by significant hormonal fluctuations that profoundly influence a woman's physical and mental health. As estrogen and progesterone levels plummet to their pre-pregnancy states, new mothers may experience a range of symptoms, including mood swings, fatigue, and even conditions such as postpartum depression, affecting approximately one in nine parents. Concurrently, hormonal changes associated with lactation, such as increased levels of prolactin and oxytocin, play critical roles in milk production and maternal bonding, highlighting the complex interplay between hormonal regulation and maternal well-being during this transitional phase [8].

However, the postpartum hormonal landscape can bring challenges. A decrease in estrogen and progesterone following childbirth may contribute to postpartum mood swings, and some women experience postpartum depression, often linked to these hormonal adjustments. Relaxation techniques, such as breathing exercises and mindfulness, have been shown to reduce stress and anxiety during lactation, promoting a more positive breastfeeding experience and improving milk supply. By managing stress and promoting relaxation, these interventions can enhance oxytocin release and overall lactation outcomes.

After childbirth and during lactation, hormonal shifts trigger a series of physical changes that support breastfeeding and recovery from pregnancy. Here's an in-depth look at these changes [9]:

2.4.1 Milk production and lactation

Prolactin: The primary hormone responsible for initiating and maintaining milk production is prolactin. Following delivery, prolactin levels rise sharply, stimulating the mammary glands to produce milk. This is critical for breastfeeding success. The amount of milk produced is directly related to the frequency of breastfeeding, as prolactin levels fluctuate based on demand.

Oxytocin: Often referred to as the "love hormone," oxytocin plays a significant role in the milk ejection reflex, helping to release milk from the glands into the nipple during breastfeeding. It also helps contract the uterus post-delivery, promoting uterine involution (the return of the uterus to its pre-pregnancy size).

2.4.2 Breast changes

Increased size and tenderness: Under the influence of progesterone and estrogen during pregnancy, the breasts undergo significant changes in preparation for breastfeeding, including increased size and tenderness. After birth, the release of prolactin ensures that milk production is established, further changing the size and feel of the breasts as they become engorged with milk.

Areolar and nipple changes: The areola and nipples darken during pregnancy and after birth, which helps the infant locate the breast for feeding. This color change can remain post-lactation, even after weaning.

2.4.3 Uterine involution and hormonal regulation

After delivery, the uterus contracts to shrink back to its pre-pregnancy size, a process influenced by oxytocin. This contraction helps control bleeding, but can also lead to postpartum cramps, particularly during breastfeeding when oxytocin levels surge. The uterus undergoes this process for about 6–8 weeks post-delivery.

2.4.4 Skin and hair changes

Skin elasticity and stretch marks: During pregnancy, the skin stretches to accommodate the growing fetus, and while much of this returns to normal postpartum, some women experience lingering stretch marks. Hormonal changes after childbirth can also influence skin pigmentation, sometimes causing conditions such as melasma (dark patches of skin), which typically fade over time.

Hair loss: Many women experience a condition called "postpartum hair loss" due to hormonal fluctuations, particularly the sudden drop in estrogen levels after childbirth. This usually leads to thinning hair, especially around the temples and crown. Hair typically regrows within a few months, but this process can be distressing for some women.

2.4.5 Metabolic and cardiovascular adjustments

Return of menstrual cycles: Hormonal shifts influence the return of menstruation after childbirth. For women who breastfeed, prolactin levels remain elevated, which can suppress ovulation and delay the return of menstruation. For non-breastfeeding women, ovulation typically returns within a few months.

Body weight and fat distribution: Pregnancy leads to increased fat storage for energy reserves during breastfeeding. After childbirth, metabolism begins to return to pre-pregnancy levels, though it can take several months to return to baseline. Breastfeeding also increases energy expenditure, helping some women return to their pre-pregnancy weight.

These physical changes illustrate how the body adapts to support both the newborn and the mother's recovery after pregnancy. Each of these processes is influenced by the complex hormonal environment that is established after childbirth, and it is key to supporting new mothers physically and emotionally.

2.5 Menopause

Menopause typically occurs between 45 and 55 years. These hormonal changes become more pronounced. Before this stage, estrogen and FSH levels start to become variable, with menstrual cycles remaining regular or becoming slightly irregular [10].

2.5.1 Early perimenopause

Here, estrogen and FSH levels become increasingly erratic, leading to more noticeable irregularities in menstrual cycles and the onset of menopausal symptoms such as hot flashes and mood changes.

2.5.2 Late perimenopause

In the late perimenopause stage, estrogen levels decrease, while FSH levels increase, signaling the body's transition away from regular menstruation. This phase may bring heightened symptoms that affect a woman's overall health. Understanding these hormonal changes is crucial for addressing their implications for women's health, particularly in managing conditions that can arise from hormonal fluctuations.

The decline in estrogen leads to symptoms such as hot flashes, night sweats, and changes in mood. These fluctuations can also affect bone density and cardiovascular health. Hormonal changes during menopause are linked to increased risks of osteoporosis and heart disease due to the protective effects of estrogen being reduced [10].

Throughout a woman's life, hormonal fluctuations are normal and can significantly impact physical health, emotional well-being, and overall quality of life. Understanding these changes can help in managing symptoms associated with different life stages.

3. Hormonal changes effects on oral condition

Hormonal fluctuations throughout a woman's life can lead to various oral health issues, particularly during critical periods such as puberty, menstruation, pregnancy, and menopause. These hormonal changes influence biological functions that directly impact oral health, including blood circulation to the mouth and saliva production. So hormonal fluctuations can significantly impact oral health in women at various life stages. Here is how these changes manifest:

3.1 Puberty and oral health

During puberty, increased levels of hormones can cause heightened sensitivity in the gums, leading to conditions such as gingivitis, which is characterized by swollen and bleeding gums. The surge in hormones can also result in increased inflammation and a greater susceptibility to bacterial infections within the oral cavity. On the other hand, mood swings and changes in routine during puberty may affect oral hygiene practices. Interestingly, gingival inflammation does not always correlate directly with the amount of plaque present; instead, it may be more significantly influenced by variations in hormonal levels. This observation suggests that hormonal fluctuations could play a crucial role in the inflammatory response of the gums [11, 12].

Contrary to this notion, research indicates that maintaining good oral hygiene has a more positive impact on the gingival health of adolescents than the increasing levels of steroid hormones during puberty. This finding highlights the importance of effective oral care practices in managing gingival conditions, particularly in younger populations. During puberty, the changes in microbial composition within the oral cavity are largely driven by the gingival tissue's reaction to sex hormones. These hormones modify the local environment, allowing certain bacterial species to thrive in response to the elevated hormone levels, which can further influence gingival health.

Progesterone and estrogen hormones can lead to periodontis causing bacteria to grow. Thus, periodontis is more common in the pubertal age in comparison with others in their prepubertal stage. Also, it has been reported that there is a higher population of bacteria in subgingival pockets is present during puberty, which may selectively accumulate estradiol and progesterone [11–13].

3.2 Menstrual cycle and oral health

Some women experience gingival inflammation and sensitivity just before menstruation due to hormonal changes. Symptoms may include swollen gums and increased bleeding. Hormonal fluctuations can alter taste perception, potentially affecting dietary choices and oral care habits.

The menstrual cycle also introduces hormonal fluctuations that can affect oral health. The increase in progesterone during certain phases can cause gums to become bright red and swollen, contributing to discomfort and increased bleeding. This phenomenon, often referred to as menstruation gingivitis, highlights the intricate link between hormonal changes and oral health [12].

The menstrual or reproductive cycle is marked by a cyclical increase in the production and secretion of estrogen and progesterone, which begins at puberty. Researches has shown that significant inflammatory changes in the gums can occur during this cycle, particularly when there is an imbalance in sex hormones. These hormonal fluctuations can exacerbate existing gingival conditions, leading to increased inflammation. During menstruation, variations in the flow of gingival crevicular fluid (GCF) are primarily observed in individuals with pre-existing gingivitis, as opposed to those with healthy gums. Studies have indicated that levels of inflammatory cytokines, such as interleukin 1β (IL1β), exhibit notable changes, with a consistent rise in GCF from the onset of menstruation to the peak of progesterone levels. This increase may be attributed to the role of progesterone in stimulating inflammatory cells to produce higher amounts of IL1β.

Furthermore, other inflammatory cytokines, including interleukin 6 (IL6) and tumor necrosis factor alpha, may also play a role in the gingival inflammatory changes that occur throughout the menstrual cycle. These cytokines contribute to the overall inflammatory response, highlighting the complex interplay between hormonal fluctuations and oral health during this period. Understanding these dynamics is crucial for managing gingival health in individuals affected by hormonal changes [11].

3.3 Pregnancy effects on oral condition

Pregnancy triggers significant hormonal shifts that affect various physiological systems, including the endocrine and oral health systems. The two primary hormones involved are estrogen and progesterone, which undergo dramatic increases during gestation. Estrogen, in particular, is produced in quantities exceeding those seen throughout a woman's non-pregnant life, playing a crucial role in uterine and placental development, as well as fetal maturation. The rise in estrogen levels peaks in the third trimester and is linked to symptoms such as nausea during the first trimester and breast development during the second trimester [14].

Studies indicate that 30 to 100% of pregnant women may suffer from gum inflammation, which can progress to periodontitis if untreated. If inflammation is not addressed, it can lead to the deterioration of tooth support and, ultimately, tooth loss [12]. Some women develop benign growths called pyogenic granulomas on the gums during pregnancy due to hormonal changes and increased blood flow. Also, it has been reported that morning sickness can lead to acid exposure from vomiting, increasing the risk of dental erosion.

During pregnancy, alterations in the oral microbiome are evident, with total viable microbial counts significantly higher than those observed in non-pregnant women. These changes may be influenced by hormonal fluctuations that affect bacterial growth, highlighting a bidirectional relationship between microbiota and hormonal levels. The hormonal changes during pregnancy can lead to a heightened risk of periodontal disease. The increased blood flow and hormonal variations may exacerbate pre-existing conditions or contribute to new issues in oral health. Women experiencing periodontal disease during pregnancy have been observed to have a higher risk of pregnancy complications, suggesting a significant interplay between oral and systemic health [15].

Moreover, the modifications in hormone levels can also influence dental caries development, potentially affecting the Decayed, Missing, and Filled Teeth (DMFT) status of pregnant women. As insulin sensitivity decreases later in pregnancy, the body's ability to regulate blood glucose is impaired, which can lead to increased sugar levels in the mouth—contributing to a higher risk of dental caries. Researches have indicated a bidirectional relationship between periodontal disease and adverse pregnancy outcomes, including preterm birth and low birth weight [16].

The hormonal changes that lead to gingival inflammation can create an inflammatory environment that may affect overall health, underscoring the importance of dental care during and after pregnancy [17]. Elevated systemic inflammation and increased periodontal pathogens can disrupt homeostasis in the fetal-placental unit, potentially leading to complications [18].

In summary, pregnancy involves significant hormonal fluctuations, notably increases in estrogen and progesterone, which can have profound effects on the oral cavity. These hormones can alter the immune response, leading to an increased risk of gum disease and other oral health issues. Here is a detailed breakdown of the primary effects:

3.3.1 Pregnancy gingivitis

Pregnancy gingivitis is a common condition characterized by swollen, red, and bleeding gums, particularly around the second trimester. The increased levels of progesterone during pregnancy can cause the gums to become more sensitive to plaque, leading to inflammation. The condition is often worsened by poor oral hygiene. Pregnant women may experience changes in their saliva composition, contributing to the increased susceptibility of the gums to bacterial infections [19].

3.3.2 Periodontal disease

Untreated gingivitis can develop into more severe periodontal disease, which leads to the destruction of the supportive tissues around the teeth, including the alveolar bone. The disease may result in clinical attachment loss, deepening of the periodontal pockets, and bone loss, particularly in women who already have periodontal risk factors before pregnancy. There is still some controversy about the relationship between periodontal disease and adverse pregnancy outcomes, but numerous studies have shown a significant association between periodontal disease and preterm birth or low birth weight [20].

3.3.3 Microbial changes

Pregnancy can shift the microbial balance in the oral cavity, promoting the growth of harmful bacteria. The resulting dysbiosis (imbalance of the oral microbiome) can contribute to the progression of gingivitis and periodontitis. Increased levels of bacteria such as *Porphyromonas gingivalis* and *Fusobacterium nucleatum* during pregnancy can exacerbate periodontal conditions. These bacteria are implicated not only in local oral inflammation but also in systemic effects, such as the risk of preterm labor or low birth weight. The presence of certain bacteria in the mouth, like *P. gingivalis*, can increase the levels of inflammatory cytokines, which are linked to preterm births and low-birth-weight babies. Studies are needed to understand how *P. gingivalis* affects pregnancy, particularly by disrupting early processes like uterine artery remodeling, which impacts adverse pregnancy outcomes (APOs). Early oral treatments, ideally starting before conception, may help mitigate this. While *P. gingivalis* causes imbalances in oral bacteria, further research is required to see if this contributes to systemic health issues, including APOs. Additionally, *P. gingivalis* potentially invading the maternal-fetal interface and causing placental dysbiosis related to APOs is an interesting area for future investigation.

Current literature supports the link between *F. nucleatum* and preterm birth, intra-amniotic infection, stillbirth, neonatal sepsis, and hypertensive disorders of pregnancy. *F. nucleatum* possesses key virulence mechanisms that allow it to attach and disseminate across endothelium, enabling its hematogenous spread [21, 22].

3.3.4 Alveolar bone health

Pregnancy hormones may influence bone metabolism and decrease the body's ability to regenerate alveolar bone. Increased bone resorption and a reduction in bone density can make the alveolar bone more susceptible to destruction from periodontal disease. The combination of hormonal effects and periodontal disease progression can thus increase the risk of tooth mobility and eventual tooth loss [23].

3.3.5 Best timing for dental treatment during pregnancy

The second trimester (weeks 13–27) is considered the safest time for most dental treatments during pregnancy. At this stage, the risk of miscarriage is lower, and the baby's organs have already formed. Dental treatments such as fillings, crowns, and even certain extractions are generally considered safe, but non-essential treatments, such as cosmetic procedures, should be avoided [24].

First trimester: During the first trimester, dental treatments that are not urgent should be postponed to avoid any potential risks to fetal development. The first 12 weeks are critical for the development of the baby's organs and tissues, and the risk of teratogenic effects from medications, anesthetics, or radiation is higher [24].

Third trimester: The third trimester is a less ideal time for dental procedures due to the physical discomfort that may accompany lying back in the dentist's chair and the potential for higher blood pressure or gestational hypertension. However, necessary treatments such as tooth extractions or infection control may still be performed if urgent [24].

Appropriate supplementation of a variety of nutrition during pregnancy has become an effective way to prevent periodontal disease and adverse pregnancy outcomes the management of periodontal infection during pregnancy should follow relevant treatment principles, and the ideal time for periodontal treatment is the second trimester (14–27 weeks). If intervention for infection is absolutely necessary, emergency treatment can be performed throughout pregnancy [20].

3.3.6 Considerations during pregnancy

Dental X-rays should be avoided unless absolutely necessary. If an X-ray is required, a lead apron should be used to shield the abdomen. Modern digital X-rays expose the body to much lower levels of radiation than traditional methods, which reduces risks, but it is still advisable to postpone elective X-rays during pregnancy.

Local anesthetics such as lidocaine with epinephrine are commonly used during dental procedures and are generally considered safe during pregnancy. However, care should be taken to avoid excessive amounts of epinephrine, as it may cause vasoconstriction, affecting blood flow to the fetus.

Penicillin and its derivatives (such as amoxicillin) are considered safe during pregnancy and are commonly prescribed for oral infections; also, the metronidazole has similar condition. Clindamycin is another safe alternative for treating infections. Tetracyclines should be avoided during pregnancy as they can affect fetal bone development and teeth discoloration. As an analgesics, the acetaminophen is the safest pain killer during pregnancy, and the ibuprofen is safe also except in the 3th trimester [24].

3.4 Postpartum period and lactation effects on oral health

The hormonal changes during lactation not only facilitate milk production but also induce physiological adaptations in various maternal tissues. For example, there is an increased demand for calcium and other minerals, which can lead to a transient loss of bone minerals.

After weaning, hormonal levels revert to pre-pregnancy states, and bone remineralization becomes a priority, highlighting the dynamic interplay between lactation and maternal health. These hormonal shifts also have implications for oral health. Changes in hormone levels can affect the composition of saliva and the immune response in the oral cavity, potentially increasing susceptibility to dental issues during the postpartum period Thus, understanding the hormonal changes during lactation is essential for both maternal and child health, including aspects related to oral care.

During the postpartum period and lactation, significant hormonal fluctuations can profoundly impact oral health. The hormonal changes that occur, particularly involving estrogen and progesterone, can lead to alterations in the oral environment, resulting in various oral health issues.

Following childbirth, women experience a significant drop in estrogen levels, which can affect oral health in several ways. The decrease in estrogen is associated with reduced blood flow and changes in the immune response, making the gums more susceptible to inflammation and infection. This can lead to an increased risk of periodontal diseases, such as gingivitis and periodontitis, particularly if oral hygiene is not adequately maintained [25].

Additionally, women may experience symptoms such as dry mouth during this period, which can exacerbate plaque buildup and increase the risk of cavities and periodontal disease. Saliva plays a crucial role in neutralizing acids produced by plaque and in maintaining oral health; therefore, reduced saliva can lead to halitosis and increased dental issues [25].

Lactation also introduces changes in hormone levels, particularly increases in prolactin and oxytocin, which can further influence oral health. While breastfeeding may have protective effects against tooth decay due to the beneficial properties of breast milk, hormonal changes can still affect the gums. Some women may experience swollen or bleeding gums during this time due to elevated levels of estrogen and progesterone, similar to what occurs during pregnancy. The inflammation of the gums can lead to more severe conditions if left untreated, emphasizing the importance of maintaining good oral hygiene practices during lactation [26, 27]. Also, trabecular rich sites of the mandible were found affected by lactation and it should be considered in advanced dental treatments [28].

In summary, lactation can influence dental and oral health in various ways, both directly and indirectly, due to hormonal shifts, dietary changes, and the physiological demands of breastfeeding. Here are some key ways lactation may affect oral health [29]:

3.4.1 Dry mouth

Hormonal impact: During lactation, prolactin levels increase to stimulate milk production, but this can also decrease saliva production, leading to dry mouth (xerostomia). Saliva is essential for neutralizing acids in the mouth and protecting against cavities and gum disease. Reduced saliva flow increases the risk of tooth decay and bad breath impact on Oral Health: Saliva plays a crucial role in maintaining the balance of bacteria in the mouth. When saliva production is low, harmful bacteria thrive, potentially leading to issues such as tooth decay, gingivitis, and even infections like thrush, which is more common in breastfeeding women due to hormone changes.

3.4.2 Gum sensitivity

Hormonal influence: Just as pregnancy can affect gum health due to hormonal fluctuations, lactation can also contribute to gum sensitivity. Elevated levels of progesterone and estrogen postpartum can lead to an increased blood flow to the gums, making them more susceptible to irritation and inflammation. Gingivitis, characterized by swollen, bleeding gums, may become more noticeable during lactation.

3.4.3 Oral hygiene difficulties

During breastfeeding, women may experience difficulty maintaining oral hygiene due to fatigue or time constraints. This can worsen gum issues if plaque accumulates on teeth, exacerbating gingival problem. Also, lactating women often require extra calories to meet the energy demands of breastfeeding. If this caloric increase includes sugary or acidic foods and drinks, it can affect oral health. Sugary snacks or beverages can feed harmful bacteria in the mouth, contributing to plaque buildup and the formation of cavities. Dehydration during lactation can not only exacerbate dry mouth but also affect overall oral health. Dehydration can reduce saliva production, leading to an increased risk of tooth decay and gum disease.

3.4.4 Tooth erosion

The dietary habits of a lactating mother can sometimes include more acidic foods and beverages, such as citrus fruits and juices, which can erode tooth enamel over time. While lactation itself does not directly cause tooth erosion, dietary choices can contribute to enamel wear, especially when combined with dry mouth.

3.4.5 Periodontal diseases

After childbirth, the rapid hormonal fluctuations associated with breastfeeding can affect the health of both soft and hard oral tissues. The decrease in estrogen and progesterone after delivery might increase the risk of periodontal diseases if the individual was already susceptible.

Therefore, lactation, through hormonal shift and special habits, can influence various aspects of oral health, making good oral hygiene and regular hydration important during this period. If you have specific concerns about oral health while breastfeeding, consulting a dentist is recommended.

3.4.6 Considerations in dental treatments

Most local anesthetics, including lidocaine, are safe during lactation, as they have minimal secretion into breast milk. However, it is always best to consult with a healthcare provider regarding any concerns. Also, most antibiotics are safe for breastfeeding mothers, but medications like tetracycline can be excreted in breast milk and should be avoided. Penicillin, amoxicillin, and clindamycin are generally considered safe and effective for managing oral infections during lactation.

3.5 Menopause and its impact on oral health

Menopause is characterized by significant hormonal changes that impact various bodily functions, including oral health. As women approach their late 30s and into their 40s, the ovaries gradually produce less estrogen and progesterone, which are essential for regulating the menstrual cycle and reproductive health. This hormonal decline can result in a variety of symptoms that extend beyond the reproductive system and can significantly affect oral health.

One of the notable effects of decreased estrogen levels is the reduction in saliva production. Estrogen receptors are present in the oral mucosa and the salivary glands, and as estrogen levels drop, saliva production may decline. A lower saliva flow can lead to dry mouth (xerostomia), which not only affects comfort but also increases the risk of dental issues such as cavities and gum disease, as saliva plays a crucial role in washing away food particles and aiding digestion. Effective management strategies include using over-the-counter products like saliva substitutes, chewing sugar-free gum, and increasing water intake [30].

Hormonal fluctuations during menopause can also render the gums more sensitive and prone to inflammation. Women may experience conditions such as gingivitis or periodontitis more frequently during this time, as hormonal changes can lead to increased gum sensitivity Another consequence of hormonal changes is the potential alteration in taste perception. Women may experience a metallic taste or a reduced sense of taste, which can further complicate the experience of eating and enjoying food during menopause [31].

A 2023 survey indicated that a large majority of women over 50 are unaware of these risks, with 84% not realizing that menopause can affect oral health, and nearly 90% unaware of specific risks like increased tooth decay and gum disease [32].

The decline in estrogen during menopause can compromise oral health, heightening the likelihood of conditions such as gingivitis and periodontitis, which can lead to attachment loss and tooth loss. Many women report heightened tooth sensitivity during menopause, often linked to the loss of enamel and exposure of dentine, which can lead to pain and discomfort. This sensitivity may also arise from changes in oral hygiene routines or dietary habits that women adopt during this period. Menopausal women are at an increased risk of developing periodontal disease due to hormonal changes. This condition manifests as swollen, bleeding gums, and can progress to more severe forms if not managed appropriately Changes in gum health are also prevalent during menopause. Symptoms may include changes in gum color, increased bleeding, gum recession, and inflammation, with studies suggesting that up to 60% of women may experience periodontal symptoms. Chronic gum disease, or periodontitis, can lead to tooth loss and is associated with other systemic health issues, such as heart disease and diabetes [30].

Burning mouth syndrome (BMS) is another oral health concern affecting approximately 15% of menopausal women. This condition involves a burning sensation in the mouth, which may affect the tongue, gums, and lips, and can also alter taste perception, especially for salty or spicy foods. The risk of tooth loss increases during menopause, with studies showing that more than one in four post-menopausal women may experience this within 5 years. This heightened risk is often linked to bone density loss in the jaw, a common consequence of menopause, which can destabilize teeth and make them more prone to becoming loose or falling out [33].

4. Preventive measures and management for women

To mitigate the effects of hormonal fluctuations on oral health, particularly regarding conditions such as gingivitis, women can adopt several preventive measures and management strategies. These include maintaining proper oral hygiene, making healthy lifestyle choices, and seeking regular dental care. Regular dental check-ups: Regular dental visits are essential for the early detection and treatment of gum disease. Dentists can identify the initial signs of gingivitis and recommend appropriate interventions to prevent its progression into more severe forms of gum disease, such as periodontitis. It is advisable for women to schedule professional cleanings and check-ups at least twice a year. In the following, we mention the most important ways to maintain oral health during hormonal changes [34–36].

5. Proper oral hygiene practices

Establishing a consistent oral hygiene routine is critical for preventing gum disease. Women should brush their teeth at least twice daily with fluoride toothpaste, floss daily, and consider using an antiseptic mouthwash to further reduce plaque and bacteria in the mouth. Additionally, utilizing a soft-bristled toothbrush can help prevent damage to gums and enamel.

5.1 Healthy lifestyle

A balanced diet rich in vitamins and minerals can support immune function and gum health. Consuming fruits, vegetables, whole grains, and lean proteins while avoiding excessive sugars and acidic foods is vital in minimizing the risk of plaque buildup and inflammation. Furthermore, avoiding smoking and limiting alcohol intake can significantly reduce the risk of developing gum disease.

5.2 Stress management

Hormonal fluctuations can lead to increased stress, which may adversely affect oral health by weakening the immune system. Women should engage in stress-reducing activities, such as exercise, meditation, or hobbies, to maintain both mental and oral health. Adequate sleep is also crucial in managing stress and promoting overall wellbeing.

5.3 Hormonal balance

Women experiencing hormonal changes, especially during pregnancy or menopause, should consult healthcare providers for guidance on managing these fluctuations. Hormonal imbalances can impact saliva production, increasing the risk of dry mouth, which in turn elevates the likelihood of developing gum disease. Maintaining open communication with healthcare professionals about any changes can help in adopting effective preventive measures.

Another method is also suggested for postmenopausal women such as hormone replacement therapy (HRT). Hormone replacement therapy (HRT) can be considered to alleviate various menopausal symptoms, including those affecting oral health. Although HRT has its risks, some studies suggest that it may help improve oral conditions by stabilizing fluctuating hormone levels. It is advisable for women to consult with healthcare providers to evaluate the benefits and potential side effects of HRT. However, studies on the dangers of using them have not reached a definitive conclusion; for example, Yuk et al. reported that menopausal hormone therapy increases the risk of oral cavity cancer in postmenopausal women [37]. Also, many women explore alternative treatments such as herbal remedies, acupuncture, and relaxation techniques to manage menopausal symptoms. Acupuncture, for example, has been shown to reduce the frequency and intensity of hot flashes. However, the effectiveness of these treatments can vary, and further research is needed to establish their safety and efficacy in relation to oral health.

6. Conclusion

Hormonal fluctuations throughout a woman's life can significantly influence oral health. Understanding these effects is crucial for maintaining good oral hygiene practices and seeking timely dental care when necessary. Regular dental check-ups are important for managing these changes effectively.

However, the above findings from various studies all indicate the impact of hormonal changes on women's oral and dental health. The cohort studies that evaluated the participants during a long term have reported different results, which show that by removing confounding factors, it cannot be definitely stated that there is a relationship between these hormonal changes and oral and dental problems. A cohort study conducted by Romandi et al. showed periodontitis was directly associated with a longer duration of breastfeeding and was inversely associated with artificial menopause and early and late menopausal ages [38]. But Rafiei et al. reported after adjusting for all potential confounders, no correlation was found between hormonal fluctuations and periodontal status, even in pregnancy and lactation [39]. Therefore, due to the many variables that can affect this phenomenon, it is not possible to reach a definite conclusion, but it is clear that hormonal changes change the conditions of the mouth, but the destructive results of these effects can be prevented by planning. Therefore, it can be concluded that routine dental visits, training from an early age, and educating the oral hygiene and proper nutrition for each period of lifetime can help women in preventing oral and dental complications caused by hormonal changes.

Author details

Mehrad Rafiei[1,2]

1 Maxillofacial Surgery and Implantology and Biomaterial Research Foundation, Tehran, Iran

2 Student Research Committee, Rafsanjan University of Medical Sciences, Rafsanjan, Iran

*Address all correspondence to: mehradr1374@gmail.com

References

[1] Zacur HA. Hormonal changes throughout life in women. The Journal of Headache and Pain. 2006;**46**:S50-S55

[2] Lee PA, Houk CP. Puberty and its disorders. Pediatric Endocrinology. 2007;**2**:273-304

[3] Fehring RJ, Schneider M, Raviele K. Variability in the phases of the menstrual cycle. Journal of Obstetric, Gynecologic, and Neonatal Nursing. 2006;**35**:376-384

[4] Kazma JM, van den Anker J, Allegaert K, Dallmann A, Ahmadzia HK. Anatomical and physiological alterations of pregnancy. Journal of Pharmacokinetics and Pharmacodynamics. 2020;**47**(4): 271-285

[5] Brik M, Sandonis M, Temprado J, et al. Anxiety during pregnancy and low birth weight: An observational cohort study. Authorea. 2023;**2023**:1-8. DOI: 10.22541/au.167895543.37653507/v1

[6] Soma-Pillay P, Nelson-Piercy C, Tolppanen H, Mebazaa A. Physiological changes in pregnancy: Review articles. Cardiovascular Journal of Africa. 2016;**27**:89-94

[7] Chauhan A, Potdar J. Maternal mental health during pregnancy: A critical review. Cureus. 2022;**14**:e30656. DOI: 10.7759/cureus.30656

[8] Zourladani A, Zafrakas M, Chatzigiannis B, Papasozomenou P, Vavilis D, Matziari C. The effect of physical exercise on postpartum fitness, hormone and lipid levels: A randomized controlled trial in primiparous, lactating women. Archives of Gynecology and Obstetrics. 2015;**291**:525-530

[9] Martin C, Rokibullah R, Sofinia H. The physiological changes in the postpartum period after childbirth. Asian Journal of Social and Humanities. 2022;**1**(03):105-118

[10] Talaulikar V. Menopause transition: Physiology and symptoms. Best Practice & Research. Clinical Obstetrics & Gynaecology. 2022;**81**:3-7

[11] Sathish AK, Varghese J, Fernandes AJ. The impact of sex hormones on the periodontium during a woman's lifetime: A concise-review update. Current Oral Health Reports. 2022;**9**(4):146-156

[12] Boyapati R, Cherukuri SA, Bodduru R, Kiranmaye A. Influence of female sex hormones in different stages of women on periodontium. Journal of Mid-life Health. 2021;**12**(4):263-266

[13] Rashidi Maybodi F, Jalali Pandary M, Rahaei Z, Nikniaz S. Awareness of the effect of fluctuations in female sex hormone levels on periodontal health among obstetricians. Journal of Advanced Periodontology & Implant Dentistry. 2018;**10**:29-34

[14] Costantine MM. Physiologic and pharmacokinetic changes in pregnancy. Frontiers in Pharmacology. 2014;**5**:65

[15] Wu M, Chen SW, Jiang SY. Relationship between gingival inflammation and pregnancy. Mediators of Inflammation. 2015;**2015**(1):623427

[16] Patil SR. Oral changes in pregnant and nonpregnant women: A case-control study. Journal of Orofacial Sciences. 2013;**5**(2):118-122

[17] Figuero E, Carrillo-de-Albornoz A, Martín C, Tobías A, Herrera D. Effect

of pregnancy on gingival inflammation in systemically healthy women: A systematic review. Journal of Clinical Periodontology. 2013;**40**(5):457-473

[18] Mariam S, Hasan S, Shinde M, Gupta J, Buch SA, Rajpurohit KS, et al. Pregnancy outcomes and maternal periodontal diseases: The unexplored connection. Cureus. 2024;**16**(6)

[19] Talebessy R, Cecilia S. Gingivitis and oral health diseases related to pregnancy. Crown: Journal of Dentistry and Health Research. 2023;**1**(1):1-5

[20] Nannan M, Xiaoping L, Ying J. Periodontal disease in pregnancy and adverse pregnancy outcomes: Progress in related mechanisms and management strategies. Frontiers in Medicine. 2022;**9**:963956

[21] Reyes L, Phillips P, Wolfe B, Golos TG, Walkenhorst M, Progulske-Fox A, et al. Porphyromonas gingivalis and adverse pregnancy outcome. Journal of Oral Microbiology. 2017;**10**(1):1374153

[22] Vander Haar EL, So J, Gyamfi-Bannerman C, Han YW. Fusobacterium nucleatum and adverse pregnancy outcomes: Epidemiological and mechanistic evidence. Anaerobe. 2018;**50**:55-59

[23] Shoji K, Shimauchi H, Shinoda H. Effects of pregnancy, lactation and dietary calcium on alveolar bone loss. Clinical Calcium. 2002;**12**(7):992-996

[24] Hemalatha V, Manigandan T, Sarumathi T, Aarthi Nisha V, Amudhan A. Dental considerations in pregnancy-a critical review on the oral care. Journal of Clinical and Diagnostic Research. 2013;7(5):948-953

[25] Gürsoy M, Pajukanta R, Sorsa T, Könönen E. Clinical changes in periodontium during pregnancy and post-partum. Journal of Clinical Periodontology. 2008;**35**(7):576-583

[26] Aghazadeh Z, Behroozian A, Najafi H, Faramarzi M. Comparison of gingival and dental indices in lactating and non-lactating mothers during first 6 month after delivery. Pesquisa Brasileira em Odontopediatria e Clínica Integrada. 2019;**19**:e4586

[27] Öztürk L, Akyüz S, Garan A, Yarat A. Salivary and dental-oral hygiene parameters in 3rd trimester of pregnancy and early lactation: The effect of education. Marmara Dental Journal. 2013;**1**(1):1-8

[28] Coşgunarslan A, Canger EM, Soydan Çabuk D, Kış HC. The evaluation of the mandibular bone structure changes related to lactation with fractal analysis. Oral Radiology. 2020;**36**:238-247

[29] Peres KG, Chaffee BW, Feldens CA, Flores-Mir C, Moynihan P, Rugg-Gunn A. Breastfeeding and Oral health: Evidence and methodological challenges. Journal of Dental Research. 2018;**97**(3):251-258

[30] Dutt P, Chaudhary SR, Kumar P. Oral health and menopause: A comprehensive review on current knowledge and associated dental management. Annals of Medical and Health Sciences Research. 2013;**3**(3):320-323

[31] Shigli KA, Giri PA. Oral manifestations of menopause. Journal of Basic and Clinical Reproductive Sciences. 2015;**4**(1):4-8

[32] Thomas N, Peters K, Reilly KO, Sousa MS, George A. Oral health care among women in perimenopause or menopause: An integrative review. Journal of Midwifery & Women's

Health. 2024;**13668**:1-15. DOI: 10.1111/jmwh.13668

[33] Dahiya P, Kamal R, Kumar M, Gupta R, Chaudhary K. Burning mouth syndrome and menopause. International Journal of Preventive Medicine. 2013;**4**:15

[34] Basha FY, Ganapathy D, Venugopalan S. Oral hygiene status among pregnant women. Research Journal of Pharmacy and Technology. 2018;**11**(7):3099-3102

[35] Rukmini JN, Sachan R, Sibi N, Meghana A, Malar CI. Effect of menopause on saliva and dental health. Journal of International Society of Preventive and Community Dentistry. 2018;**8**(6):529-533

[36] Hambire C, Hambire U. Oral health care and treatment needs in postmenopausal women. Journal of Oral Health and Community Dentistry. 2021;**15**(1):24-29

[37] Yuk JS, Kim BY. Relationship between menopausal hormone therapy and oral cancer: A cohort study based on the health insurance database in South Korea. Journal of Clinical Medicine. 2022;**11**(19):5848

[38] Romandini M, Shin HS, Romandini P, Laforí A, Cordaro M. Hormone-related events and periodontitis in women. Journal of Clinical Periodontology. 2020;**47**(4):429-441

[39] Rafiei M, Salarisedigh S, Khalili P, Jamali Z, Sardari F. Hormonal fluctuations and periodontal status in postmenopausal women. International Journal of Dentistry. 2022;**2022**(1):9990451

Chapter 14

The Impact of Estrogen Deficiency Symptoms on Health-Related Quality of Life in Menopausal-Aged Women in China

Martin Downes, Kyoo Kim, Marcelo Graziano Custodio, Igor Solev, Tommaso Simoncini and Qi Yu

Abstract

Menopausal symptoms are a critical health issue as they can have a substantial detrimental effect on women's physical and mental health and substantially impair health-related quality of life (HRQoL). Vasomotor symptoms (VMS) such as hot flushes, sweating, sleep disturbances, irritability, anxiety, and depression are often considered the cardinal symptoms of menopause. Among Chinese women of menopausal age, the symptom burden is high, with hot flushes/sweating, sleep disorders, mood disorders, and fatigue reported to be prevalent. In this chapter, we describe the available data on the burden of menopausal symptoms across pre-, peri-, and postmenopausal phases among Chinese women and the impact of these symptoms on HRQoL. We provide an overview of the recommendation for estrogen-based menopausal hormone therapy for the treatment of estrogen deficiency symptoms, given in combination with progestogen for non-hysterectomized women. We also describe the benefits of estradiol plus dydrogesterone among postmenopausal women of Chinese ethnicity, which include consistent improvements in symptom frequency and severity and improvements in HRQoL. Finally, we highlight the importance of timely identification and management of menopausal symptoms among Chinese women and the need to increase awareness of menopausal hormone therapy in this population.

Keywords: menopause, symptoms, health-related quality of life, China, menopausal hormone therapy, estradiol, dydrogesterone

1. Introduction

The adult female life is made up of three broad phases: reproductive, menopausal transition, and postmenopause [1]. According to the STRAW staging system [1], updated 10 years later as STRAW+10 [2], these three phases include a total of seven stages which are centred on the final menstrual period (Stage 0) [1, 2]. The reproductive phase is made up of early (Stage −5), peak (Stage −4), and late (Stage −3) stages and is followed by the menopausal transition phase, which consists of early (Stage −2) and late (Stage −1) stages [1]. Following Stage 0, the postmenopause phase includes early (Stage +1) and late (Stage +2) stages [1, 2]. The perimenopausal phase extends from early (Stage −2) through late (Stage −1) menopausal transition to early post menopause (Stage +1), lasting up to four years [2].

Vasomotor symptoms (VMS) such as hot flushes, sweating, sleep disturbances, irritability, anxiety, and depression [3–5] are often considered the cardinal symptoms of menopause and are "likely" and "most likely" during perimenopausal Stages −1 and + 1, respectively, according to the STRAW+10 criteria [2, 3, 6–9]. The postmenopausal period is associated with genitourinary syndrome of menopause (GSM), with vaginal dryness, burning and irritation, sexual symptoms including lack of lubrication and dyspareunia and urinary issues including increased urgency, dysuria and recurrent urinary tract infections comprising the key symptoms [10]. Menopausal symptoms at all stages are a critical health issue as they can have a substantial detrimental effect on women's physical and mental health and substantially impair health-related quality of life (HRQoL) [11–16]. **Figure 1** illustrates the effects of estrogen deficiency in the female body.

The frequency of VMS due to estrogen deficiency symptoms of menopause can vary based on ethnicity [17–19]. Women of Asian ethnicity often report fewer hot flushes and a shorter duration of VMS than those from other ethnic backgrounds, with reasons for these variations including lifestyle, genetics, body weight, and psychosocial and perceptual differences [17, 18, 20]. In China, there are currently almost 168 million women aged 45 to 59 years, highlighting the large number potentially

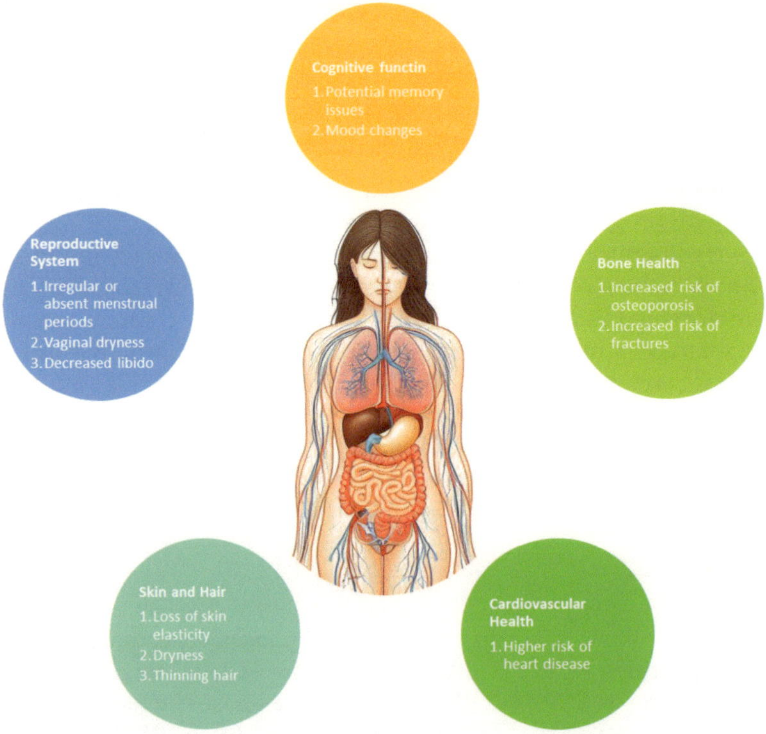

Figure 1.
The effects of estrogen deficiency.

experiencing menopausal symptoms and requiring healthcare services to alleviate their symptoms [3, 5, 8, 21–24]. Furthermore, research has shown the symptom burden among Chinese women of menopausal age to be high, with hot flushes/ sweating, sleep disorders, mood disorders, and fatigue reported to be prevalent [25], However, additional robust research into the prevalence and impact of menopausal symptoms or HRQoL among menopausal-aged women in China, particularly during the perimenopausal phase, is needed.

Patient-reported outcome (PRO) tools are increasingly being recognized by regulators and healthcare professionals as valuable in collecting unique, patient-centred information on the impact of health conditions and treatments [26], with PRO research using digital technology offering a promising alternative to time-consuming, resource intense paper-based research [27]. PROs are regularly used in clinical trials of menopausal women and can provide important insights into the patient journey and need for support and treatment. Popular tools include the 5-item European Quality of Life Dimension Five Level (EQ-5D-5L), the Menopause-Specific Quality of Life (MENQOL) questionnaire, a 29-item, 4-domain questionnaire assessing menopause-specific QoL, and the 11-item, 3-scale, Menopause Rating Scale (MRS), a self-administered questionnaire that measures the severity of a range of menopause-related symptoms in aging women with high reliability and validity [28–30].

2. Symptoms and health-related quality of life among pre-, peri- and post-menopausal women

Cost utility models are playing an increasingly important role in decision making in China, with health state utility values (HSUV) measured by the preferred, validated and widely used EQ-5D-5L being a key requirement [31]. With this in mind, a cross-sectional study by Rautenberg et al. measured symptoms and health-related quality of life in a cohort of menopausal-aged women in China, with the purpose of parameterising for a cost utility model to inform healthcare services in China [32]. As perimenopause has previously been associated with more somatic symptoms than other menopause stages [33], Rautenberg et al. also looked to explore utility by stage. In the cross-sectional study, around 30,000 females were invited to a survey link via SMS or WeChat, with the first 2000 females over 45 years included. Participants completed screening questions and the EQ-5D-5L, programmed in a personal digital assistant (PDA) format for smartphone. Utility tariffs were converted to EQ-5D-5L raw scores using Chinese value sets [34].

Respondents were classified as either premenopausal, perimenopausal and postmenopausal using the STRAW+10 criteria [2] and based upon a reported four-year median duration of perimenopause [4]. Premenopausal was defined as respondents with a uterus, regular menstruation and reporting last menstrual period up to the study date [December 2020]; perimenopausal was defined as respondents reporting irregular menstruation at the time of the study and up to four years prior to the study; and postmenopausal was defined as women with a uterus reporting the date of last menstrual period ≥ four years prior to the study [2, 4].

Among the 2000 included women (mean age: 49 years, 732 (37%) were premenopausal (mean age: 47 years), 798 (40%) were perimenopausal (mean age: 49 years) and 470 (23%) were postmenopausal (mean age: 53 years). A higher proportion of women reported an effect on the mobility, self-care, pain/discomfort and anxiety/ depression domains of the EQ-5D-5L in the perimenopausal group compared with the premenopausal and postmenopausal groups. The proportion reporting effects was 25, 9 and 22% for mobility, 14, 3 and 14% for self-care, 60, 40 and 57% for pain/ discomfort and 71%, 50% and 59% for anxiety/depression in the perimenopausal, premenopausal and postmenopausal groups, respectively. Additionally, symptomatic perimenopausal women with intact uterus had significantly lower HRQoL (health state utility value: 0.864) than symptomatic premenopausal (0.919, $p < 0.05$) and postmenopausal (0.877, $p < 0.05$) women (assessed using ANOVA with adjustment by the Tukey method). HRQoL was also significantly lower among symptomatic versus asymptomatic women within each group (premenopausal: 0.919 vs. 0.977 [$p < 0.05$]; perimenopausal: 0.864 vs. 0.956 [$p < 0.05$]; postmenopausal: 0.877 vs. 0.966 [$p < 0.05$]).

Overall, 83% of respondents reported experiencing menopausal symptoms. A significantly higher proportion of perimenopausal women (in the menopausal transition phase) reported symptoms (91%) compared with premenopausal (77%, $p < 0.05$) and postmenopausal (81%, $p < 0.05$) women. Nine of the 11 symptoms assessed (sleep problems, irritability, exhaustion, anxiety, hot flushes, depression, heart discomfort, loss of interest in sexual activity and vaginal dryness) were reported in significantly more women in the perimenopausal group compared with the premenopausal group. Two symptoms (joint pain and bladder problems) were reported in numerically more perimenopausal women but the differences did not reach statistical significance. Compared with the postmenopausal group, five of the 11 symptoms were reported in significantly more perimenopausal women (sleep problems, irritability, anxiety, hot flushes, depression), with no significant between-group difference in the other six symptoms (exhaustion, joint pain, heart discomfort, loss of interest in sexual activity, bladder problems and vaginal dryness).

HRQoL was significantly lower in the perimenopausal group compared with the premenopausal (with uterus) group for several symptoms of varying impact on daily life; this included sleep problems and anxiety (ranging from little or no impact to large impact), exhaustion (ranging from little or no impact to moderate impact), irritability (ranging from moderate to large impact), hot flushes, heart discomfort and loss of interest in sexual activity (moderate impact) and depression (large impact) (**Table 1**). HRQoL was also significantly lower for one symptom having a large impact on daily life (loss of interest in sexual activity) in the perimenopausal group compared with the postmenopausal (with uterus) group.

Overall, the study demonstrated that symptom burden is high across the menopausal stages, with perimenopausal women experiencing significantly more symptoms and having significantly lower HRQoL compared with premenopausal and postmenopausal women. One of the key strengths of the study was timely, smartphone-based electronic data collection in a large cohort that was representative of the general population in China [34–39]. Utilizing smartphones for data collection in this study also resulted in no missing values when completing the EQ-5D-5L survey, as there was a requirement for each question to be completed before a respondent could move onto the next question. Furthermore, the EQ-5D-5L used during the study is more sensitive to changes in HRQoL than the EQ-5D-3L, which was used in a prior study by Liu et al. that measured HSUV in premenopausal (0.810) and postmenopausal (0.800) women in China but did not report HSUV for perimenopausal women [24]. The authors did highlight that many of the symptoms assessed during the study may occur independently of menopause and that due to the nature of the study, causality and relationship with hormone levels could not be assessed. Moreover, detailed socio-demographic characteristics that may have confounded outcomes were not

Symptom	Premenopausal mean ± SD	Perimeno pausal mean ± SD	Postmen opausal mean ± SD	Perimenopausal vs. premenopausal; mean difference; 95% CI	Perimenopausal vs. postmenopausal; mean difference; 95% CI
No or little impact on daily life					
Anxiety	0.92 ± (0.08)	0.85 ± (0.11)	0.89 ± (0.08)	−0.07*; (0.11, −0.03)	−0.04; (−0.09, 0.01)
Bladder problems**	0.91 ± 0.03	0.77 ± 0.14	0.89 ± 0.10	−0.14; −0.34, 0.06	−0.12; −0.29, 0.06
Depression	0.9 ± 0.12	0.9 ± 0.09	0.89 ± 0.08	0.00; −0.05, 0.05	0.01; −0.05, 0.08
Exhaustion	0.93 ± 0.07	0.9 ± 0.07	0.88 ± 0.10	−0.03*; −0.06, 0.00	0.03; −0.01, 0.06
Heart discomfort	0.9 ± 0.1	0.85 ± 0.15	0.86 ± 0.14	−0.05; −0.13, 0.03	−0.01; −0.1, 0.08
Hot flushes	0.92 ± 0.08	0.89 ± 0.09	0.87 ± 0.12	−0.03; −0.06, 0	0.01; −0.02, 0.05
Irritability	0.91 ± 0.11	0.88 ± 0.10	0.9 ± 0.07	−0.04; −0.08, 0.00	−0.02; −0.07, 0.03
Joint discomfort	0.91 ± 0.11	0.89 ± 0.11	0.87 ± 0.16	−0.02; −0.08, 0.04	0.02; −0.06, 0.09
LOI sexual activity	0.91 ± 0.07	0.88 ± 0.12	0.88 ± 0.11	−0.03; −0.07, 0.01	0.00; −0.04, 0.04
Sleep problems	0.95 ± 0.07	0.90 ± 0.11	0.93 ± 0.07	−0.05*; −0.08, −0.02	−0.03; −0.07, 0.00
Vaginal dryness	0.9 ± 0.06	0.87 ± 0.10	0.88 ± 0.15	−0.03; −0.09, 0.02	−0.01; −0.07, 0.05
Moderate impact on daily life					
Anxiety	0.88 ± 0.09	0.84 ± 0.12	0.85 ± 0.13	−0.04; −0.07, 0.00	−0.01; −0.05, 0.04
Bladder problems	0.86 ± 0.12	0.82 ± 0.11	0.76 ± 0.13	−0.04; −0.18, 0.1	0.06; −0.1, 0.23
Depression	0.88 ± 0.09	0.83 ± 0.13	0.83 ± 0.15	−0.05; −0.1, 0.00	0.01; −0.05, 0.06
Exhaustion	0.90 ± 0.08	0.84 ± 0.12	0.86 ± 0.12	−0.06*; −0.09, −0.02	−0.01; −0.05, 0.03
Heart discomfort	0.88 ± 0.06	0.75 ± 0.22	0.82 ± 0.06	−0.14*; −0.27, −0.01	−0.07; −0.25, 0.10
Hot flushes	0.91 ± 0.09	0.83 ± 0.15	0.84 ± 0.12	−0.08*; −0.14, −0.03	−0.02; −0.09, 0.05
Irritability	0.90 ± (0.08)	0.84 ± (0.13)	0.83 ± (0.16)	−0.06*; (−0.1, −0.02)	0.01; (−0.04, 0.05)
Joint discomfort	0.86 ± 0.10	0.81 ± 0.15	0.84 ± 0.12	−0.05; −0.1, 0.00	−0.03; −0.09, 0.03
LOI sexual activity	0.90 ± 0.07	0.83 ± 0.14	0.82 ± 0.16	−0.07*; −0.13, −0.01	0.01; −0.06, 0.08
Sleep problems	0.91 ± 0.07	0.86 ± 0.11	0.86 ± 0.13	−0.04*; −0.07, −0.02	0.00; −0.03, 0.03
Vaginal dryness	0.89 ± 0.10	0.85 ± 0.13	0.87 ± 0.10	−0.04; −0.11, 0.03	−0.02; −0.09, 0.06
Large impact on daily life					
Anxiety	0.88 ± 0.08	0.80 ± 0.16	0.84 ± 0.14	−0.09*; −0.16, −0.01	−0.04; −0.13, 0.05
Bladder problems**	0.95 ± 0.08	0.73 ± 0.13	0.68 ± 0.27	−0.21; −0.65, 0.22	0.05; −0.33, 0.44

Symptom	Premenopausal mean ± SD	Perimeno pausal mean ± SD	Postmen opausal mean ± SD	Perimenopausal vs. premenopausal; mean difference; 95% CI	Perimenopausal vs. postmenopausal; mean difference; 95% CI
Depression	0.89 ± 0.05	0.74 ± 0.19	0.82 ± 0.15	−0.15*; −0.23, −0.08	−0.08; −0.18, 0.01
Exhaustion	0.87 ± 0.09	0.82 ± 0.13	0.80 ± 0.19	−0.05; −0.12, 0.02	0.01; −0.07, 0.09
Heart discomfort**	0.81 ± 0.07	0.67 ± 0.18	0.62 ± 0.20	−0.14; −0.38, 0.11	0.05; −0.10, 0.21
Hot flushes	0.87 ± 0.13	0.79 ± 0.23	0.72 ± 0.21	−0.07; −0.25, 0.1	0.08; −0.09, 0.24
Irritability	0.88 ± 0.08	0.79 ± 0.16	0.85 ± 0.14	−0.09*; −0.15, −0.03	−0.06; −0.12, 0.01
Joint discomfort	0.86 ± 0.09	0.78 ± 0.16	0.76 ± 0.16	−0.08; −0.18, 0.01	0.02; −0.07, 0.11
LOI sexual activity	0.90 ± 0.09	0.84 ± 0.10	0.92 ± 0.07	−0.06; −0.11, 0.01	−0.08*; −0.15,-0.01
Sleep problems	0.89 ± 0.09	0.81 ± 0.15	0.86 ± 0.13	−0.08*; −0.12, −0.03	−0.05; −0.1, 0.00
Vaginal dryness	0.91 ± 0.08	0.83 ± 0.12	0.83 ± 0.17	−0.08; −0.17, 0.01	0.00; −0.1, 0.1

CI, confidence interval; and SD, standard deviation. *$p < 0.05$.
***low sample size to detect differences.*

Table 1.
Health state utility values according to symptoms with varying impact on daily life (respondents with uterus) reported by Rautenberg et al. *[32] Reuse licensed under a Creative Commons Attribution 4.0 International License.*

measured. Respondents were also restricted to women with digital literacy and access to a smartphone. Despite the limitations, the findings provide important insights into the symptom and HRQoL burden among menopausal-aged women in China.

3. Untreated symptom burden remains high in post-menopausal women

Symptom burden during the postmenopausal phase remains substantial, as shown by the high proportions of postmenopausal women experiencing symptoms in the Rautenberg study [32]. Furthermore, a secondary analysis of data from the Women Health Needs Survey 2018 involving 3199 women aged 40–55 years in China found that high proportions of women suffered from insomnia (48.0%), fatigue (42.7%) and mood swing (39.8%), with 19.3% suffering from depressive symptoms [40]. Notably, postmenopause increased the risk of depressive symptoms [40]. The high symptom burden during postmenopause is also highlighted by baseline data from a pooled analysis of two phase 3, double-blind, randomized, placebo-controlled studies assessing the impact of low (E1mg/D5mg) and ultra-low (E0.5mg/D2.5mg) estradiol plus dydrogesterone versus placebo on treating vasomotor symptoms in postmenopausal women [41]. The first study was conducted in France, Poland, Romania and Russia and the second was conducted in China. Patients enrolled in the European study were randomized 2:1:2 to receive oral continuous E0.5mg/D2.5mg, E1mg/D5mg or placebo for 13 weeks. Women enrolled in the Chinese study were randomized 1:1 to receive continuous combined E0.5mg/D2.5mg or placebo once daily for 12 weeks [42]. At baseline, despite having a lower number of hot flushes, the Chinese population had

	European		Chinese	
	E0.5mg/D2.5mg (n = 122)		E0.5mg/D2.5mg (n = 163)	
Domain	Baseline	EOT	Baseline	EOT
1- Hot flushes, sweating	2.82 (0.79)	1.20 (0.81)*	2.39 (0.73)	1.18 (0.82)*
2- Heart discomfort	1.18 (1.04)	0.78 (0.78)	1.01 (1.04)	0.60 (0.78)*
3- Sleep problems	2.19 (1.25)	1.16 (1.02)	1.95 (1.31)	1.17 (1.07)*
4- Depressive mood	1.68 (1.21)	0.92 (0.94)	1.33 (1.13)	0.77 (0.82)*
5- Irritability	1.86 (1.11)	1.04 (0.99)	1.62 (1.19)	0.95 (0.88)*
6- Anxiety	1.58 (1.21)	0.77 (0.90)	1.32 (1.06)	0.68 (0.86)*
7- Physical and mental exhaustion	1.86 (1.00)	1.23 (0.86)	2.06 (1.08)	1.29 (0.87)*
8- Sexual problems	1.20 (1.19)	0.72 (0.98)	1.67 (1.30)	1.08 (1.14)
9- Bladder problems	1.02 (1.11)	0.66 (0.91)	0.90 (1.02)	0.56 (0.87)*
10- Dryness of vagina	1.24 (1.19)	0.74 (0.96)	1.70 (1.29)	1.04 (1.10)*
11- Joint and muscular discomfort	2.22 (1.00)	1.72 (0.98)	1.88 (1.23)	1.40 (0.97)*
Somato-vegetative (1 + 2 + 3 + 11)	8.41 (2.89)	4.86 (2.51)	7.22 (3.10)	4.34 (2.57)*
Psychological (4 + 5 + 6 + 7)	6.93 (3.78)	3.94 (3.08)	6.33 (3.83)	3.70 (2.96)*
Urogenital (8 + 9 + 10)	3.47 (2.65)	2.12 (2.18)	4.27 (3.00)	2.68 (2.56)*
TOTAL	18.81 (7.50)	10.92 (6.59)	17.82 (8.47)	10.72 (6.99)*

D, dydrogesterone; E, estradiol; and EOT, end of treatment. $^*p < 0.05$ *versus placebo.*

Table 2.
Menopause Rating Scale score across treatment groups [41]. Reuse licensed under a Creative Commons Attribution 4.0 International License.

similar average MRS total scores compared with the European population (**Table 2**). Among the 11 MRS domains, "hot flushes and sweating" was the most negatively impacted domain at baseline (as shown by the highest score), while "sleep problems", "irritability", "physical and mental exhaustion" and "joint and muscular discomfort" were also strongly impacted at baseline for both populations. The Chinese population presented a higher baseline score in the "sexual problems" and "dryness of vagina" domains. In the European population, the baseline "somato-vegetative" subscale was higher than in the Chinese population, while the "psychological" subscores were similar and the "urogenital" subscore was lower in the European population than in the Chinese population. These data highlight the need for effective treatment spanning all symptomatic stages of menopause.

4. Estradiol plus dydrogesterone improves symptom frequency and severity among postmenopausal women

Estrogen-based menopausal hormone therapy is the foundation of treatment for estrogen deficiency symptoms, including VMS, and has been shown to reduce symptom frequency and severity and improve HRQoL [43–46]. Guidelines recommend tailoring menopausal hormone therapy to individual patients' symptoms and circumstances using the most appropriate dose of estrogen and, in some cases, selecting the most suitable route of estrogen administration [43, 46–51].

For non-hysterectomized women, estrogen is given in combination with progestogen in either a cyclic or continuous form [43, 47, 48]. Progestogens have different affinity to receptors including the glucocorticoid receptors, androgen receptors and mineralocorticoid receptors in addition to their affinity for the progesterone receptor [52]. Dydrogesterone, a progestogen from a natural source, has the most neutral metabolic and side-effect profile of the progestogens [40, 52].

Femoston Conti®, low-dose estradiol plus dydrogesterone (1 mg 17β-estradiol combined with 5 mg dydrogesterone [E1mg/D5mg]) was approved in Europe in 2000 for the treatment of estrogen deficiency symptoms and prevention of osteoporosis in postmenopausal women at least 12 months since last menses [53]. In 2010, an ultra-low estradiol plus dydrogesterone (Femoston-mini®; 0.5 mg 17β-estradiol continuously combined with 2.5 mg dydrogesterone [E0.5mg/D2.5mg]) was approved for the treatment of estrogen deficiency symptoms in postmenopausal women at least 12 months since last menses [53]. Femoston is the only single fixed dose menopause hormone therapy containing dydrogesterone. Dydrogesterone, like the micronized progesterone, comes from a natural source (e.g. yam and soy) [54, 55]. Its unique molecular features are obtained through a photochemical process [53], creating a bent molecular conformation, conferring a high selectivity for progesterone receptors [54, 55], with better oral bioavailability compared with oral micronized progesterone [56–58]. Dydrogesterone presents a biological progestogenic, anti-estrogenic, anti-androgenic and anti-mineralocorticoid activity with no anti-gonadotrophic, estrogenic, androgenic, or glucocorticoid actions [55]. Unlike other progestogens, dydrogesterone is non-thermogenetic, non-sedative, does not inhibit gonadotropin release or ovulation, does not influence central nervous system function and psyche, and does not antagonize various central effects of estrogens [59].

The ultra-low dose formulations have been shown in several randomized, placebo-controlled clinical studies to reduce VMS, including hot flushes and moderate-to-severe hot flushes, in postmenopausal women compared with placebo, with no safety concerns [42, 60–62]. Additionally, patient-reported improvements have been shown with ultra-low estradiol plus dydrogesterone based on improved scores on the MRS [42, 62].

The 2024 pooled analysis by Yu et al., included data from 574 women who had received either E0.5mg/D2.5mg (n = 285) or placebo (n = 289) [41]. Similar to previous studies [17, 18, 20], the mean number of hot flushes per day at baseline was higher in the European population than in the Chinese population (**Figure 2**). In both the European and Chinese populations, women receiving E0.5mg/D2.5mg experienced greater reductions from baseline in the mean daily number of hot flushes at Weeks 4, 8 and end of treatment compared with women who received placebo (**Figure 2**). The absolute mean (95% confidence interval [CI]) daily number of hot flushes, measured weekly, was lower in women treated with E0.5mg/D2.5mg compared with placebo at each time point in the Chinese population and from Week 2 onwards in the European population (**Figure 2**). The reduction in absolute mean daily number of hot flushes with E0.5mg/D2.5mg treatment occurred more rapidly in the European population than in the Chinese population, in which the reduction was more gradual (**Figure 2**). Nevertheless, by end of treatment the absolute mean number of hot flushes per day in the E0.5mg/D2.5mg treatment arms had reached a similar level in the European and Chinese populations (**Figure 2**).

The same pattern was evident in the daily number of moderate-to-severe hot flushes. At baseline, the mean number of moderate-to-severe hot flushes per day was higher in the European population than in the Chinese population. Women receiving E0.5mg/D2.5mg experienced greater reductions from baseline in mean number of

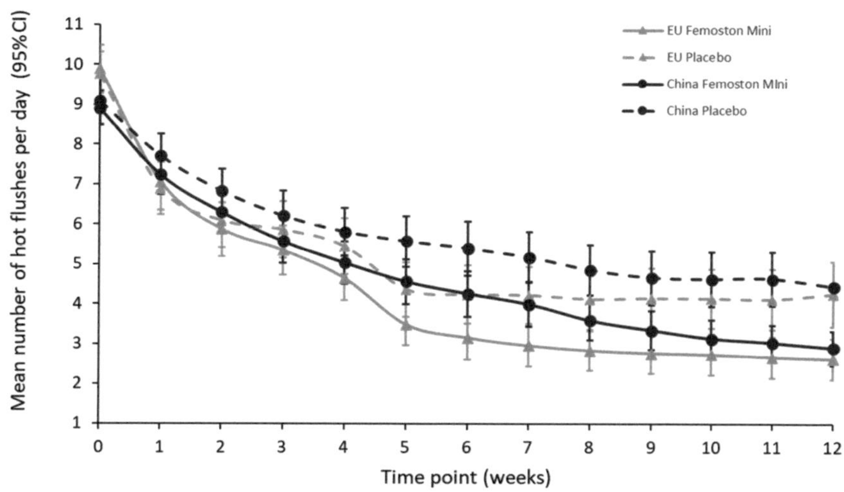

Figure 2.
Absolute number of hot flushes per day [41]. Reuse licensed under a Creative Commons Attribution 4.0 International License. CI, confidence interval; D, dydrogesterone; E, estradiol; and EU, European.

moderate-to-severe hot flushes per day at Weeks 4, 8 and end of treatment compared with women who received placebo, both in the European and Chinese populations.

By end of treatment, European women treated with E0.5mg/D2.5mg reported significant improvement in the 'Hot flushes, sweating' item score versus placebo. In the Chinese population, women receiving E0.5mg/D2.5mg reported significant improvements at end of treatment in all item scores except 'Sexual problems' and in the three subscale scores and the total score versus placebo (**Table 2**).

The pooled analysis had several strengths including the placebo-controlled, double-blind, randomized nature of the included studies and the individual data analysis. However, the authors noted that it was a *post hoc* analysis, therefore definitive conclusions from the results require further confirmation. Despite the limitations, the data provide clinically valuable information on the benefits of E0.5mg/D2.5mg among postmenopausal women of different ethnicities, building upon the favorable impacts shown in previous studies of ultra-low-dose estradiol plus dydrogesterone in postmenopausal women [42, 60–62]. Overall, the study showed consistent improvements in VMS with ultra-low-dose estradiol plus dydrogesterone versus placebo, in both European and Chinese postmenopausal women.

5. Conclusions

Menopause symptoms are a consequence of estrogen deficiency and can have a substantial detrimental effect on Chinese women's HRQoL, as shown by the Rautenberg et al. study which demonstrated impaired HRQoL across all phases of menopause, with perimenopausal women experiencing significantly more symptoms and significantly lower HRQoL compared with premenopausal and postmenopausal women [31]. As such, timely identification and management of menopausal symptoms in this cohort is paramount. Recognition of symptoms associated with the perimenopausal stage should be pursued to ensure timely intervention before HRQoL is substantially impaired. Global medical societies recommend estrogen treatment for the efficacious management of estrogen deficiency symptoms, with decisions about dose made on an individualized basis with no arbitrary limits placed on the duration of use [43, 50, 63]. It is reported that Asian women can be less likely than Caucasian women to use menopausal hormone therapy, in part due to a lack of awareness of the treatment and in part due to uncertainty about the risks and benefits of such a therapeutic strategy within specific ethnic groups [25, 64, 65]. The benefits shown in the Chinese population of the pooled analysis described above include improved VMS and a consistently positive impact on HRQoL. These benefits are of real clinical relevance and can be used to support patients in their decision-making surrounding the use of menopausal hormone therapy.

Acknowledgements

Editorial assistance was provided by Metamols Ltd., funded by Abbott Established Pharmaceuticals.

Conflict of interest

IS, KK, and MGC are employees of Abbott Products Operations AG, Allschwil, Switzerland and own shares in Abbott. MD works for Griffith University on projects funded by the Australian Government Department of Health and Aged Care, Queensland Health, Abbott Products Operations AG, and Illumina.

QY declares no conflicts of interest.

TS reports having received in the past three years consulting fees from Astellas, Gedeon Richter, Mitsubishi Tanabe, Sojournix, Estetra, Actavis, Abbott, Medtronic, Applied Medical, Johnson and Johnson and speaker's honoraria from Shionogi, Gedeon Richter, Theramex, Abbott, Intuitive Surgical, and Applied Medical.

Author details

Martin Downes[1*], Kyoo Kim[2], Marcelo Graziano Custodio[2], Igor Solev[2], Tommaso Simoncini[3] and Qi Yu[4]

1 School of Medicine and Dentistry, Griffith University, Queensland, Australia

2 Abbott Products Operations AG, Switzerland

3 Division of Obstetrics and Gynecology, Department of Clinical and Experimental Medicine, University of Pisa, Pisa, Italy

4 Gynecological Endocrinology and Reproduction Center, Peking Union Medical College Hospital, Beijing, China

*Address all correspondence to: m.downes@griffith.edu.au

References

[1] Soules MR, Sherman S, Parrott E, et al. Executive summary: Stages of reproductive aging workshop (STRAW). Climacteric. 2001;**4**:267-272

[2] Harlow SD, Gass M, Hall JE, et al. Executive summary of the stages of reproductive aging workshop + 10: Addressing the unfinished agenda of staging reproductive aging. The Journal of Clinical Endocrinology and Metabolism. 2012;**97**(4):1159-1168

[3] Huang Z, Shi J, Liu W, et al. The influence of educational level in peri-menopause syndrome and quality of life among Chinese women. Gynecological Endocrinology. 2020;**36**(11):991-996

[4] Delamater L, Santoro N. Management of the Perimenopause. Clinical Obstetrics and Gynecology. 2018;**61**(3):419-432

[5] Li L, Wu J, Pu D, et al. Factors associated with the age of natural menopause and menopausal symptoms in Chinese women. Maturitas. 2012;**73**(4):354-360

[6] Menopause Subgroup. Chinese Society of Obstetrics and Gynecology, Chinese Medical Association. Chinese guideline on menopause management and menopause hormone therapy (2018). Zhonghua Fu Chan Ke Za Zhi. 2018;**53**(11):729-739

[7] Wang X, Ran S, Yu Q. Optimizing quality of life in perimenopause: Lessons from the east. Climacteric. 2019;**22**(1):34-37

[8] Sun N, Xing J, Li L, et al. Impact of menopause on quality of life in community-based women in China: 1 year follow-up. Archives of Psychiatric Nursing. 2018;**32**(2):224-228

[9] Chou MF, Wun YT, Pang SM. Menopausal symptoms and the menopausal rating scale among midlife Chinese women in Macau, China. Women Health. 2014;**54**(2):115-126

[10] Kim H-Y, Kang S-Y, Chung Y-J, et al. The recent review of the genitourinary syndrome of menopause. Journal of Menopausal Medicine. 2015;**21**(2):65-71

[11] Freeman EW, Sherif K. Prevalence of hot flushes and night sweats around the world: A systematic review. Climacteric. 2007;**10**(3):197-214

[12] Khan SJ, Kapoor E, Faubion SS, et al. Vasomotor symptoms during menopause: A practical guide on current treatments and future perspectives. International Journal of Women's Health. 2023;**15**:273-287

[13] Pinkerton JV, Santen RJ. Managing vasomotor symptoms in women after cancer. Climacteric. 2019;**22**(6):544-552

[14] Whiteley J, Wagner J-S, Bushmakin A, et al. Impact of the severity of vasomotor symptoms on health status, resource use, and productivity. Menopause. 2013;**20**(5):518-524

[15] Nappi RE, Siddiqui E, Todorova L, et al. Prevalence and quality-of-life burden of vasomotor symptoms associated with menopause: A European cross-sectional survey. Maturitas. 2023;**167**:66-74

[16] Tamlyn Anne R, Downes M, Simoncini T, et al. Evaluating the cost utility of estradiol plus dydrogesterone for the treatment of menopausal women in China. Journal of Medical Economics. 2024;**27**(1):16-26

[17] Avis NE, Crawford SL, Green R. Vasomotor symptoms across the menopause transition: Differences among women. Obstetrics and Gynecology Clinics of North America. 2018;**45**(4):629-640

[18] Boulet MJ, Oddens BJ, Lehert P, et al. Climacteric and menopause in seven south-east Asian countries. Maturitas. 2008;**61**(1-2):34-53

[19] Gold EB, Sternfeld B, Kelsey JL, et al. Relation of demographic and lifestyle factors to symptoms in a multi-racial/ethnic population of women 40-55 years of age. American Journal of Epidemiology. 2000;**152**(5):463-473

[20] Haines CJ, Chung TK, Leung DH. A prospective study of the frequency of acute menopausal symptoms in Hong Kong Chinese women. Maturitas. 1994;**18**(3):175-181

[21] Dunneram Y, Greenwood DC, Burley VJ, et al. Dietary intake and age at natural menopause: Results from the UK women's cohort study. Journal of Epidemiology and Community Health. 2018;**72**(8):733-740

[22] United Nations World Population Prospects 2019 [Internet]; 2019. Available from: https://population.un.org/wpp/ [Accessed: July 14, 2021]

[23] Zhang L, Ruan X, Cui Y, et al. Menopausal symptoms among Chinese peri- and postmenopausal women: A large prospective single-center cohort study. Gynecological Endocrinology. 2021;**37**(2):185-189

[24] Liu K, He L, Tang X, et al. Relationship between menopause and health-related quality of life in middle-aged Chinese women: A cross-sectional study. BMC Women's Health. 2014;**14**:7

[25] You Y, Lin L, Yu Q. Exploring menopausal symptoms, attitudes, and behaviors among menopausal women in China: An online research perspective. Menopause. 1 Nov 2024;**31**(11):1006-1013

[26] Mercieca-Bebber R, King MT, Calvert MJ, et al. The importance of patient-reported outcomes in clinical trials and strategies for future optimization. Patient-Related Outcome Measures. 2018;**9**:353-367

[27] Trojan A, Huber U, Brauchbar M, et al. Consilium smartphone app for real-world electronically captured patient-reported outcome monitoring in cancer patients undergoing anti-PD-L1-directed treatment. Case Reports in Oncological. 2020;**13**(2):491-496

[28] Coon C, Bushmakin A, Tatlock S, et al. Evaluation of a crosswalk between the European quality of life five dimension five level and the menopause-specific quality of life questionnaire. Climacteric. 2018;**21**(6):566-573

[29] Schultz NM, Morga A, Siddiqui E, et al. Psychometric evaluation of the MENQOL instrument in women experiencing vasomotor symptoms associated with menopause. Advances in Therapy. 2024;**41**(6):2233-2252

[30] Heinemann K, Ruebig A, Potthoff P, et al. The menopause rating scale (MRS) scale: A methodological review. Health and Quality of Life Outcomes. 2004;**2**:45

[31] Liu GE, Hu SL, Wu JH, et al. China Guidelines for Pharmacoeconomic Evaluations. Beijing: China Market Press; 2020

[32] Rautenberg TA, Ng SKA, Downes M. A cross-sectional study of symptoms and health-related quality of life in menopausal-aged women in China. BMC Women's Health. 2023;**23**:563

[33] Matthews KA, Bromberger JT. Does the menopausal transition affect health-related quality of life? The American Journal of Medicine. 2005;**118**:25-36

[34] Luo N, Liu G, Li M, et al. Estimating an EQ-5D-5L value set for China. Value in Health. 2017;**20**(4):662-669

[35] Bot BM, Suver C, Neto EC, et al. The mPower study, Parkinson disease mobile data collected using ResearchKit. Scientific Data. 2016;**3**:160011

[36] Fan X, Wang D, Hellman B, et al. Assessment of health-related quality of life between people with Parkinson's disease and non-Parkinson's: Using data drawn from the '100 for Parkinson's' smartphone-based prospective study. International Journal of Environmental Research and Public Health. 2018;**15**(11):2538

[37] Gwaltney CJ, Shields AL, Shiffman S. Equivalence of electronic and paper-and-pencil administration of patient-reported outcome measures: A meta-analytic review. Value in Health. 2008;**11**(2):322-333

[38] Rutherford C, Costa D, Mercieca-Bebber R, et al. Mode of administration does not cause bias in patient-reported outcome results: A meta-analysis. Quality of Life Research. 2016;**25**(3):559-574

[39] Bushnell DM, Reilly MC, Galani C, et al. Validation of electronic data capture of the irritable bowel syndrome–quality of life measure, the work productivity and activity impairment questionnaire for irritable bowel syndrome and the EuroQol. Value in Health. 2006;**9**(2):98-105

[40] Fu J-X, Luo Y, Chen M-Z, et al. Associations among menopausal status, menopausal symptoms, and depressive symptoms in midlife women in Hunan Province, China. Climacteric. 2020;**23**(3):259-266

[41] Yu Q, Stevenson JC, Tatarchuk T, et al. Ultra-low-dose estradiol and dydrogesterone for treatment of vasomotor symptoms in Europe and China. Climacteric. 2024 Jul;**30**:1-7

[42] Ren M, Ruan X, Gu L, et al. Ultra-low-dose estradiol and dydrogesterone: A phase III study for vasomotor symptoms in China. Climacteric. 2022;**25**(3):286-292

[43] Baber RJ, Panay N, Fenton A, Group IMSW. 2016 IMS recommendations on women's midlife health and menopause hormone therapy. Climacteric. 2016;**19**(2):109-150

[44] Mintziori G, Lambrinoudaki I, Goulis DG, et al. EMAS position statement: Non-hormonal management of menopausal vasomotor symptoms. Maturitas. 2015;**81**(3):410-413

[45] Nelson HD, Haney E, Humphrey L, et al. Management of menopause-related symptoms. Evidence Report/Technology Assessment (Summary). 2005;**120**:1-6

[46] "The Hormone Therapy Position Statement of The North American Menopause Society" Advisory Panel. The 2022 hormone therapy position statement of the North American Menopause Society. Menopause. 2022;**29**(7):767-794

[47] Cobin RH, Goodman NF, Committee ARES. American Association of Clinical Endocrinologists and American College of endocrinology position statement on Menopause-2017 update. Endocrine Practice. 2017;**23**(7):869-880

[48] de Villiers TJ, Hall JE, Pinkerton JV, et al. Revised global consensus statement

on menopausal hormone therapy. Maturitas. 2016;**91**:153-155

[49] Hamoda H, Panay N, Pedder H, et al. The British menopause society and Women's health concern 2020 recommendations on hormone replacement therapy in menopausal women. Post Reproductive Health. 2020;**26**(4):181-209

[50] Lambrinoudaki I, Armeni E, Goulis D, et al. Menopause, wellbeing and health: A care pathway from the European menopause and Andropause society. Maturitas. 2022;**163**:1-14

[51] Menopause Subgroup. Chinese Society of Obstetrics and Gynecology, Chinese Medical Association. [the 2023 Chinese menopause symptom management and menopausal hormone therapy guidelines]. Zhonghua Fu Chan Ke Za Zhi. 2023;**58**(1):4-21

[52] Vigneswaran K, Hamoda H. Hormone replacement therapy - current recommendations. Best Practice & Research. Clinical Obstetrics & Gynaecology. 2022;**81**:8-21

[53] Femoston-Conti 0.5 mg/2.5 mg and 1 mg/5 mg Film-Coated Tablets. Summary of Product Characteristics. Abbott Laboratories

[54] Al-Jasem Y, Malik MMK, Taha A, et al. Preparation of steroidal hormones with an emphasis on transformations of phytosterols and cholesterol - a review. Mediterranean Journal of Chemistry. 2014;**3**:796-830

[55] Griesinger G, Tournaye H, Macklon N, et al. Dydrogesterone: Pharmacological profile and mechanism of action as luteal phase support in assisted reproduction. Reproductive Biomedicine Online. 2019;**38**(2):249-259

[56] Schindler AE, Campagnoli C, Druckmann R, et al. Classification and pharmacology of progestins. Maturitas. 2008;**61**(1-2):171-180

[57] Rižner TL, Brožic P, Doucette C, et al. Selectivity and potency of the retroprogesterone dydrogesterone in vitro. Steroids. 2011;**76**(6):607-615

[58] Stanczyk FZ, Hapgood JP, Winer S, et al. Progestogens used in postmenopausal hormone therapy: Differences in their pharmacological properties, intracellular actions, and clinical effects. Endocrine Reviews. 2013;**34**(2):171-208

[59] Kuhl H. Pharmacology of estrogens and progestogens: Influence of different routes of administration. Climacteric. 2005;**8**(Suppl. 1):3-63

[60] Notelovitz M, Lenihan JP, McDermott M, et al. Initial 17beta-estradiol dose for treating vasomotor symptoms. Obstetrics and Gynecology. 2000;**95**(5):726-731

[61] Notelovitz M, Mattox JH. Suppression of vasomotor and vulvovaginal symptoms with continuous oral 17beta-estradiol. Menopause. 2000;**7**(5):310-317

[62] Stevenson JC, Durand G, Kahler E, et al. Oral ultra-low dose continuous combined hormone replacement therapy with 0.5 mg 17beta-oestradiol and 2.5 mg dydrogesterone for the treatment of vasomotor symptoms: Results from a double-blind, controlled study. Maturitas. 2010;**67**(3):227-232

[63] Genazzani AR, Divakar H, Khadilkar SS, et al. Counseling in menopausal women: How to address the benefits and risks of menopause hormone therapy. A FIGO position paper.

International Journal of Gynaecology and Obstetrics. 2024;**164**(2):516-530

[64] Gupta S, Forbes N, Kirkman R. Attitudes to menopause and hormone replacement therapy among Asian and Caucasian women general practitioners. Maturitas. 2001;**39**(2):169-175

[65] Harris TJ, Cook DG, Wicks PD, et al. Ethnic differences in use of hormone replacement therapy: Community based survey. BMJ. 1999;**319**(7210):610-611

Chapter 15

Women-Controlled Universal Vaginal Protection against STIs and Unintended Pregnancy

Rabeea F. Omar, Sylvie Trottier and Mathieu Leboeuf

Abstract

Men have a universal protection tool (male condom) under their control to protect themselves against sexually transmitted infections (STIs) including HIV/AIDS, and to avoid unintended pregnancy. Unfortunately, it is not consistently used. Male condom is used in only one-third of at-risk sexual intercourse by men 15–44 years of age. On the other hand, despite being up to 8 times more at risk of getting STIs during an unprotected vaginal intercourse, women have no means under their control to protect themselves as men do. In addition, they are vulnerable to unintended pregnancy that represents about 45% of all pregnancies (of more than 200 million pregnancies annually) around the globe. It is primordial to empower women with vaginal multipurpose prevention technologies (MPTs) to protect themselves during sexual intercourse when men do not use means of protection. Women need safe, effective, affordable and accessible vaginal protection. Protecting women will be beneficial, not only for them, but also for the whole society as well.

Keywords: women's sexual and reproductive health, women-controlled prevention, sexually transmitted infections (STIs), unintended pregnancy, non-hormonal contraceptives

1. Introduction

Women are men's partners in life. They are also friends, colleagues, mothers, spouses, daughters, grandmothers. It is important for the society to keep women healthy and well. Furthermore, women should have control over their reproductive and sexual health, as men do. In fact, a fair share of new medical technologies should be adapted to better address women's health needs. Empowerment of women with means of protection against vaginal and systemic infections and unintended pregnancy that are under their control will be beneficial for them and for the whole society as well. It is also important that women be involved in decision-making for the development of such protective women-controlled products. The first step is that women around the globe get sufficient education, so this will make them less vulnerable to exploitation. Women represent half (49.6%) of the world population, yet they have not enough protection under their control despite the fact that they are more vulnerable to certain diseases compared to men. Of the nearly 4 billion women worldwide, there are 1.9 billions who are of reproductive age (15–49 years old) [1]. Based on United Nations population (UNFPA) report, there are about 257 million women worldwide who have *unmet need* for safe, affordable and accessible modern contraceptive [2]. This translates to the fact that nearly half (about 45%) of all pregnancies worldwide are unintended representing a critical global crisis [2, 3].

Adding to this crisis, is the increase in sexually transmitted infections (STIs) worldwide. In 2020, there were an estimated 374 million new cases of the four curable STIs– chlamydia (129 million), gonorrhea (82 million), syphilis (7.1 million) and trichomoniasis (156 million)- in adolescents and adults aged 15–49 years [4]. Furthermore, according to the World Health Organization (WHO), there are 1 million STIs acquired every day around the world [5]. One of the main reasons for that is the remarkable decline in condom use. To support this, news just came out from the WHO on 29 August 2024 of an urgent report from its Regional Office for Europe which revealed that condom use among sexually active adolescents has declined significantly since 2014, with rates of unprotected sex in Europe worryingly high. The proportion of sexually active adolescents who used a condom during the last intercourse fell from 70% to 61% among boys and 63% to 57% among girls between 2014 and 2022. This large study surveyed more than 242,000 adolescent 15-year-olds across 42 European countries and regions in 2014–2022. This puts teens at significant risk of acquiring STIs and having unintended pregnancy [6]. Similarly, in the United States of America (USA), adolescents and young adults aged 15–24 years represented half (50%) of the 26 million new cases of STIs in 2018. Furthermore, the STDs surveillance report for 2019 from the US-Centers for disease control (CDC) published in April 2021 showed that, among the same age group of 15–24 years old, gonorrhea increased by 56%, Chlamydia increased by 19% and syphilis increased by 74% [7] since 2015. This is an unsettling increase of STIs among young people over the last several years. Outside Europe and USA, the situation is much worse in less developed countries/regions.

HIV/AIDS alone claimed the lives of 40 million humans worldwide over the last 4 decades since the start of the epidemic in the early 1980s [8]. Women mortality due to cervical cancer that is caused by sexually-transmitted human papilloma virus (HPV) infection climbed from 273,000 in 2007 to 342,000 in 2020 [9, 10]. For herpes, almost half of the world population aged 50 years and under has cold sore- *Herpes simplex* virus-1 (HSV-1) infection [11]. There are also 536 million people aged 15–49 years living with HSV-2 genital herpes infection worldwide; women and adolescent girls make more than half of all genital herpes infections [12]. Moreover, more than 75% of all Chlamydia infection occur in women. The majority of Chlamydia infections in women are asymptomatic (silent infection), thus increasing the risk for complications such as infertility and pelvic inflammatory diseases (PID) [13]. On the other hand, pregnancy complications claim the lives of more than 500,000 women every year worldwide [14]. These are all compelling facts that demonstrates the urgent need to protect and empower women.

2. Women at the center of social structure

Women count for about half of any society. Strong, healthy, happy and well-educated women will build strong, happy families and a stronger, prosperous society. Women-specific medical issues such as pregnancy, menstruation, menopause, sexually transmitted infections, etc. should receive fair attention from the scientific and medical community and should be addressed adequately. Depriving women, especially pregnant ones, from adequate women-adapted medical care and screening not only put their health at risk, but also that of their children to be born (see real life example in Section 3 below).

3. Women's sexual and reproductive health and their well-being

Because of their anatomy and physiology that are different than men, women have specific vulnerabilities and health risks. For example, sexual intercourse impacts women more than men in many ways. It's women who face and live with unintended pregnancy and its consequences. It's also them who are at higher risk of getting STIs including HIV in unprotected vaginal intercourse. Here is an example of the price the society could pay for not paying close attention to women sexual and reproductive health. In a recently published study (July 2024) [15], women aged 15–44 living in Australia had a worrying increase in infectious syphilis over the last 10 years (between 2011 and 2021) with a subsequent rise in transmission from infected pregnant women to their children (congenital syphilis). The study showed that the notification rate for syphilis in Aboriginal and Islander women rose from 56 (95% confidence interval [CI], 45–65) cases per 100,000 in 2011 to 227 (95% CI, 206–248) cases per 100,000 population in 2021. For non-Indigenous women, it rose from 1.1 (95% CI, 0.8–1.4) to 9.2 (95% CI, 8.4–10.1) cases per 100,000 population [15]. Moreover, a WHO recent report noted a surge in adult and maternal syphilis (1.1 million) and associated congenital syphilis (523 cases per 100,000 live births per year) during the COVID-19 pandemic. Furthermore, in 2022, there were 230,000 syphilis-related deaths [4]. This shows a sluggish and insufficient screening of pregnant women. Antenatal screening of pregnant women should be greatly improved and followed by prompt treatment for infectious syphilis when diagnosed to avert congenital syphilis that is easily preventable [15]. Such improved intervention would save hundreds of thousands of human lives and millions of dollars in related medical care and treatment cost.

4. Pre-exposure prophylaxis (PrEP) to prevent HIV transmission

Pre-Exposure prophylaxis (PrEP) uses antiretrovirals and only protects against HIV infection, but not against other STIs and this represents an important disadvantage. We have previously discussed in details the difference between offering women protection against only HIV or universally protecting them against all STIs including HIV [16]. In July 2012, the US-food and drug administration (FDA) approved the use of tenofovir disoproxil fumarate/emtricitabine (TDF/FTC) as the first PrEP for HIV negative people who are at high risk of acquiring HIV [17]. Both antiretroviral drugs prevent HIV infection by inhibiting the enzyme reverse transcriptase of the virus. Few years later, in October 2019, Tenofovir alafenamide fumarate/emtricitabine (TAF/FTC) received an indication for HIV prophylaxis [18], the second PrEP drug to do so. This improved second medication is less nephrotoxic compared to TDF/FTC.

Very recently (in July 2024), Lenacapavir (HIV-1 capsid inhibitor) investigated as PrEP was demonstrated to provide total protection against HIV with no infection among 2134 participants in the Lenacapavir group in Phase III trial (PURPOSE 1 study, trial registration number NCT04994509) among young women and adolescent girls in Africa [19]. This prompted advocates to immediately call upon investigators and regulators for accelerated timeline for widespread access to this twice-yearly injectable Lenacapavir as PrEP for prevention of HIV. Here are the detailed results of this landmark trial: among 5338 participants who were initially HIV-negative, 55 incident HIV infections were observed: 0 infection among 2134 participants in the Lenacapavir group (0 per 100 person-years; 95% CI, 0.00 to 0.19), 39 infections among 2136 participants in the TAF/FTC group (2.02 per 100 person-years; 95% CI, 1.44 to 2.76), and 16 infections among 1068 participants in the once-daily oral TDF/FTC group (1.69 per 100 person-years; 95% CI, 0.96 to 2.74) [19]. Background HIV incidence in the screened population (8094 participants) was 2.41 per 100 person-years (95% CI, 1.82 to 3.19). These are excellent results for a new and improved PrEP for prevention of HIV infections that would help with patients' compliance as it is administered only twice a year. This strategy will re-define HIV prevention landscape, a real game-changer if access to it would be adequate. However, it remains as protection against only HIV, and it has a price tag of about $45,000 per person per year.

5. It's all about women control of their own protection

It is crucial to empower women for control of their own protection. Many barriers remain to condom use (**Figure 1**) including reduced excitement, sensation, allergy, male willingness, etc. Despite their wide availability and affordability, male condoms are used globally in only one-third of at-risk sexual intercourse such as sex with infected partner, sex with multiple partners, sex with partner who has multiple partners, sex with partner with history of unprotected sex, sex with partner who injects illicit drugs and shares needles, etc. [20]. Furthermore, the use of female condoms (**Figure 1**) has been slow because it is cumbersome to use, has limited access and high price, especially for women in low-income countries. It may also collapse inside the vagina as it is difficult to hold in place properly inside the vagina during intercourse.

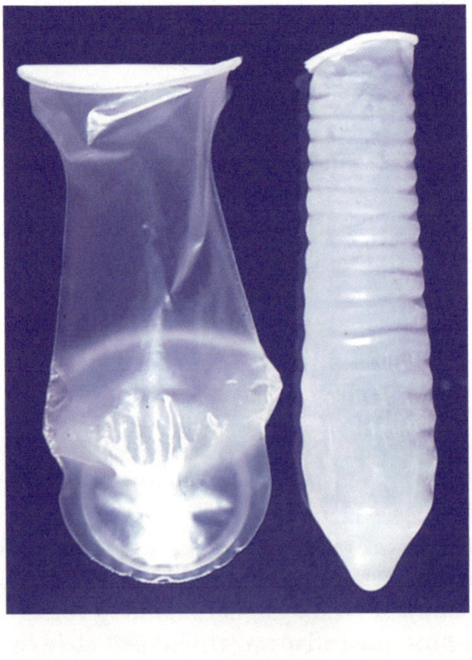

Figure 1.
Female condom and male condom.

Women need proper and easy to use protection, under their own control, against not only STIs (HIV, HSV, HPV, gonorrhea, Chlamydia, syphilis, trichomoniasis, etc.), but also against unintended pregnancy as well. Vaginal products that offer dual protection would be ideal to give women the same universal protection and control men have with the male condom. An ideal women-controlled product should have as many as possible of the following characteristics: (i) offer dual protection against pregnancy and STIs as explained above, (ii) be safe, effective and acceptable, (iii) be affordable and accessible, (iv) offer immediate vaginal protection upon application, (v) not adversely affect normal vaginal flora, (vi) be compatible with male condom, (vii) not accumulate in vagina, and give no vaginal leak after vaginal application. Furthermore, it is better to be discrete and unnoticed/unfelt (imperceptible) by the woman's male sexual partner. An effective women-controlled dual protection product could avert millions of infections and unwanted pregnancies around the globe. The gain for the whole society in lives saved, complications and cost avoided will be enormous.

6. Multipurpose prevention technologies (MPTs)

It is important to continue developing protective means against HIV infection, other STIs and unintended pregnancies that are tailored to the needs of women of reproductive age [21]. This includes the development of women-controlled multipurpose prevention technologies (MPTs) [21–23]. Women-controlled MPTs are vaginal products offering dual protection that act as microbicides against STIs including HIV and as contraceptives against unintended pregnancy. Women should receive medical care adapted to their health situation and needs. For example, offering pregnant women with HIV a personalized clinical approach to diminish the risk of infection for themselves and their newborn [24].

Over the last 2–3 decades, many researchers have been racing to develop vaginal microbicide/contraceptive products (See reference [16] for further reading about previously investigated products). Until today, no approved dual protection vaginal product exists to protect women broadly against STIs and unintended pregnancy. However, there are some advances in this area; here they are: Thus far, VivaGel® a vaginal product which is a dendrimer-based vaginal microbicide gel made from poly-l-lysine, has the European union (EU) marketing approval for prevention of bacterial vaginosis (BV) [25]. Furthermore, a first on-demand 'prescription' vaginal gel made of (lactic acid, citric acid and potassium bitartrate) (Phexxi®) has been approved by the US-FDA to prevent unintended pregnancy [26]; this product is also being tested in advanced clinical trial for prevention of STIs such as gonorrhea and Chlamydia. A different product, Annovera® is a vaginal ring (soft, flexible silicone ring) releasing ethinyl estradiol and segesterone acetate that can be used for up to one year (13 cycles) to prevent unwanted pregnancy [27]; an option that can help easing access to those women in low-income settings.

Finally, the *Invisible Condom®* (IC) is a woman-controlled microbicide/ non-hormonal contraceptive vaginal gel that can be used for dual protection against sexually transmitted infections (STIs), including HIV and unwanted pregnancies as demonstrated in the laboratory [28–31]. Phase I and Phase II safety and acceptability clinical studies were successfully carried out in Québec City, Canada and in Cameroon with the contribution of more than 500 women who had ~30,000 vaginal gel applications, and their male sexual partners [32–34]. The *Invisible*

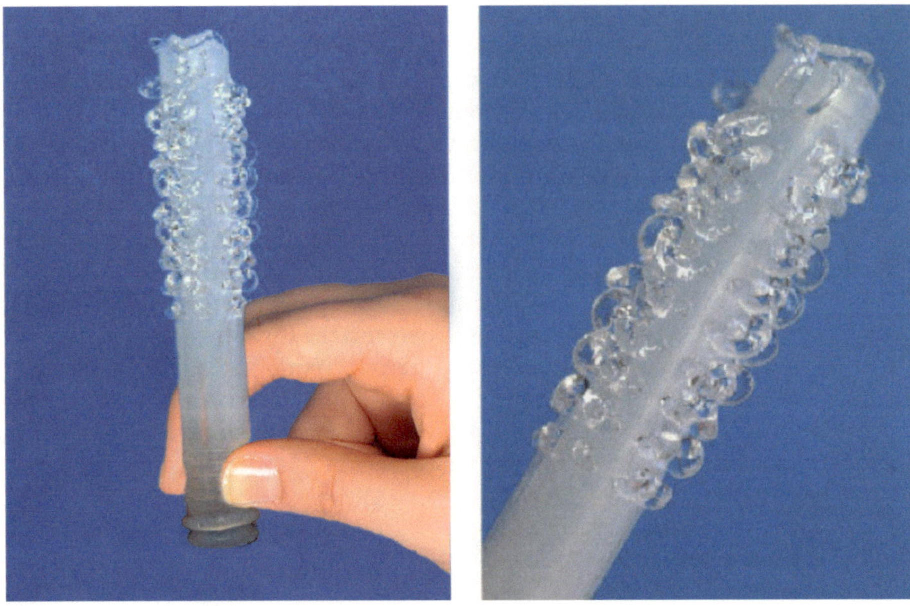

Figure 2.
The INVISIBLE CONDOM® and its special vaginal applicator.

Condom® is a sustained release system that is also discrete (imperceptible to sexual partner), affordable, and user-friendly. Women do not need to remove the product after vaginal intercourse as it mixes with natural vaginal secretions and is gradually eliminated (within a few hours after application) without leakage due to the rheological characteristics of the gel polymer of the product that adheres to vaginal and cervical mucosa [35]. A special vaginal applicator with multiple apical and lateral holes (See photo in **Figure 2**) was also developed for intra-vaginal use and delivery of this gel for homogenous distribution to the cervix and the vaginal walls to offer optimal mucosal coverage for better protection [35]; uncovered mucosa = unprotected mucosa = risk of infection. In addition to offering protection against STIs, the Invisible Condom® also offers a non-hormonal (on-demand) family planning method that does not interfere with the physiology of the menstrual cycle, and does not have the systemic side effects usually associated with hormonal contraceptives. The Invisible Condom® was recently tested in a Phase II B spermicidal and early contraceptive efficacy trial. Results demonstrated that, for *in vitro* spermicidal effect, 98% of sperms were immotile in presence of the Invisible Condom®. For post-coital test (sperm viability in cervical mucous), 99% of sperms were immotile in presence of IC. For contraceptive efficacy, among 30 couples, overall, 410 vaginal intercourses in 95 menstrual cycles were protected during 3-month period of IC use before each vaginal intercourse with probability of 24 conceptions prevented according to Wilcox's table. Four women became pregnant; two during unprotected vaginal intercourse around ovulation time, and two were user failure [36]. This typical-use pregnancy rate (about 13%) is similar to that of the approved vaginal contraceptive gel Phexxi that is normal for these barrier methods. Furthermore, perfect-use contraceptive efficacy is usually higher around 93% (i.e. 7% pregnancy rate). Larger Phase III contraceptive efficacy trial is being planned as well as other efficacy trials against STIs.

7. Inclusion, equity and access

7.1 Inclusion

Women are the end-users of such vaginal protective products in development. To successfully fulfill their protection needs, women should be involved in key steps of product development such as design, characteristics, acceptability, safety and efficacy testing, etc. It is important for the developers to include women's feed-back and remarks to improve and optimize such products.

7.2 Equity

For many decades, in heterosexual (vaginal-penile) intercourse, men have been controlling protection against STIs including HIV, and sometimes unintended pregnancy. Women who cannot negotiate protected sexual intercourse with their male partners would be at risk of getting infected or becoming pregnant. Knowing that females are inherently more at risk, compared to men, of becoming infected with STIs, women need and deserve control of their own protection.

7.3 Access

In addition to being safe and effective, new vaginal products to protect women against vaginal infections and unintended pregnancy should be affordable and easily accessible by women from all walks of life. As for male condoms, women-controlled prevention products should be available over-the-counter (OTC). Ease of access will greatly help reduce STIs including HIV, and unintended pregnancy around the globe. In addition to saving women lives, it will save millions of dollars used to address such important medical issues.

8. Conclusion

To sustain the development of women-controlled protective products, especially against infections that are sexually transmitted, sufficient and continuous funding is needed. Women's health, particularly sexual and reproductive health is classically low funded field [21]. It is important that more funds get allocated to this vital area. The time to act is now to empower women with proper and novel medical technologies for prevention, diagnosis and treatment that are adapted to their health needs. Scientists and clinicians should be relentless in pursuing advanced applied medical research that will, at the end, lead to having richness of products and tools to protect women and improve their sexual and reproductive health. It is important to keep a cap on prices for such innovative products. If too expensive, they would not be adequately accessible to all, especially to those from low-income countries/regions. This would exclude the most vulnerable and will undermine the good protective effect of such products. It is always better to prevent than to treat diseases. What we cannot do is wait. The need for safe, effective, affordable and accessible products for prevention of STIs/HIV and unwanted pregnancies under the control of women is too great [37]. Such affordable prevention products will save millions of lives of women who will actively help the world to prosper. The end result would be having whole winning society, not just winning women.

Acknowledgements

The authors would like to thank Jean-Luc Simard for his help with the references. The authors would also like to thank all women who participated in clinical trials to help make available new medical technologies and new medications for prevention and treatment of infections to save human lives, especially those of women.

Conflict of interest

The authors declare no conflict of interest.

Notes/thanks/other declarations

The authors would like to dedicate this book chapter to Prof. Michel G. Bergeron, and to the Infectious Diseases Research Centre (IDRC) of Laval University on its 50th anniversary. IDRC was founded by Dr. Bergeron in 1974. Thank you Michel for dedicating 50 years of your life to help save human lives from infectious diseases!

Nomenclature

HIV	Human Immunodeficiency Virus
AIDS	Acquired Immune Deficiency Syndrome
STIs	sexually transmitted infections
BV	bacterial vaginosis
PID	pelvic inflammatory diseases
MPTs	multipurpose technologies
WHO	World Health Organization
UNFPA	United Nations population fund
US-FDA	United States-food and drug administration
US-CDC	United States- centers for disease control and prevention
EU	the European union
CI	confidence interval
IC	invisible condom®
OTC	over-the-counter
IDRC	infectious diseases research centre

Author details

Rabeea F. Omar[1,3]*, Sylvie Trottier[1,3] and Mathieu Leboeuf[2]

1 Department of Microbiology, Infectious Diseases and Immunology, Faculty of Medicine, Laval University, Quebec City, Quebec, Canada

2 Department of Obstetrics and Gynecology, Faculty of Medicine, Laval University, Quebec City, Quebec, Canada

3 Infectious Diseases Research Centre, Laval University Hospital Centre (CHUL), Quebec City, Quebec, Canada

*Address all correspondence to: rabeea.omar@crchudequebec.ulaval.ca

References

[1] United Nations, Department of Economic and Social Affairs, Population Division. World Family Planning 2022: Meeting the changing needs for family planning: Contraceptive use by age and method. Available from: https://population.un.org/wpp/Publications/Files/WPP2022_Methodology.pdf

[2] United Nations Population Fund. UNFPA State of world population 2023. 8 billion lives, infinite possibilities: the case for rights and choices. Available from: https://www.unfpa.org/sites/default/files/swop23/SWOP2023-ENGLISH-230329-web.pdf [Accessed: 6 August 2024]

[3] Bearak J, Popinchalk A, Alkema L, Sedgh G. Global, regional, and subregional trends in unintended pregnancy and its outcomes from 1990 to 2014: Estimates from a Bayesian hierarchical model. The Lancet Global Health. 2018;**6**(4):e380-e3e9. DOI: 10.1016/S2214-109X(18)30029-9

[4] WHO. Implementing the global health sector strategies on HIV, viral hepatitis and sexually transmitted infections, 2022-2030—Report on progress and gaps. Available from: https://iris.who.int/bitstream/handle/10665/376814/9789240094925-eng.pdf [Accessed: 6 Aug 2024]

[5] WHO. Sexually transmitted infections (STIs). Fact sheets. 2024. Available from: https://www.who.int/news-room/fact-sheets/detail/sexually-transmitted-infections-(stis) [Accessed: 6 Aug 2024]

[6] WHO. Alarming decline in adolescent condom use, increased risk of sexually transmitted infections and unintended pregnancies, reveals new WHO report. 2024. Available from: https://www.who.int/europe/news/item/29-08-2024-alarming-decline-in-adolescent-condom-use--increased-risk-of-sexually-transmitted-infections-and-unintended-pregnancies--reveals-new-who-report#:~:text=An%20urgent%20report%20from%20the,(STIs)%20and%20unplanned%20pregnancies [Accessed: 2 September 2024]

[7] Centers for Disease Control and Prevention. Sexually Transmitted Disease Surveillance 2019. Available from: https://www.cdc.gov/std/statistics/2019/std-surveillance-2019.pdf [Accessed: 6 August 2024]

[8] Swinkels HM, Justiz Vaillant AA, Nguyen AD, Gulick PG. HIV and AIDS. Treasure Island (FL): StatPearls; 2024

[9] Singh D, Vignat J, Lorenzoni V, Eslahi M, Ginsburg O, Lauby-Secretan B, et al. Global estimates of incidence and mortality of cervical cancer in 2020: A baseline analysis of the WHO global cervical cancer elimination initiative. The Lancet Global Health. 2023;**11**(2):e197-e206. DOI: 10.1016/S2214-109X(22)00501-0

[10] WHO/ICO Information Centre on HPV Cervical Cancer. HPV and cervical cancer in the world. 2007 report. Vaccine. 2007;**25**(Suppl 3):C1-C230. DOI: 10.1016/S0264-410X(07)01183-8

[11] Looker KJ, Magaret AS, May MT, Turner KM, Vickerman P, Gottlieb SL, et al. Global and regional estimates of prevalent and incident herpes simplex virus type 1 infections in 2012. PLoS One. 2015;**10**(10):e0140765. DOI: 10.1371/journal.pone.0140765

[12] Looker KJ, Garnett GP, Schmid GP. An estimate of the global prevalence and

incidence of herpes simplex virus type 2 infection. Bulletin of the World Health Organization. 2008;**86**(10):805-812. DOI: 10.2471/blt.07.046128

[13] WHO. Chlamydia. Fact sheets. 2024. Available from: https://www.who.int/news-room/fact-sheets/detail/chlamydia [Accessed: 6 August 2024]

[14] WHO. The global burden of disease: 2004 update. Available from: https://iris.who.int/bitstream/handle/10665/43942/9789241563710_eng.pdf [Accessed: 4 September 2024]

[15] Hengel B, McManus H, Monaghan R, Mak DB, Bright A, Tolosa X, et al. Notification rates for syphilis in women of reproductive age and congenital syphilis in Australia, 2011-2021: A retrospective cohort analysis of national notifications data. The Medical Journal of Australia. 2024;**221**(4):201-208. DOI: 10.5694/mja2.52388

[16] Omar RF, Bergeron MG. The future of microbicides. International Journal of Infectious Diseases. 2011;**15**(10):e656-e660. DOI: 10.1016/j.ijid.2011.05.001

[17] Celum C, Baeten JM. Tenofovir-based pre-exposure prophylaxis for HIV prevention: Evolving evidence. Current Opinion in Infectious Diseases. 2012;**25**(1):51-57. DOI: 10.1097/QCO.0b013e32834ef5ef

[18] Gilead. U.S. Food and Drug Administration Approves Descovy® for HIV Pre-Exposure Prophylaxis (PrEP) [press release]. 2019. Available from: https://www.gilead.com/news-and-press/press-room/press-releases/2019/10/us-food-and-drug-administration-approves-descovy-for-hiv-preexposure-prophylaxis-prep [Accessed: 7 August 2024]

[19] Bekker LG, Das M, Abdool Karim Q, Ahmed K, Batting J, Brumskine W, et al. Twice-yearly lenacapavir or daily F/TAF for HIV prevention in cisgender women. The New England Journal of Medicine. 2024;**391**:1179-1192. DOI: 10.1056/NEJMoa2407001

[20] Copen CE. Condom use during sexual intercourse among women and men aged 15-44 in the United States: 2011-2015 National Survey of family growth. National Health Statistics Reports. 2017;**105**:1-18

[21] Omar RF, Leboeuf M, Bergeron MG. Time to put women-controlled multipurpose prevention technologies for their protection in full gear. Archives of Gynecology and Obstetrics. 2023;**4**(4):99-101. DOI: https://doi.org/10.33696/Gynaecology.4.052

[22] Dohadwala S, Politch JA, Barmine JH, Anderson DJ. A brief history and advancement of contraceptive multipurpose prevention technology (cMPT) products. Open Access Journal of Contraception. 2023;**14**:83-94. DOI: 10.2147/OAJC.S375634

[23] Soh C, van der Straten A, Hemmerling A, Turpin JA, Young HB. Editorial: Multipurpose prevention technologies: Call for innovative strategies to address critical priorities and gaps. Frontiers in Reproductive Health. 2024;**6**:1417974. DOI: 10.3389/frph.2024.1417974

[24] Clarke DF, Penazzato M, Capparelli E, Cressey TR, Siberry G, Sugandhi N, et al. Prevention and treatment of HIV infection in neonates: Evidence base for existing WHO dosing recommendations and implementation considerations. Expert Review of Clinical

Pharmacology. 2018;**11**(1):83-93. DOI: 10.1080/17512433.2018.1393331

[25] Businesswire. EU Marketing Approval Granted for VivaGel® BV. 2015. Available from: [https://www.businesswire.com/news/home/20150924005411/en/EU-Marketing-Approval-Granted-for-VivaGel%C2%AE-BV [Accessed: 6 August 2024]

[26] Drugs.com. Phexxi FDA Approval History. 2021. Available from: https://www.drugs.com/history/phexxi.html [Accessed: 6 August 2024]

[27] Population council. FDA Approves the First One-Year Contraceptive Fully under a Woman's Control. 2018. Available from: https://popcouncil.org/media/fda-approves-the-first-one-year-contraceptive-fully-under-a-womans-control/#:~:text=August%208%2C%202018%E2%80%94The%20Population,entire%20year%20of%20protection%20against [Accessed: 6 August 2024]

[28] Bestman-Smith J, Piret J, Desormeaux A, Tremblay MJ, Omar RF, Bergeron MG. Sodium lauryl sulfate abrogates human immunodeficiency virus infectivity by affecting viral attachment. Antimicrobial Agents and Chemotherapy. 2001;**45**(8):2229-2237. DOI: 10.1128/AAC.45.8.2229-2237.2001

[29] Piret J, Omar RF. The invisible condom: A unique mode of action with a low toxicity profile. In: Proceedings of the XV International AIDS Conference, Bangkok, Thailand, July 11-16. 2004

[30] Piret J, Gagne N, Perron S, Desormeaux A, Tremblay MJ, Gourde P, et al. Thermoreversible gel as a candidate barrier to prevent the transmission of HIV-1 and herpes simplex virus type 2. Sexually Transmitted Diseases. 2001;**28**(8):484-491. DOI: 10.1097/00007435-200108000-00012

[31] Piret J, Lamontagne J, Bestman-Smith J, Roy S, Gourde P, Desormeaux A, et al. In vitro and in vivo evaluations of sodium lauryl sulfate and dextran sulfate as microbicides against herpes simplex and human immunodeficiency viruses. Journal of Clinical Microbiology. 2000;**38**(1):110-119. DOI: 10.1128/JCM.38.1.110-119.2000

[32] Mbopi-Keou FX, Trottier S, Omar RF, Nkele NN, Fokoua S, Mbu ER, et al. A randomized, double-blind, placebo-controlled phase II extended safety study of two invisible condom formulations in Cameroonian women. Contraception. 2010;**81**(1):79-85. DOI: 10.1016/j.contraception.2009.07.002

[33] Omar RF, Guilbert E, Gallo MF, Leboeuf M, Boissinot M, Sellam A, et al. Empowerment of women: Closing the medical technologies gender gap. Journal of Obstetrics and Gynaecology Canada. 2018;**40**(1):78-83. DOI: 10.1016/j.jogc.2017.07.009

[34] Trottier S, Omar RF, Desormeaux A, Drouin J, Gagnon MT, Vezina F, et al. Safety, tolerance and acceptability of the invisible condom and its vaginal applicator in healthy women and their male sexual partners. Contraception. 2007;**76**(2):117-125. DOI: 10.1016/j.contraception.2007.04.015

[35] Omar RF, Trottier S, Brousseau G, Lamarre A, Alexandre G, Bergeron MG. Distribution of a vaginal gel (invisible condom) before, during and after simulated sexual intercourse and its persistence when delivered by two different vaginal applicators: A magnetic resonance imaging study. Contraception. 2008;**77**(6):447-455. DOI: 10.1016/j.contraception.2008.01.015

[36] Omar RF, Leboeuf M, Lemyre M, Chabot I, Trottier S, Ulmann A, et al. A pre-phase III efficacy trial of the

spermicide/contraceptive effect of the invisible condom, a non-hormonal vaginal gel, in women from Canada. Journal of Obstetrics and Gynaecology Canada. 2022;**44**(2):175-181. DOI: 10.1016/j.jogc.2021.09.018

[37] Harrison P, Mellors JW, Richardson B, Masse BR, Abdool Karim Q, Abdool Karim SS, et al. Challenges in HIV-prevention microbicide research. Science. 2008;**321**:532-534. DOI: 10.13140/2.1.4519.4888